CW01483718

Best Wishes Craig
Andrea
2003

Love, Luck or Miracle

A Factual Account of the Diaries Recording Derek's Return Back to Life

Andrea Craig

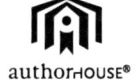

authorHOUSE®

AuthorHouse™ UK Ltd.
500 Avebury Boulevard
Central Milton Keynes, MK9 2BE
www.authorhouse.co.uk
Phone: 08001974150

© 2009 Andrea Craig. All rights reserved.

No part of this book may be reproduced, stored in a retrieval system, or transmitted by any means without the written permission of the author.

First published by AuthorHouse 7/23/2009

ISBN: 978-1-4389-9413-0 (sc)

This book is printed on acid-free paper.

'COLD IS THE LIFE OF THE MAN WHO
DOES NOT BELIEVE IN LOVE,

UNFORTUNATE IS THE LIFE OF THE MAN
WHO DOES NOT BELIEVE IN LUCK

AND SAD IS THE LIFE OF THE MAN
WHO DOES NOT BELIEVE IN MIRACLES.'

ACKNOWLEDGEMENTS

I would like to offer my heartfelt thanks to the two young ladies working at the B&Q store, who having just recently completed their C.P.R. training course, attended to Derek immediately at the scene of his collapse, their continued efforts undoubtedly saved his life. I offer my thanks to the dentist, nurse and doctor who arrived on the scene at the same time as the paramedics who took over on their arrival and kept Derek's life going until he reached hospital. These people will never know how often my silent thanks go out to them.

I wish to acknowledge my sincerest thanks to Doctor Chambers and his very fine team of doctors for their incredible expertise in the operation of the Intensive Treatment Unit, not forgetting of course the dedication of the unit's nursing staff. I do not know the individual names of each member of staff but I will certainly remember each of them in person.

I wish to thank Doctor Oates who was present from Derek's admittance into I.T.U. until his discharge from Ward 37 six months later. I wish to express a special thank-you to her, for not only her complete dedication as a doctor overseeing Derek's medical recovery throughout, but also the patience and understanding shown to myself at all times.

My sincere thanks go to the Ward Manager and the nurses of Ward 37, who took such special care of Derek day in and day out, always showing patience and understanding for his unusual needs. To the domestic staff who always had a cheery word of encouragement and a welcome cup of tea, I would like to say thank-you for bringing a little sunshine into the ward even on the many dark and rainy days we spent there.

I say a special thank-you to the patients in Arrowe Park Hospital for looking out for Derek when he was first admitted onto Ward 37, especially John, Harry, Mike, Bob and his lovely wife Norma.

I would like to thank his Cardiologist, Doctor Newall for his time and detailed explanations of Derek's condition and Doctor Palmer of Broadgreen Hospital for his valued second opinion and ongoing six monthly reviews. I wish to thank Doctor Colin Pinder for his neurological expertise and the invaluable help and advice he gave to me and a huge thank-you to the staff of Wirral 'Neuro' Rehabilitation Unit for the two months specialized care given when Derek was finally admitted.

A huge thank-you to all the therapists who worked diligently to bring Derek so far along his pathway, and to those who still work with him, we met many very special people during Derek's recovery and neither Derek nor I will ever forget anyone of you.

My deepest thanks go to that special small group of family and friends, who have walked the journey with us both, upholding, supporting and encouraging us along the way. This has been a journey we would have found almost impossible without the love, thoughts and prayers of so many wonderful people, who sadly were unable to visit Derek, but kept our spirits up with your many cards and words of encouragement.

Derek and I wish to offer our sincerest thanks to George, Sarah and Max for simply always being there and to especially express my own gratitude for all the help given to me, often after you had completed a full day's work. My demands must have been quite considerable at times and yet all were met without complaint.

Finally I would like to say a very special thank-you to Sarah without whose help I could not have completed the reproducing of these diaries and to Derek himself for the patience and understanding shown during the many hours it took of my time.

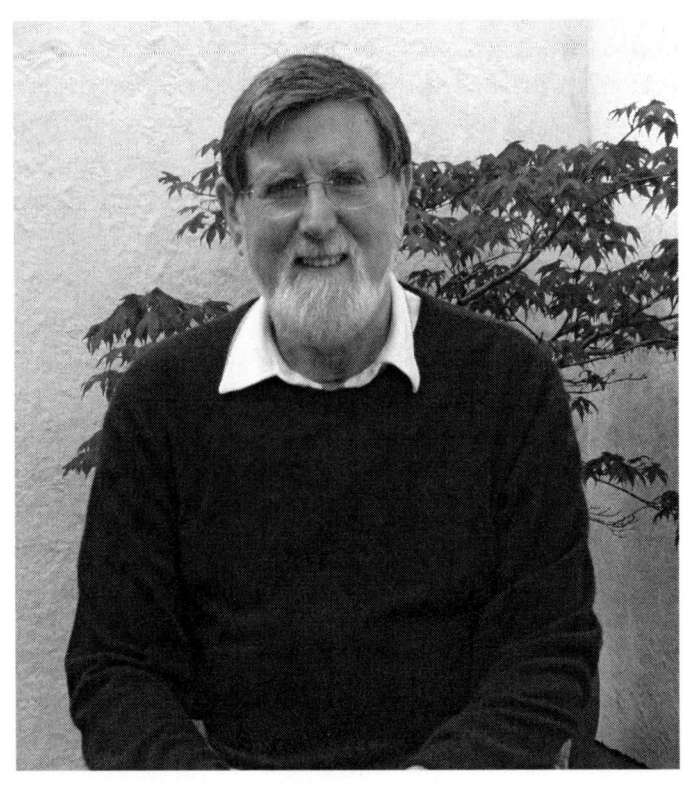

Derek

INTRODUCTION

The writing and reproducing of Derek's daily diaries is my way of helping to piece together for my husband, a part of his life that was wiped from his memory in one cruel moment of time when an out of hospital cardiac arrest so very nearly robbed him of his life. For anyone else who may read this account I hope it will serve as a sincere and genuine warning to never neglect your own health and early warning signs.

We live in a time when fitness, health and heart awareness is being brought to the public's attention as never before but sadly there are still far too many who are, just as Derek was, too afraid to face the early warning signs. Fear itself is one of the greatest dangers, for the symptoms and their cause are nearly always treatable if caught in time and on the rare occasions when they are not, then what have you got to lose, turning away from the symptoms will not make the condition go away. Face it, the relief of knowing more than makes up for the sure niggling fear you will undoubtedly live with if you do not.

Derek tried to ignore his early warning signs in the belief that they would go away or tried to convince himself that they did not exist. He left it too late. Had he not done so then much could have been done to avoid the brain damage he is now left struggling with. A healthy lifestyle is vitally important to keeping fit and well but it is not always enough, Derek was a fit man who took plenty of exercise and ate a good nutritionally balanced diet but he was afraid of all things medical and what he felt would be an invasion of his personal privacy, so having regular check-ups was a definite no-no for him.

If Derek's account can convince one person of the importance of taking control of their own health then his experience will not have been in vain and for those of you who may in the future have to travel the same pathway as Derek, finding themselves with the same formidable mountain to climb then I hope his diaries will give you and those closest to you a little help and encouragement as you struggle along your own individual journey.

We are all becoming so called 'experts' on anything and everything 'Google' can throw up today. We live in a highly technological and supposedly more efficient world. A factual world with all knowledge at our fingertips with merely the press of a few computer keys but sadly, I believe, a much more isolated world in which the modern man and woman is so busy with their careers and keep fit lifestyles that sharing and even caring for anyone outside of their own insular world is a thing of the past.

As the modern world we live in appears to be crashing at present with proclaimed banking efficiency proving itself to have been truly inefficient, the word of government ringing hollow with each fresh promise and many thousands of people finding themselves without work and wondering what life will hold for them, we find ourselves without any sense of security and standing upon very uncertain ground. These are indeed frightening times and circumstances which man cannot choose to turn away from as he can his own health, but the fear can be equally as strong if not stronger and we ignore the warning signs at our peril.

A cold outlook of what I believe is becoming an increasingly cold world. An equation set to equal disaster is enveloping us and all mathematical equations are cold, calculated, seemingly indisputable facts. Derek's own personal experience tells of such a cold calculated equation equalling a near fatal disaster but it also tells of the one thing that is capable of cutting across it and cancelling it out, 'the power of love.'

Whatever pathway in life you are struggling along, no matter how hopeless a situation you may find yourself to be in, remember that you can travel that road alone in fear and isolation or you can open your heart to love and share it with those nearest and dearest to you or in some cases those you simply meet along the way. In Derek's story I share how I believe God's Love cut directly across what could factually have been a fatal passing. I believe it was the Power of God's Love working through the presence of two female shop assistants and the expertise of a fine medical team which saved Derek's life and it was the love of his family which gave Derek the encouragement to face a mountain he once believed too high to climb.

The power of love should never be underestimated, not just in our personal relationships but in our outlook to all things about us in the living out of our daily lives. We need to start looking through the eyes of love at the world in which we live with fresh hope, even when all seems quite hopeless, and most importantly I believe is to soften our hearts with renewed love, even though they may have been hardened over considerable time.

The medical profession claimed that Derek had been an extremely lucky man with the exception of one doctor who did declare that a miracle had truly taken place and another declaring that a medical recovery of global proportions had taken place.

Love, luck or miracle, the health of our world is in great need of all three and I share Derek's story in the hope that the reading of it may help each person to discover that all three will help you in your individual quest for true fitness, health and happiness.

CHAPTER ONE

I knew it was a lovely Spring day even before I had opened my eyes, the room was alight with a brilliance which could only radiate from an early morning sun in a cloudless sky, its radiance not only penetrated the still drawn curtains but also straight through my eyelids as only a bright light could.

"Good morning", I murmured. "It's another beautiful morning. What do you think we should do today?"

My husband rolled over onto his back, "what time is it?" he queried, and before I could reply he continued, "It must still be quite early. I think I might enjoy lying here a little longer."

"Have you any preference for what you think we might do or where we might go", I persisted.

"Not fussy at all, you decide," he replied," whatever you wish to do will be o.k. with me."

"Are you alright?" I asked.

"Of course I am, why do you ask?"

"No reason," I said not wishing to add that I thought he sounded a little flat and that it was not like him to want to lie in bed, especially on such a beautiful day.

"O.K. you stay here, I'm going to get up. Lie here for as long as you like but I don't want to waste this glorious sunshine," and with that I jumped out of bed and went straight into the bathroom. By the time I came out Derek was up and already in the shower having first been downstairs to open the curtains and lay the table for breakfast. I could not help but chuckle to myself knowing that he would not lie in once I was up.

Our conversation that morning was much the same as it had always been over the five years since Derek's retirement. I think he enjoyed the freedom from the pressures that always accompanied the running of a business and the fact that he could now choose to lie-in if he desired to do so, but he never did.

Our day had begun much the same as any other except we were in exceptionally high spirits due to it being such a beautiful sunny day. A day which lay spread out before us like a clean new sheet, inviting us to do with it whatever we should choose. I went downstairs ahead of Derek and put a light under our usual breakfast of porridge. Oats help to keep the arteries clear and had become a regular part of our healthy daily diet. Apart from student days, holidays and celebratory lapses, we had eaten healthily most of our lives. Derek had also kept himself reasonably fit and active through racket sport and walking, all the activities he partook in were played with a very competitive streak which kept Derek, and many others around him, driven and on their toes.

The porridge was ready and while waiting for Derek I went and opened the French windows situated at the far end of the kitchen where we had a small dining area. I walked out onto the miniature patio which is not overlooked and offers a wide expansive view over the River Dee. I closed my eyes and turned my face to the early morning sun. It was April and spring seemed to have been by-passed by the arrival of an early summer which had brought with it a Mediterranean feel of hot but beautifully fresh morning air. It was perfect weather which we had been fortunate to have enjoyed for several days in a row.

I found myself wondering what time our daughter, Sarah would arrive home. She had spent the night with Victoria, a lifelong friend. Life had parted them for several years and having recently met up they had a lot of catching up to do. Derek and I were so pleased that they had made contact once again and hoped that the girls had spent a pleasant time together.

I heard Derek moving about in the kitchen behind me and walked back in to find him placing two bowls of porridge on the table. We sat besides the open windows making small talk as we ate. The air was very relaxed between us, a little different to what it had been of late as Derek had been acting very oddly and extremely tense for some time, but although he seemed quite relaxed this morning I could not dismiss the fact that he seemed to be more subdued than usual.

"Isn't this the most wonderful day, what about a drive out into Wales? We can pack a picnic for lunch," I ventured.

"O.K.," came the reply from the other side of the table.

"Derek, you would tell me if anything was troubling you, wouldn't you. I really don't mind staying at home if you would rather."

"Really I'm fine, couldn't feel better. Why do you keep going on?"

"It's just because you seem to be so quiet, that's all."

"I'm just sitting here enjoying the sun. It's so warm we could be on holiday abroad somewhere."

"Talking about holidays are you looking forward to Lake Como?" I asked.

"Not really."

"Why ever not"? I asked, unable to keep the surprise from my voice.

Had I heard correctly, both Derek and I adored Italy and had been excitedly looking forward to our planned trip ever since Marlene and Glyn had invited us to join them for two weeks in May.

"I don't know, can't say but I do have a very strong feeling that I'm not meant for Lake Como."

I was a little shocked. "You're being so silly, why say such a thing when we've been looking forward to it so much."

Only the previous week we had spent a day shopping for the holiday. Derek had been reluctant as ever to spend on himself, but nevertheless excited that he had been able to purchase a new linen jacket to replace an old faithful one which I had threatened to throw away if he should ever wear it again. We had talked about little else that day and he had expressed, quite strongly, how he felt we both needed this forthcoming break.

"Take no notice of me," he said, believing that he had upset me. "It's just that I wish you and I were going off somewhere on our own for a little while."

"We can be on our own today for the whole day, I can have a cold lunch prepared and packed in no time at all and we could make an early start."

"That would be nice," he replied," but how about a quick walk around the marina before-hand, there'll be few people there this time of the morning."

"Yes I'd love that," I said standing up gathering the dishes together. As I washed them, Derek closed and locked the French windows and came across to help dry.

Half an hour later we were in the car heading towards our local marina. Derek had been right when he had said there would be no traffic, what bliss, but then seven forty-five on a Saturday morning never saw very much traffic on the road, not the same as a week-day when it would have been building up towards peak hour.

The drive along the Peninsula was as beautiful as we had ever witnessed it. No mist or haze, which would normally have been the case, to obscure the landscape. We had clear uninterrupted views across the fields of green and vivid yellow crops. Blue sea surrounded us on three sides reflecting a cloudless, brilliant blue sky. We both agreed that this Mediterranean morning was as beautiful, if not more so, than anything we had experienced abroad. It felt fresh and vibrant and this was our doorstep where we were fortunate to live, a place we had never taken for granted, we simply counted our blessings each day for the beauty which surrounded us, and never more so as on that Saturday morning of April 28th.2007.

We arrived to find ourselves the only two people there and marvelled at how the early morning sun danced across the sands reflecting a shimmering light of dazzling pinks. The tide was coming in rapidly and as we walked around the marina the early morning sun blended together the blue of the sky and the aqua-marine of the sea and somehow merged and softly diffused them with the pink of the sand and nearby rocks, turning our immediate world into the most magical of places.

We walked that morning as we did many mornings hand-in-hand along the narrow pathway with the marine lake on our left-hand side and the rising sea from an incoming tide gently lapping around our feet on our right. The sea was calm and the air was still.

Derek spoke softly afraid that he might disturb the peace, "I remember when you once described to me how you felt when the tide was in and you walked alone around here with water lapping all around you and how on that occasion you told me that the experience had helped to save your sanity and had given you the strength to carry on."

"I remember well," I whispered. Like Derek I too was afraid to disturb the peace that had enveloped us both.

"I never ever fully appreciated the depth of meaning behind your words until this very moment," he confessed. "This really is magical. But don't you find it strange that there is absolutely no-one else about, not even anyone out walking their dog."

Derek was talking as though he really was afraid of breaking a spell which had been cast, holding us both in that moment of something very special. I had often found myself walking alone there during the past years of my life and the marina had forged a special place within my heart and so the happiness I felt at that simple, (oh so simple,) moment in time is indescribable. To be sharing the magic that I had once discovered whilst on my own, now with the dearest and most wonderful man I had ever known, goes deeper than my words can express. We walked on in silence totally at one with each other and the world about us.

We arrived back at the car and Derek suggested we spend a little longer breathing in the beauty and freshness of it all. We leaned against the rail looking out over the marina towards the estuary. I followed the antics of two seagulls who could not decide whether they should be floating on the water or walking upon it. They were so funny to watch and I remember thinking how sad that people often do not have the time or the inclination to watch such simple things in life. It was a moment of pure enjoyment and genuine entertainment watching them.

The seagulls flew off as Derek announced that he had never felt as happy in his entire life as he did at that moment.

"As strong as that," I teased.

"Please believe how serious I'm being," he said. "It's more than a feeling of happiness," he continued, "it's more like a feeling of inner peace. Yes that's it, I feel a deep sense of inner peace for the first time in my life and it's filling my entire being."

Turning to him I gently leaned over and kissed him lightly, "You'll never know how long I have waited to hear you say that." I knew that the moment was in some way special, everything suddenly felt so different and the most wonderful part of it was that we had the rest of the beautiful, magical day ahead of us to share and enjoy together. He put his arms around me and gave me a great warm hug.

"We're so lucky," he whispered, "so very lucky to have each other."

"For now and always," I replied.

Derek indicated that it was time we should be heading back and as he drove us home, I closed my eyes and gave thanks that perhaps now we could at last finally put the past behind us. An unpleasant past, a past he had found difficult in laying to rest.

Before retiring Derek had run several small companies within the construction industry, an industry which had sadly, during the latter years of his working life, managed to turn itself into a ruthless and somewhat immoral body of bullies. Giant companies within the industry had begun to with-hold payments irrespective of how this procedure affected lesser companies than themselves.

Derek's companies were amongst those hit very badly, forcing him into an earlier than planned retirement.

During the five years since he had retired, he had been so pleased to escape from it all but had been unable to free himself of the nasty taste and deep felt sense of injustice it had left him with. There were times during those years when I had felt as though I had been supporting a broken man. A man who's sensitivity had never been meant for the industry in which he had served his entire working life. A spiritual man, although he would never claim to be a religious one, who felt a deep sense of what was considered ethically and morally correct and had no time for those who practiced deceit and wrong doing. He had cared deeply for those who had worked for him. I

Andrea Craig

had always considered him a shining example in a somewhat grubby industry. His latest remarks had instilled in me the hope that perhaps from this day on we could now live without those demons from the past. I silently thanked God that Derek had at long last found his peace and would now be free to enjoy the rest of his life.

Arriving home, Derek asked whether or not I thought we should perhaps wait for Sarah's return in case she would like to come with us.

"We'll never get out at this rate," I said with a little irritation creeping into my voice, "she'll not be home until ten or later. You know what the girls are like when they get together, it could easily be later than that if they have slept-in.

"No, she definitely said she would be home early and by the time you have everything ready we shouldn't have long to wait."

"In that case I'm going to finish off the ironing from yesterday."

"And I'll water these tubs," he shouted from the back patio.

I decided to first wash the salad greens and prepare some foodstuff for packing and was just finishing when Derek walked back into the kitchen and over to the cupboard where the ironing-board was kept and lifted it out.

"Would you like me to put the ironing-board up for you," he asked, already placing it in position.

"Thank-you, sweetheart, these few bits won't take long to iron."

"While you're doing that I think I might run along to B&Q and buy that last piece of wood I need for the shed extension."

"I thought you were watering the pots," I said feeling rather surprised that he should even consider it, "you loathe B&Q., why today of all days." I suddenly experienced the feeling that our planned picnic was beginning to slide away from us.

"I won't be long and can water the plants later," he said, "I only need that one piece of wood and if I can get it and give it a coat of preservative before we go out then I'll be able to place it in position tomorrow ready for me to begin nailing the sides together first thing Monday morning."

"OK, but please be quick, we'll need to be ready to go just as soon as Sarah gets back."

"Shan't be long, straight there and back." He leaned over the ironing board, gave me a little kiss and was gone.

"Bye, be careful and take care," I called after him. Words I called out every time either Derek or Sarah left the house. I must have believed they formed a sort of safety net around each of them whenever they left the security of their home.

I continued ironing and seconds later looked up to find Derek looking at me in a way that pierced straight through to my heart.

"What on earth are you doing?" I laughed but was nevertheless startled to see him there.

"Looking at you," he whispered.

"Don't be silly," I gently scolded, "You gave me such a fright. I thought you had left."

"Andrea, could I have a great big hug before I go?" he asked very quietly.

I placed the iron down feeling slightly taken aback. Derek and I often gave each other lots of spontaneous hugs and kisses but this time something I saw in his eyes rang a little alarm bell somewhere deep down inside of me. I walked around to stand directly in front of him and placing my arms about him I told him that he could have as many as he wished.

"Just one special one will do," he uttered holding me tightly, so tight I had to gently push him away.

"Be off or we'll never get out,"

He closed the kitchen door behind him and I picked up the iron once more. Just a few shirts to go I thought hanging up a blouse I had just finished belonging to Sarah which was always very tricky to press. Turning back to the board I was once again startled to see Derek standing in the doorway which he had supposedly closed behind him some minutes earlier.

"Gosh you're determined to frighten the life out of me this morning," I exclaimed, "what have you forgotten?"

"Nothing," he replied

"Derek what on earth is the matter with you?"

"Andrea, I don't want to go."

Laughing a little nervously I told him he had no need to go.

"No," he interrupted, "you don't understand. I mean I don't want to leave you now, not ever, but I know that I must."

"In that case stop being so silly and go," and with those words I walked across the kitchen and gently pushed him out of the door adding, "The quicker you go the quicker you'll be back again."

By this time I was beginning to feel a little uneasy and thinking perhaps we should not be going out for the day, maybe Derek would rather continue with his work on his shed project. Dismissing these thoughts I picked up the first of the remaining two shirts still waiting to be pressed and carried on, only to discover that I could not clear the strange image I had seen upon Derek's face as he had stood in the doorway silently watching me.

I had finished and was clearing away the ironing when Sarah walked into the kitchen commenting on the glorious weather.

"Derek's off to B&Q I believe. He gave me such a lovely big hug before he left and said that you'd both already walked around the marina. He seems very happy with himself this morning."

We decided to have a coffee and took them out onto the patio where we chatted pleasantly about how Sarah had enjoyed her evening with Victoria. I looked at my watch, it was eleven-thirty. Too late to take a packed lunch I thought, might as well have lunch at home before we set off, there would still be plenty of time for a leisurely drive afterwards. Sarah had arranged to spend her week-end visiting Anglesey so it would only be myself and Derek going for a drive.

As Sarah cleared the cups away I found myself looking up at the kitchen clock feeling strangely uneasy. I told myself to stop this nonsense and tried to hold onto the conversation we had shared earlier that morning when Derek had spoken of his newly discovered sense of peace but in spite of this I could no longer deny the feeling of alarm bells ringing somewhere inside of me.

Trying to keep control I turned and began slicing the tomatoes. Sarah was sitting at the kitchen table preoccupied reading the newspaper.

"I wonder where he is?" a question I was asking myself rather than Sarah.

"Who?" queried Sarah.

"Derek," I answered, "I was wondering where he could have got to. He said he wouldn't be long." I looked at my watch with a nervousness I had never experienced before. Eleven-forty five, something had gone wrong, I could feel it.

"Give him time. It will take half an hour to drive there, half an hour to drive home again and another half hour to browse through B&Q. You know what he's like. He'll be back anytime now you'll see."

Whilst I could not argue with what Sarah was saying, I was experiencing an almost overpowering sense of foreboding. To calm myself I began filling the kettle and although it was too early to switch it on I thought I would get the cups out and set the table. As I reached into the cupboard for the tea-cups I suddenly felt a sharp shock as though a bolt of lightning had struck me, everything went black and I heard myself shouting, "Something's wrong Sarah, something is so terribly wrong. Why isn't he home? I want him home here right now!"

"Mum, stop it. What on earth is the matter with you? He won't be long, come and sit down," pleaded Sarah.

I turned once again to look up at the clock. It was twelve noon and I felt that the world, my world had stopped. I could not sit down. I paced about trying to control the feeling of panic that was fighting to take over.

"Don't be daft," rationalized Sarah, "do come and sit down."

"I'm not being daft, Sarah, I know something's wrong and I want him home,"

"Mum, calm down, he won't be long now. For the last time do come and sit down."

I looked at the time once again as though some meaning of what was going on inside of me would be discovered there.

"He must have gone on somewhere else." I was merely voicing my thoughts out aloud as I found things to do whilst waiting.

"You're just being silly," spoke a voice from behind the paper. Deciding that I was being too ridiculous for words Sarah had sought normality in the printed events of the day.

"I'm telling you Sarah, something is not right. I know he should be home by now," I whispered once again turning to look at the clock.

"I have such a strange feeling." I was simply stating a fact and not talking to anyone in particular. I felt trapped within some kind of time warp. Time was all I had to focus upon for some strange reason that eluded me. Joining Sarah at the kitchen table I finally sat down.

"What time is it," I asked.

"Just gone past twelve-thirty," replied Sarah and immediately the phone rang out startling us both. With an overwhelming sense of foreboding I picked it up to hear a clear distinctive female voice asking if she may speak to Mrs. Craig.

"Speaking," I murmured trying to sound in control.

"Hello, Mrs. Craig, this is Arrowe Park hospital here, the A & E department. Can you please confirm that you are Mrs. Andrea Craig."

"You're speaking to Andrea Craig," I replied, surprised to hear how strong my voice sounded for I felt strangely weak.

"Mrs. Craig I have to inform you that your husband was brought into A & E a short time ago."

"Just tell me is he alive or dead," I uttered. What a foolish thing to say. I could not believe I had just asked that, but it was the only thing that seemed to matter.

"He is still alive Mrs.Craig, but your husband has suffered a cardiac arrest, he has been resuscitated but I would ask that you get here as quickly as you can. Please do not drive yourself and it would be better if you did not come alone.

If there is no-one who can drive you, would you please take a taxi, the voice sounded kind and gentle but very factual, I respect factual. I am a factual person myself.

"Mrs. Craig, do you understand? Do you have anyone with you?" the kind voice went on.

"Yes," I replied. "My daughter is with me and will run me in immediately. "

I replaced the receiver. Sarah was already on the move, remaining very calm and organized. I also respect organized, as I am an organized person as well as being a factual one. A person who is able to cope and remain calm in most circumstances so why on this occasion was I experiencing a strange tremor travelling throughout my entire body? Why did my mind feel as though it had gone into free fall, leaving all that was normal far behind, suddenly nothing felt real, I seemed to be moving through a world without substance

The hospital was no more than a ten minute drive away but the journey seemed to take forever. I sat quietly in the passenger seat and all I could hear was the beat of my heart as it went thump, thump, thump…, and all I could see was the look on my husband's face as he had stood in the kitchen doorway a little earlier that morning watching me in a way that had pierced my heart and left me with a slightly strange feeling.

"Please God take care of him and help me to remain strong." I prayed as the thump, thump, thump continued.

"Be careful, Pops but do hurry," I instructed Sarah, who was offering me words of comfort at the same time as reassuring herself that all would be well.

"Please God do not let him suffer." I did not know what to pray for as I have always believed that to ask anything for oneself was a selfish request, to even ask anything of God was to doubt His ability to know what was best for each of us. "Please forgive me," I can remember asking, "and just take care of him within Your Will." I knew then that I had handed Derek over into God's care and could face whatever had to be faced. Nevertheless my heart continued to race with the thump, thump, thump threatening to deafen me with every pounding beat and the tremor I first experienced five minutes ago still had a hold.

Finally, we arrived at the hospital and Sarah found an empty space to park the car. We ran towards the entrance of A and E and not quite sure of where we should be going we stopped an ambulance man who was walking towards us. "Excuse me," I said, "my husband has just been brought in here, where can we find him".

"What's his name, love?" he asked. I told him and he quickly disappeared around a corner asking us both to wait where we were until he came back. I remember thinking how quiet everywhere was. I had never been into this department of the hospital before and I was surprised to see so little activity. In no more than two or three minutes the ambulance-man reappeared.

"Mrs. Craig, the doctor would like to have a word with you and your daughter," and with that he moved away leaving a theatre gowned young lady standing before us. I just managed to thank him before we were ushered into a small room. It was square in shape with painted white walls. Several chairs were positioned around a coffee table which stood in the middle of the room with a cooling-water machine placed on another table in one corner.

The doctor closed the door behind her creating the sense of feeling one experiences when sitting in the cabin of an aero-plane when the doors are closed just before take-off. As well as feeling a little shakey I began to feel slightly claustrophobic. This is the room where people are brought to receive bad news I found myself thinking. She walked across the room and sat down next to me speaking very gently, "Hello Mrs. Craig, might I ask if this is your daughter?"

I introduced Sarah and went on to say that we wished to see Derek immediately but was interrupted,

"Mrs. Craig, please do sit down, we need to have a little chat before you see your husband. You see I am afraid the news is not good." The doctor went on to inform us of what had taken place.

Gosh, I thought, she doesn't look any older than Sarah and how attractive she is. What on earth had this to do with the explanation being delivered at that particular moment, concentrate Andrea I told myself. Listen hard…

"Do you understand Mrs. Craig?" I heard myself being asked.

"Yes, yes I do." I replied. Why did she think me incapable of understanding her, why did she not simply take us to see him, I should be at his side, all this wasted time, I did not understand why we were being kept waiting.

"……… very lucky to have had a doctor in the store who was able to work on your husband until the paramedics arrived," continued the doctor.

"How long did it take for them to reach him?" this was Sarah now speaking.

"Please may we see him, I must see him," I said rudely breaking into their conversation.

"My Colleague would like to come in and have a word with you both first. There are several facts you must be made to understand before you are taken through to see your husband. Have you understood any of what I have been explaining to you so far, Mrs. Craig?"

The room was still, the only sound was that of my heart still pounding in my ears. I felt a sense of the unreal, that none of this was really happening. I could at that moment so easily have either laughed or cried at the sense of absurdity.

"Mr. Craig has suffered an out-of-hospital cardiac arrest and we now know for certain that he has sustained massive damage," she continued. Massive damage I remember thinking, damage to what, as far as I was concerned the only thing that mattered at that moment was whether he was alive or dead and they had said that he was alive and I wanted desperately to see him, to be with him.

How can I accurately recall the uncontrolled thoughts rushing around inside of my head at such a moment, when I really should have been at home having lunch, Derek should have coated his one piece of wood with preservative ready for to-morrow and we should have been sitting around our table deciding finally how we were going to spend the rest of the afternoon. I would no doubt have scolded him for being late and told him it was too late to drive into Wales.

Now here I was sitting in this little room with its' painted white walls in Arrowe Park hospital being told that my husband was massively damaged… oh my goodness me what is that…looking down I had suddenly discovered two rather large reddish stains right in the front of my white shirt, tomato stains acquired whilst preparing lunch. What a mess, how could I have left home without first changing into something else? Silly inane thoughts which refused to be shut out, my hands made them-selves busy in an unsuccessful attempt to hide them.

"Will you both be alright if I go to see if doctor is ready now?" we were asked.

"Yes we'll be fine." Fine, would we ever be fine again I wanted to scream. Then I found myself wanting to laugh again for it all felt weirdly bizarre. I must get a grip, I told myself.

Sarah had just come back into the room, when did she leave it, I could not remember her going out.

"John's on his way, mum," she announced, "I thought I'd better let him know what's happened." John was Sarah's current boy-friend. There was a knock on the door and a young looking man walked in dressed in green theatre overalls. Goodness me everyone looks so young I thought.

"Hello, Mrs. Craig, my name is Tony Alderman and I would like to go over all that my colleague has, I believe, already explained to you and your daughter. We are now preparing your husband for I.T.U. which means Intensive Treatment Unit."

"I would like to see my husband," I said," I need to see him please," I begged.

"All in good time Mrs. Craig, but right now there are one or two things I must first go over to make sure that you both understand what has happened to Derek and what a serious situation we have here." Sarah and I sat and listened intently to Dr. Alderman's explanation of Derek's cardiac arrest.

Apparently Derek had been shopping in our local B&Q store when he collapsed in aisle fifty two where he had been looking for his piece of wood.

"He would never have known what was happening as it would have happened so quickly. There was a gentleman standing next to him at the time who had tried to prevent him from falling but with Derek being such a big man, he had been unable to do so, Derek went down hitting the floor hard, catching his head as he fell but that is only a superficial injury causing no concern at all."

Another knock on the door caused me to jump, John had arrived and asked if he could come in or should he wait outside. He was told to come in and the doctor continued. Two female assistants who had only completed a CPR (Cardio Pulmonary Resuscitation) training course a few days before had been in the same aisle stacking shelves when the incident took place and were able to begin resuscitation on him immediately.

"Mrs. Craig, this prompt action undoubtedly contributed to your husband being alive at this moment. They continued working on him until the paramedics arrived and who, as luck would have had it, had been on stand-by only minutes away from the store when they received the call-out. On arrival at the scene they quickly injected adrenalin and had to shock three times, a pulse was finally detected and maintained but there was no spontaneous breath."

Dr. Alderman continued to further explain how the ambulance crew had to keep working on him in the ambulance and had got him to A&E as quickly as they possibly could.

To me they were just words but not the words I needed to hear.

"Please tell me," I murmured, "is he going to be alright? I simply want to see him. Can we not go over this a little later," I pleaded to be allowed to go through, that we might be losing valuable minutes.

"Mrs. Craig there are several things which we have to make clear to you before you do go in to see your husband, certain things we have to be sure that you and your daughter fully understand before you see him. You see, we believe Derek may have sustained massive damage to both his heart and his brain, he is no longer breathing for himself. Do you understand what we are saying?"

As I sat, I began to witness the man addressing me as growing younger before my eyes, or was it I suddenly growing so much older? All I wanted to do was pick Derek up and take him home for lunch and I needed to do it right at that very moment. If only I could do that, then none of this would be happening.

"I shall leave you for a moment whilst I go and see if it is possible to take you through, please be patient a little while longer, I shall be as quick as I can", and with that Dr. Alderman was gone.

I could hear voices, not the doctors I realized, for he had left the room, must be Sarah or John talking. The world which had stopped for me earlier that morning felt as though it was now managing to slip away from me completely. I could see and I could hear, but that part of myself which was known as the inner me, had discovered a place that was neither light nor dark or cold nor warm but simply detached. Everything was taking place outside of it and nothing seemed to be real.

Dr. Alderman returned to the room and handed me a hospital bag containing Derek's belongings including his wallet and car keys. Unfortunately his shirt was not saved because it had been cut away by the ambulance crew enabling them to carry out vital work on him. The shirt was really not important but nevertheless I found myself wondering what shirt he had been wearing that morning. I hoped that it had been a good one and yet what a complete waste if it had been. What a ridiculous thing to think about but from my newly discovered place of detachment I had begun to believe that all things were ridiculous. I had even questioned as to how could Derek possibly have collapsed on such a beautiful day, as if he had chosen to do so himself, how ridiculous was that.

"Would you and your daughter like to come through now, Mrs. Craig? Please just the two of you."

John stood up taking the bag of belongings from me stating that he would look after everything.

"You will have to hurry as we are waiting to take him through to ITU as quickly as possible," spoke the doctor. Leaving the quiet of the room behind us, Sarah and I followed closely behind Dr. Alderman, moving swiftly through double doors we entered into a world of much activity. People everywhere, many of them with worried faces as they anxiously paced up and down, or sat awaiting news of their own particular relative. We passed patients lying about on bed-trollies. We knew that patients were lying in beds behind curtained-off cubicles with many nurses and doctors practicing their own expertise on each one. This was the A.&

E. Majors department and it was busy, extremely busy.

We were brought to a sudden halt as Dr. Alderman turned and told us that we would have to prepare ourselves for what we were about to witness. He warned that we would have to be very careful of the many wires and tubes around Derek and explained that the doctors and medical technicians were still working on him. He asked if we were up to facing this and I assured him that we were.

"Then in we go, just in here, once again please be careful, we can only give you one or two minutes with him", although he spoke very gently I could sense the urgency behind his words and not wishing to detain the medical staff longer than necessary, Sarah and I entered the cubicle which was like no other either of us had ever been in before.

Two doctors had spent time explaining to us in detail all that had led up to this moment but nothing could have prepared us for the sight which greeted us.

We found ourselves having to step over endless coils of wire which were feeding the life-saving equipment being used by several doctors. Gently encouraged by Dr. Alderman I carefully approached one side of the bed as Sarah made her way around to the other.

Lying on the bed in-front of us Derek appeared almost unrecognizable. The biggest shock to me was to see how blown his body was but this was very quickly explained to be due to the high levels of oxygen being pumped into him. He lay with his poor body twisted and strangely contorted, blood was everywhere. This person could not be Derek, this body lying before me did not resemble him at all. His hair and beard were matted with blood, he appeared to be bleeding from his ears, eyes and nose and his flesh was pulled back taught over his face revealing blooded teeth. There was such a pained expression etched upon his face I wished Sarah had never had to witness. Having seen him, Sarah quickly left. I asked if I might touch him and was told that I could with extreme care and could if I wished, have two minutes alone with him.

It was then that I felt something, a force perhaps, but I really cannot explain what that force was except that it was strong enough to pull me from my place of detachment and back into the present. Having already handed Derek over into God's care I knew that I must now place my full trust in that same God and these doctors who were fighting to save my husband's life. Placing a hand on his exposed, twisted arm and the other over his head I silently asked for God to keep him safe. I prayed for any healing power that I was capable of giving, be given in accordance with His Divine Will and that if He should wish to take my husband at this time then so be it.

"Good-bye, my darling," I whispered, "Follow the light, but if God does not want you just yet then please fight your way back to us, we are right here beside you."

"Are you ready, Mrs. Craig? We must move quickly," the doctor spoke kindly, "would you please wait in the room with your daughter once again. We are taking Derek through for an MRI scan and as soon as we are ready to take him through to I.T.U. we will let you know.

As we sat, Sarah related to John how shocked we had both been on seeing Derek.

"Such pain, did you ever see so much pain on anyone's face," cried Sarah, "and why was his poor body so contorted?" I could not give her the answers she was seeking instead I looked at my watch, twelve-thirty, my watch has stopped I remember noting.

The door opened and Dr. Alderman asked hurriedly if we would follow him as they took Derek through to intensive care. Everything was happening at break-neck speed and as we ran to keep up I heard the doctor quoting visiting times but was assured these did not apply to us at this present moment. On reaching the unit we were asked to wait in a small waiting-room, which was situated immediately outside of the unit. Once Derek had been settled, we were told somebody would come out to call us.

This room was even smaller than the previous one we had occupied and also had white painted walls. I believe all hospital walls should be painted, so much cleaner and far more practical than wallpaper, which I loathe to see just as much as I loathe to see carpets laid in a hospital which I consider to be most unhygienic. Chairs were positioned tightly along three walls of this room and one small table occupied space along the fourth wall, upon which someone had left a half-drunk cup of what appeared to be very strong coffee and a half-eaten sandwhich. There were no windows to allow natural daylight in or offer much needed fresh-air but it was clean and offered temporary respite.

During this waiting period I began to have my first rational thoughts since receiving the telephone call earlier and it dawned on me that there were other people who would have to be notified quickly. Derek's son Paul who lived in Germany, his sister and her family who lived no more than a couple of miles away from the hospital, next there were his close friends and the rest of our family, all would have to be told of what had happened.

Sarah in her ever caring and at the same time wonderfully efficient way which is hers informed me she had already made contact with Elaine, his sister and her family and they were on their way as we spoke. Not knowing Paul's address she asked if I could tell her where to find it. I explained where his e-mail address would be found and was assured that she would go home shortly and contact him. But first she and John would go and pick up Derek's car from where he had left it parked at B&Q. and drive it back home, at the same time checking that all had been left in order. Before returning she said she would pick up a wash-bag and change of clothes for me.

"Not forgetting a clean shirt," I quickly added. I really could not believe I had just said that, not to forget a clean shirt, did anyone really care? I found myself worrying about a clean shirt when my husband lay fighting for his life somewhere beyond those double doors.

Doors, so many doors we had passed through since first entering the hospital just after lunch, except of course we had not had any lunch. I had been attending hospitals for most of my life and never once noticed the amount of doors separating one department from another. Sitting in that overly warm and airless room I found my gaze riveted upon the double doors opposite willing them to open and my name to be called. I was soon to discover that these two doors were kept locked at all times and a buzzer had to be rung to gain admittance. I found myself wondering what I would find on the other side, peace and quiet or a hive of activity similar to A & E.

The minutes, which felt like hours, ticked by, Elaine and her family had arrived at some point and we sat drinking coffee and chatting. I really was unable to take very much in of what was being said as my whole attention lay on the other side of those doors and what might be happening. Someone had said that George had left stating he would return later.

Sarah and John arrived back to say that Paul had been contacted and arrangements had been made to pick him up on arrival from the airport on just as soon as the time of his flight was confirmed.

Sarah was in the process of telling me that she had also rung my mother and that arrangements were being made for a member of the family to run her over to the hospital, when suddenly one of the doors opened and a nurse called out for the relatives of Derek Craig, but only two at a time could be allowed in. Sarah and I walked into the unit and I was surprised to discover it to be much larger than any other I had visited before. There were at least twelve beds and most of them were occupied. Everywhere was spotlessly clean with a brightness that was very welcome after sitting in the dismal waiting area, and an atmosphere of calm, efficient activity filled the entire ward. We were asked if we had ever experienced an I.T unit before and then the nurse went on to explain that we should try not to be too alarmed at the sight of the many tubes and equipment we would see surrounding Derek as it was all doing the job of keeping him alive.

We were asked to disinfect our hands every time we entered and left the unit. It was beginning to feel very impersonal and clinically calculating, which obviously it had to be to function as efficiently as it did. We were then shown to a bed not far from the doors we had just walked through and as we approached the bed both my head and my heart began to pound once again, dear Lord, none of this felt real, so many people each fighting for either his or her individual life. Time held no meaning within the confines of this unit, each second was an eternity and one soon came to realize that each person's heart-beat meant life. Days ceased to have meaning, hours where either light or dark but gave no true measure of time.

As we stood at Derek's bed-side I tried to make sense of the monitoring equipment attached to him but my brain seemed unable to register anything at all. Bells and buzzers suddenly sounded from the bed adjacent to Derek's, a nurse appeared very quickly checking as she moved around her patient, curtains were pulled around the bed and two doctors materialized as if out of thin air.

Then just as suddenly as it had sounded from that other patient's bed, an alarm went off right next to my head causing me to jump.

"Don't be alarmed," reassured the nurse attending him, "you'll soon get used to the bleeps and buzzers going off, most of the time it simply means that something has to be changed."

I glanced over to the clock on the opposite wall, twelve-thirty it showed but I instinctively knew that it could not be correct. I looked back to see the nurse telling Sarah she had finished what she had been doing and that she could resume holding Derek's hand once more. Sarah was drawn to him with the caring, nurturing side of her nature taking over and I remember noting what a beautiful gift she had.

CHAPTER TWO

During that fateful day of Saturday, 28th April 2007 and the immediate days which followed, how I would have coped without Sarah, I simply do not know. I felt her deep love and courageous support. She filled me with strength and the courage to keep going, at the same time willing Derek to do the same.

I do not remember at which point I came to realize that Derek had collapsed on the anniversary of my father's birthday. It hardly seemed significant but twelve-thirty on my father's birthday registered every time I looked at my watch or a clock and it was not until the second week after his collapse that my mind began to record the correct time once again. At which point it seemed to me that life within the unit was indeed lived outside of normal recorded time, it was simply lived between the basic fact of life and death. Doctors who held out no promise of life yet totally dedicated to preserving it. They and that unit became my security for every single moment which Derek spent in it. I came to depend on these extremely dedicated male and female doctors and looked to them for confirmation of that hope I held deep within my heart.

During the time Derek spent hovering between life and death, the doctors kept us continually informed and updated on his condition and although they were always on hand to respond to, and answer any questions which we as Derek's family frequently put to them, their explanations were always very bleak and held out very little hope, if any at all for the future.

I received my first piece of bleak news when I was told that my husband's chances of surviving an out-of-hospital cardiac arrest were very slim. The test results were back and confirmed that Derek had sustained massive damage to both his heart and brain as first suspected and it was probably only a question of time. I was told I must be very brave and should prepare myself for the worst.

I recall the mention of fifty percent heart damage and eighty percent damage to the brain due to oxygen deprivation. I sat silently absorbing every word, there was nothing I could say and yet every fibre of my being was screaming out for them to make him better. I felt as though I was sitting in the side wings of a theatre watching a play being enacted which was proving too farcical for words.

I heard the word percentage once again and brought my attention back so that I could fully concentrate on what the doctor sitting facing me was saying.

He was explaining how only an extremely low percentage of out-of-hospital cardiac arrests ever survived, knowing that I had already been given this information only minutes before I realized that the doctor was stressing something home to me.

They were not expecting Derek to survive. Oh yes, I knew all about death sneaking up upon us as a thief in the night, I had endeavored to live my life with that in mind, but this seemed so unreal. No longer sitting in the side wings I now found myself caught up right in the middle of some theatrical farce from which there was no escape. I could not shake off the feeling that at any minute I was going to wake up from this nightmare which held me in its grip and all would be well once more. I found that I would fall in and out of the same nightmare for several weeks to come.

As I left the room in which I had received that devastating news and stood once again beside Derek's bed I discovered the nightmare had released its hold upon me and I found myself awakened to the cold reality of the medical news just delivered. I asked the nurse if I might stand behind the bed in order to place my hands on Derek's head. She moved the equipment to make this possible requesting that I be careful. Although I had already handed Derek over into God's care and keeping and had complete trust in the doctors and nurses who were tending him I wanted to do something, to feel that I was able to be doing my little bit. I wanted also for Derek to know that he was loved and that one way or the other all would be taken care of.

During the following hours Derek suffered what at first was thought to be fits but this was later explained to me as being the effects of nerve damage relating to his brain and not quite the same thing. Both his left arm and leg became rigid one moment and then would flay wildly about the next, he suffered respiratory infections and needed to be given a tracheotomy as well as the life support system he was already on. There was a lot going on that sadly Derek's body could not cope with and it was decided that he should be deeply sedated to give his brain and body a chance to heal. It was explained to me that this would seem as though Derek were in a coma as the sedation given would have to be extremely strong but it would be an induced state different to that of a coma.

It was also explained to me that Derek may never come out of this state and that if I thought there was anyone who should see him, then now was the time to call them. Family members came in to spend what each of them believed might be their last moments with him and all went out extremely upset.

The second piece of bleak news I received came several days later when I was told that there was were now signs to indicate that there was a slim chance of Derek surviving but if he did then he would most probably live in a vegetative state. At that moment the nightmare not only held me in its grip but I felt it squeezing the very life out of me. I then realized it was my own voice stating that if this were the case there was to be no more life-saving procedures carried out on my husband. I did not wish for him to be kept alive in this state anymore than he would wish for it himself.

As much as my life was unimaginable without Derek, I could accept death, for death had never been my enemy. I believed that death took us into a greater freedom of life and a greater sense of reality, a reality in which I knew Derek would blossom and be taken care of. Knowing that, I also knew I would be able to cope with whatever life brought upon me. But the news I had just been given was truly what nightmares were made of, neither life nor death but held trapped, imprisoned in a state too bleak to contemplate.

I walked from that same room in which my first piece of bleak news had been delivered to find I could not bring myself to go back to Derek's bedside instead I chose to walk outside for some badly needed fresh-air. I needed to try and reclaim a hold of something which was rapidly slipping away from me, my sanity. I needed to find a firm footing once more as I felt the ground beneath my feet shaking.

I needed suddenly to go home and be with all that was familiar. I wanted to be surrounded by normality and to be able to sleep, a long deep sleep that would block out all the thoughts and decisions which were beginning to weigh so heavy with me. But I could not leave Derek, I would have to stay and remain at his side. I turned away from the sunshine that held no warmth for me that day and walked back to the room we had been allocated in which we were able to eat and sleep during those first vital days.

Food, of which I ate very little, was brought into me daily but sleep alas eluded me. Derek's sister spent those early nights keeping me company, at the same time naturally, wanting to be close to her brother. We talked and reminisced most of the nights away and even had a good laugh now and then but while Elaine slept I walked the corridors of a very silent almost eerie world, a world totally unrecognizable compared to the hectic buzz of daily medical comings and goings which made up the normal pattern of hospital life.

That night was such a night, it had been an exceptionally hot day and the night felt even hotter. The room was stuffy and airless but Elaine had somehow managed to drop off and I tip-toed out of the room to begin walking aimlessly down the corridor. I sat on a window-sill at the end of the corridor from I.T.U. as it felt a little cooler there and my thoughts were of nothing in particular as I suddenly became aware of a calmness wrapping itself around me, I was awake and yet felt as though I was strangely asleep and at one with the hospital.

As the dawn cast its pinky glow in the quad-rangle outside, I made my way back to our room looking at the few prints which decorated the walls of the corridor as I walked slowly back. Suddenly I found myself attracted to one in particular hanging just outside of our room. It was a sketch depicting the original arched gateway to the park.

I stood and looked in absolute shock. To explain my reaction to this picture hanging on the wall in front of me I must go back to the evening of Tuesday 24th April, when we had been sitting in mediation attended once a week at a friend's house. During the hour long meditation I had been shown an image of this exact same arch. Having no previous knowledge of what I could now see was a gateway I could only describe it as being similar to that of the 'Arc de Triumph' only not as tall. Studying the picture on the wall, I knew with absolute conviction that this was the very gateway I had been shown, and as I continued to stand in front of it I knew with equal conviction that it symbolized Derek's gateway between life and death. How I knew this will be explained more fully later on but standing there right at that moment I experienced my first glimmer of hope.

A new day had dawned and we were asked to vacate our room as Derek, although still at very high risk, was now considered to be out of imminent danger from death. We were asked to abide by afternoon and evening visiting times only, unless requested otherwise. This was greeted by myself as a mixed blessing. Firstly it raised my hopes that Derek was at least now in with a fighting chance but secondly it meant I had to leave him to fight his battle alone for long periods of time and I did not know how I was going to cope with that. My strength and ability to do so came in the remembered realization that he was in God's care and keeping.

Sarah had been granted indefinite sick leave from her position at the University where she worked and looked after me with a caring and compassion that makes her the very special person she is. She was at a time in her life when she should have been carefree and busily cementing her own pathway not suddenly finding herself placed in such a demanding role, but in her usual efficient way, she took on the running of the household, the looking after me and running us both to and from the hospital every day completely in her stride.

When I retired to bed usually exhausted each night I found the bedcovers turned back, my bedside lamp switched on and Derek's wallet placed on his pillow next to my own. These were little touches that meant so very much to me and each night, I would go to sleep with my hand placed over that wallet feeling a little closer to him.

Looking back to that period of time, I find it strange that each and every night I slept soundly right through the night for usually I am a poor sleeper. During the weeks that followed, Sarah helped to restore my sense of sanity and grounding but unfortunately my sense of reality would never be the same again.

During our continued daily visits to I.T.U., I felt a deep conviction that we had to keep the left-hand side of Derek's body as mobile and as flexible as possible. I asked if we could massage him and we were told that we could with care. Sarah played her part and as she worked on one part of his body I would work on another or place my hands gently over his head. We would talk to him because we had been told that he might just be able to hear us and would find our voices reassuring.

During such a time when I was massaging his leg and Sarah was holding his hand and gently moving his arm she suddenly whispered,

"Mum, he's just squeezed my fingers." Her eyes filled as she continued, "quickly come around here. Now you hold his hand." Then she very quietly told him that I had hold of his hand and could he do the same for me. He did, a moment never to be forgotten.

I have read of such moments but I do not have it in me to be able to describe exactly how I felt. Excitement, joy or perhaps elation, are the words that best describe what one feels when that life force suddenly responds to you. His nurse made notes and asked that we keep talking to him but behaved as though nothing unusual had occurred, these nurses experience such happenings every day. No, this was definitely our moment and we savoured it. How could anyone who was capable of responding in the way Derek had, be declared to be a vegetable? He was coming back to us and I knew it.

Sadly our moment was to be quite simply no more than a moment for it was cut short by our third piece of bleak news. On this occasion we were asked into what I now called the Delivery Room. We sat still and listened whilst being informed that Derek was being brought around very slowly from his deep sedation and that any movements we had experienced from him were purely responsive movements and not those of reactive response.

A further explanation was given and words such as responsive, reactive, directive were floating about the room along with many other words I had no recognition of. I heard words confirming that it was the right-hand side of Derek's brain that had been severely damaged and this was the directive side that affected the left-hand side of the body.

Because of this damage Derek would never be able to walk or talk again if indeed he ever did come around from the vegetative state he was now declared to be in. I came out of the fog, which always seemed to envelope me at these deliveries and heard that they were about to take Derek off his life support system. I suddenly felt very cold with fear and apprehension. I knew that this equipment had been keeping my husband alive through the most vital episode of his life and I was being told it was about to be turned off.

"It is not quite as brutal as it sounds, Mrs. Craig," I heard a doctor addressing me, "we do it very gradually. Your husband will be taken off for short periods at a time and then put back onto it until hopefully he will be able to breathe for himself. This is a normal procedure," he continued, "but we must warn you that it will be a very crucial time and it could prove to be too big a strain for him. The next few hours or days will be extremely critical indeed.

The medical news had once again been delivered. How I longed at times to lash out at these men, for somewhere deep inside of me struggling and trapped within that inner nightmare was a woman wanting to scream out loud every time she heard each and every piece of devastating news they delivered, and yet at the same time I felt such respect and admiration for the work they did, I have so much to thank them for.

Over the next two weeks Derek had to fight a respiratory infection which we had been pre-warned might happen. It complicated his being weaned off the life-support system but thankfully he responded quite quickly to the medication administered and slowly but surely he was brought successfully off the support, which had been keeping him alive. Once again we were addressed and informed that although Derek was now breathing independently and continued to be brought out of his deep state of sedation, unfortunately he was not responding to any stimuli at all. His assessments and outlook was considered very poor. At this moment no one could be sure of how deep a vegetative state he would be in.

Derek eventually regained consciousness and there were times when we hung on to the belief that he did actually recognize us but then the realization would dawn that he was in actual fact looking straight through us. At other times, very fleetingly I would be convinced that he both saw and recognized us and nothing would convince me otherwise.

One particular afternoon sitting at Derek's bedside I was surprised to realize that the young man occupying the bed next to Derek, who had been very poorly the day before, was sitting beside his own bed fully clothed. This boy, who to me was no more than that, had been unconscious when Derek had first been admitted and yet here he was happily awaiting a relative to collect him and take him home. I was amazed at how quickly he had recovered, brought back from the brink, his own words, and just waiting to escape. I felt so pleased for him and was silently wishing him well for the future when he turned to me and said,

"Do not give up on him, don't ever give up and he'll make it, you'll see."

I asked him if he had any recollections or hearing whilst he had been un-conscious and his reply lives with me to this day.

He described his experience as being held in a dark tunnel in which he had no vision except that he could see varying shades of light and sometimes moving shapes but it was the words he could hear that meant most to him. He went on to explain how all the words spoken to him reached him in his tunnel as though they all entered at one end with most of them floating past him and straight out of the other. The important bit he went on to explain further was that a few of them stayed with him and it was to these that he clung.

"I've heard ye' talkin' to him," he said, "is 'e your fella'?"

I replied that he was just as the young man's relatives appeared and our conversation was brought to a halt but a few minutes later as they were about to wheel him out he turned and called back, "remember don't give up, keep on and on, never give up." With that he was gone. I wish him a good and healthy life and thank him for his words, if only he knew how much they helped that day.

On May 10th I was called into the Delivery Room and informed by Dr. Chambers, Head of I.T.U. that Derek was to be moved, sometime during the next day or two as there was nothing more that the unit could do for him.

"Where will my husband be moved to doctor," I asked, feeling as though the ground was beginning to move beneath my feet once again.

"We were hoping to move him into High Dependency which is next door but unfortunately we do not have the room. We are waiting for a bed to become available on one of the wards."

The shaking which threatened to take over my entire being had to be controlled and also the sudden sense of insecurity I was experiencing had to be dealt with, a feeling which had never been very far away during the past three weeks. This unit and its entire team with their expertise had kept my husband alive and were now abandoning him, or that is how it felt to me at that moment. The unit had been Derek's life-line and my security and it seemed that both were about to be severed.

"Doctor," I heard myself saying, "you have been very frank and at times quite brutal with me over the past two weeks with your delivery of my husband's condition and now it is my turn to be very frank and brutal with you when I say to you that I do not want my husband thrown onto a ward to simply languish away. I do not want him thrown onto a human scrap heap."

"Mrs. Craig," the doctor broke in, "this hospital is not in the habit of throwing any of its patients onto scrap heaps, human or otherwise."

I was later to deeply regret my choice of words but right then I meant them with the full force of my being. My safety net was being taken away leaving me feeling extremely vunerable, as though a vast ocean of black nothingness was opening up before me, my fear was not for myself but the knowing that Derek was unable to swim or keep afloat for himself.

Friday 11th May, Derek was moved onto Ward 37, a large respiratory ward which was situated on the third floor of the hospital. This ward was to become our second home for the following six months and its' staff were to become our extended family.

CHAPTER THREE

When I first walked onto Ward 37 it was as though I had entered into a whole new world. Of course it was a completely new and very different environment from that of I.T.U. and what first struck me was the activity. It was a very large ward which was arranged in six bedded bays leading off a long open corridor with the floor manager's office, conference room, staff kitchen, various patient's bath/shower rooms, toilets and sluice room running adjacent down the other side. Situated across the far end of this long ward one found the isolation rooms which offered the most wonderful views across the most beautiful countryside stretching down to the Dee estuary. This was Arrowe Park, the very park which gave this hospital its name. A park once noted for its zoo and school outings but since the closure of the zoo and the less frequent school visits it has more recently become noted for sports training events.

I recall thinking how light and bright the ward was and how taken aback I was with the number of nurses on duty. Nurses seemingly everywhere busily tending to their patients needs, one of the busiest wards I had ever experienced and this was to be the standard pattern of nursing care maintained each and every day we were to be on that same ward.

Derek arrived at approximately 3 o'clock in the afternoon in a very agitated state with his arms and legs flaying about all over the place, he was having his tracheotomy suctioned every two to four hours and having to be kept closely monitored. The next few days I spent trying to soothe him, I kept up the healing I had been administering to him on a daily basis, and continued to massage his arms and legs regularly at the same time becoming somewhat worried about his muscle wastage which was now so noticeable. I also felt it was more important than ever that his limbs should be kept flexible and mobile.

It became a full time job simply trying to keep his limbs from getting stuck in the sides of his bed which needed to be kept raised at all times. Derek had a tendency to lie with his head in one corner of the bed and no matter how many pillows where placed in position to prevent this, he would somehow manage to bury his head into them and throw them onto the bars, which made him look so uncomfortable. His body would stretch diagonally across the bed making his feet and legs fly through the bars on the opposite side. Covers were almost impossible to keep over him with his constant jerking and moving about.

Although Derek's eyes were now opening spontaneously he did not recognize anyone and was still declared to be in a vegetative state. As the days passed I noticed not only the massive weight and muscle loss but also the dry skin beginning to peel over his entire body. The nursing staff were not overly concerned and suggested that I apply a little extra moistourising cream when next massaging him.

On 14th May I was informed by Dr. Oates (Derek's Medical Consultant) that it had been confirmed Derek was indeed suffering from hypoxic brain injury and that the prognosis was not good, in fact it was extremely poor. Dr. Oates went on to further explain how prone to infection he would be whilst remaining on the ward and of the many hurdles he might have to overcome along the road to recovery.

At this point I requested a secondary neurological opinion regarding the future outcome and the possibility of rehabilitation for Derek. I went on to stress that whilst I wished for everything that was possible to be done for him at no time did I want anything to be done which might prolong his suffering. I knew that he was suffering and I dreaded the thought that he may be trapped inside a very dark place. Dr. Oates kindly agreed a secondary neurological opinion and added that it would be arranged.

Andrea Craig

As the day wore on Derek began to grow more and more distressed and it was obvious that he was fighting something, his tracheotomy was being checked and suctioned more frequently due to a greater mucus build-up and by the following day he had developed deep rasping sounds. A sputum culture was taken and sent for analysis. It was noted Derek was showing no reaction to verbal stimuli, no reaction visually and his arms and legs continued to flay and jerk, this was his medical report but I was growing more concerned with the peeling of his skin, no longer just dry I continued to wipe away large pieces of skin from both his face and body.

On the 16th May a meeting was held between Dr. Oates and myself when the possibility of a Peg tube being inserted was discussed. This meant a tube being inserted directly into the stomach to increase his food intake as he kept pulling out the feed tube already inserted via his nose and throat.

His consultant also discussed at length the legal 'letting go of life' opposed to the illegalities of euthanasia. It was decided that we all wanted what was best for Derek. It was finally concluded at that meeting that if Derek was assessed by his neurologist as being unsuitable for future rehabilitation and as being declared to be in a vegetative state then the doctors would decide if it were prudent to allow natural circumstances to run their course and if so then life prolonging treatment would cease and palliative care would keep him comfortable. That was the day my trust in his consulting medical doctor took root, a trust and respect which grew deeper each day that Derek remained in her care.

It was on the 18th May that Derek was visited and assessed by Dr. C. Pinder, Senior Neurologist and head of Wirral Neurological Rehabilitation Unit.

Dr. Pinder reported Derek to be in a vegetative state but claimed that he could not be classified as post vegetative until six to twelve months after injury, the prognosis was once again declared to be very poor after brain damage such as Derek's but it was considered too early to give a definitive prognosis. His recommendation was to commence weaning him off his tracheotomy as future care would be much easier without it and if Derek was to continue to pull out his N.G. tube then a Peg tube would be needed.

The following day was a day to remember, it was the day Derek spoke his first words. I had spent the day as I normally did and was sitting at his bedside with my head propped on my arm which I had resting along the cot-side. Derek was settled and calm although his arms and legs still continued to flay and jerk. I was tired, very tired but I kept whispering words of encouragement to him and telling him of little things we had done together, things we might one day do again when suddenly I heard those words I could hardly believe I had heard, "I……love….you…..help…. me."

Slow faltering words but words, which sounded like music to my ears although tearing my heart in two at the same time.

I looked around for a nurse but found only an empty nursing station, I turned back to see such a look of deep desperation in Derek's eyes as he lay silently mouthing those same pleading words, "Help me," over and over again, already on my feet I leaned over the bed and held him, "You are receiving more help than you will ever know, my darling," I whispered as my tears dropped onto his face.

"Oops," he murmured and closed his eyes once more. I continued talking to him and a few minutes later realized he was nodding and shaking his head to my questions and statements. I was both elated with his response and heartbroken with his obvious distress but at last he was back and knew me for that moment at least.

On 20th May Derek had once again succeeded in pulling out his NG tube, something which was developing into a regular habit. He was extremely agitated and needed a lot of soothing and although the nurses were always doing what they could for him there were times when they were unable to cope with his special needs as he fell outside of their usual nursing duties. He demanded time they did not have. It was decided that he needed twenty four hour nursing care which was introduced the following day.

Since those first words had been spoken, the nursing staff noticed that Derek was desperately trying to communicate but was unable to make sense with the few words he could use. Once again it was stressed to me that although he was now able to speak isolated words, this did not mean he had come out of his vegetative state and might still be left in a persistent and dependant state with a very poor quality of life.

Derek's tracheotomy was removed on the 21st May and replaced with a mini tracheotomy which was programmed to be removed on the Wednesday of that same week. The insertion of a PEG tube was discussed and planned hopefully for the coming Friday. The mini tracheotomy was removed on the Wednesday and a large dressing took its place. I felt Derek was very pleased with its removal.

May 24th dawned and I arrived on the ward at lunch-time to be greeted by a chorus of male voices singing forth their own rendition of "Blue Suede Shoes". Imagine my surprise when I realized that they were being led by none other than Derek himself, perhaps it was the sheer relief from having his tracheotomy tube removed the day before for the sound of his voice had returned to normal, but I must mention that his party trick had always been to take off Elvis Presley and on this occasion I was greatly impressed.

During the next couple of weeks the ward was to enjoy, or not, the male voice choir of bay one. The sound of singing and laughter was so unusual it brought a patient from the furthest bay at the end of the ward hobbling down to see what was going on. I had stepped outside from Derek's bay to allow the nurses to check his dressings and was musing to myself on the difference a few days could make when this same patient asked me what all the frivolity was about.

"I'm sorry it's my husband singing away, I hope he hasn't disturbed anyone?"

"Disturbed anyone," he roared, "this place needs bloody well disturbin' I can tell yer' that love."

I was not quite sure how to take him so said nothing further.

"I served in the Faulkland's and experienced things yer' would never have lived through without a sense of humour, and a bloody good laugh was what kept us goin'. That lot down there," he said pointing his thumb in the far direction," are such a bunch of bloody miserable sods, yer've no idea I can tell yer'. I've asked to be moved up this end, it sounds as though there's a continual party going on.

And I'll tell yer' this love, yer' should be bloody proud of 'im, it's better than any medicine what e's doing."

"I am proud of him," I said, "bloody proud."

It seemed strange to me how Derek could sing but could not express himself verbally. What was even stranger was that during the following weeks he was to sing in Gaelic, German and Italian as well as English, the nursing staff believed him to be bilingual, I believed him to be making it up as he went along. However a doctor told me that one school of thought believed it might be genetically possible to speak or sing in foreign languages under circumstances such as Derek's, I still believed he made it up and that it was only the accent which made him sound convincingly authentic. Later I was to discover that people suffering Dysphasia as Derek was, are able to sing clearly even when unable to talk but there had been no mention of singing in foreign languages.

Derek went down to theatre at 8.30a.m.on Friday of that week to have his Peg tube inserted. I was warned beforehand that some patients have to live out their entire lives with these tubes left in place. I could not even allow myself to think of what that might entail knowing how Derek was already reacting to his existing tubes by continually trying to remove them. The consequences would be much more serious if this tube was to be pulled out.

Later that same day Dr. Pinder visited and recorded an improvement but had been unable to assess him formally as Derek was still under sedation from his Peg tube insertion. The Peg procedure was straight forward and Derek tolerated it surprisingly well, although very tired and restless he still continued to throw himself around the bed. No two days were ever the same in fact no two hours were ever alike for he was still extremely poorly. He was still unable to sit himself up so his bed was kept in an almost upright position and he had to be cocooned in pillows, lots of pillows, pillows piled behind him, pillows placed down each side and along the foot of his bed, all to protect him from hurting himself against the bed-rails.

Derek sang and laughed but he also cried a lot during those early weeks into his recovery. He had a habit of singing "Danny Boy" but could never finish the first line without him breaking into huge heart rendering sobs. It was after one of these emotional renditions that he began to flay his arms and legs about more than usual and suddenly his right leg shot out between the bars of the bed. Sitting to the left side of his bed I automatically jumped up and went round to rectify the situation only to discover it was not going to be that easy. I gently tried pushing and pulling his leg first this way and then that way unfortunately to no avail.

Gently telling myself not to panic I pondered on what to do next. I could not help thinking that at any second now he was about to break his leg. Suddenly moving his leg into a certain position I thought I saw my chance and quickly pushed thinking, right that's got it, but no such luck I had missed the moment and had only succeeded in causing Derek to shout out as though I were trying to murder him. His head sank down lower into his pillows making me believe that any minute now not only would he break his leg but that he was going to suffocate as well.

I was unable to let go of his leg, yet I really needed to be sorting his head out. Next minute John from the bed opposite was at my side suggesting what I should do next.

"Never mind John, just hold his leg," I urged as I ran round to rescue Derek's head which he also seemed determined to get stuck between the bars on the other side of the bed. John held on to his leg, I held his head and Derek seemed totally confused as to what was going on when suddenly a nurse arrived on the scene.

"Goodness!" she exclaimed, "what do we have here?"

Confident that she could resolve the matter quickly she too tried gently maneuvering his leg back through the bars this way and then that way but once again no such luck, so another nurse was summoned to assist, next the ward manager appeared and then Bob from the bed at the far end of the bay arrived, each with their own opinion on how best to resolve the crisis.

"If anyone asks me, I think we should cut it off," I broke in.

Staff nurse looked up at me and with a look of sheer disbelief on her face said,

"I really don't think we can afford to damage a bed in that way, Mrs. Craig,"

"Oh I didn't mean the bed, staff," I replied, "I was referring to his leg."

At that moment I do not think my humour was appreciated but I did note how it had registered with Derek and I recalled how we had always told each other how important our weird sense of humour was to each other in most situations. A sense of relief swept over me as I realized that I still had mine and I really believed that Derek had recognized it. Needless to say Staff was efficient and superb in the moment of crisis and soon the bed-rail was released enabling other nurses to lower and adjust it to the right angle just enough to allow the leg, as if by magic, to slip back through.

That same night Derek pulled at his Peg tube bringing about the immediate introduction of drastic measures designed for his own protection and safety. A zip around bed cover, a little similar to what I thought of as a bed-straight jacket, it was brilliant and certainly kept Derek more comfortably positioned in his bed thereafter.

Derek's speech continued to improve over the next few days and his vocabulary grew more extensive by the day but he was still unable to speak in sentences or make much sense using the words he could pronounce.

May 30th saw Derek very low in spirit and more deeply emotional than I had ever seen him. Walking onto the ward that morning the other men greeted me with a 'thumbs down' sign and were indicating by wiping away a tear that Derek had been crying. John beckoned me over and explained that Derek had spent a particularly bad night emotionally and had not managed to pull himself out of it so far.

"As low as we've seen him, he cried and cried, and sobbed like a baby," was John's way of putting it. Distressed by this news I did not wish to continue with the conversation, so thanking him I returned to sit quietly beside my husband who showed no sense of humour now, only a heavy, aching heart that was almost stifling the very breath out of me. My mind went back to the Tuesday night before Derek had collapsed when during our meditation I had received a message along with the image of the park gateway and I had sat with a familiar 'Spirit' companion of great wisdom (I was so used to these beings as I had walked and worked with them all of my life) who told me I would have to be very strong and very brave and so very, very patient during the days to come. Wonderful advice and great words of truth but right at that moment I felt only weak, useless and extremely vunerable.

"Dear God please do not allow him to suffer this nightmare," I prayed. No sooner had my prayer been uttered (perhaps a silent scream would be a more fitting description), than I became aware of a commotion occurring in the bay, happenings coming from every direction caused me to look up and take note of what was going on. Mick who had hardly ever spoken since I had been visiting the ward was shouting out for the nurse as he was not feeling very well, John was kneeling on his bed with his head down, a position he took when unable to get his breath, and Bob was calling out in urgent need of his oxygen.

I found myself catapulted from my state of self-pity in a second. I felt ashamed and wished with all of my heart that I could do something for these wonderful but extremely poorly men who had been so caring and supportive towards Derek, I only hope that the realization and true contrition of my selfishness would, in some way, have played its part in a greater and much more meaningful prayer which was offered up that day.

A little later that morning I was told Derek had been given an enema for his constipation and had successfully opened his bowels several times throughout the night. I knew immediately why Derek was so distressed, since first regaining consciousness he had always been fully aware and extremely embarrassed by the sheer indignity of the lack of control he had over his bowel movements and my heart went out to him.

I continued to sit in silence and found my thoughts wandering back to the kindness shown the previous day from Bob and his lovely wife Norma. It was as the visitors were leaving after afternoon visiting that Norma came along and asked if she may have a word with me, I joined her at the foot of the bed.

"I'm so sorry to intrude," she began, "we haven't really had the opportunity to say more than hello and good-bye to each other, but Bob has been telling me so much about you both and of how in spite of your husband being so poorly he always manages to keep everyone's spirits up and I was wondering, well Bob and I were wondering if you would care to accept this little keepsake of good fortune. We would like so much for you to take it, I should really say they, for they're two old silver three-penny pieces which were given to Bob and I on our wedding day. You see Bob and I came from different parts of the world and with our individual careers we often had to travel apart from the other and so these two coins, which always had to be kept together, were a symbol of our always being side by side and that no matter where either of us where to travel we would always be brought safely back together again.

We have sat and watched you tend your husband's every need with a love and caring that has touched our hearts so deeply and we believe the time has come for us to now part with our good-luck coins which have kept Bob and I together all these many years past, and pray that they will do the same for the two of you. Please accept them with our love and our prayers that you will also be kept together through this very difficult period."

I held out my hands to receive the gift I believed to be beyond measure and as I looked at her through my blurry vision wishing to say thank-you I found that no words presented themselves. I was left standing speechless, so I simply placed my arms around her and in that moment felt totally at-one with a wonderful, compassionate woman who had, only a moment or two before been a comparative stranger. I shall never forget either Norma or Bob and I carry those two three-penny pieces with me always as my most prized and precious possessions but more importantly still is the love I carry for them both within my heart.

I was sitting thinking of the kindness often shown by others and how that kindness is somehow taken, as though by an invisible means, and changed into an energy which uplifts and at the same time gives one the strength to shoulder on, when I was pulled from my warm place of thoughts to find Derek awake, alert and watching me intently. I returned his gaze with a smile but he quickly buried his head once again in that funny but now familiar way he had of burrowing into his pillows. Sitting silently and deciding to see what he would do next I knew that the look on his face had been very different, it had been more aware than usual as though he had been really seeing for the first time.

The nurses all claimed that Derek did recognize and respond to me but in spite of the fact that he would smile, I felt that his look was blank as though he were looking straight through me. But the look on his face this time had definitely been very different. He had been looking at me and not through me.

Sliding quietly off my chair I knelt down at the corner of the bed where he had buried his head and waited. My hunch was soon rewarded, for only a few moments later, Derek maneuvered the pillows himself so that he could peep out believing himself to be unseen.

"Boo!" I whispered and as though talking to a fragile, frightened animal I pleaded, "Please don't hide away, this is a little secret spot where no-one else is allowed except you and me, no-one else to see or hear us."

Opening his eyes he whispered, "Andrea… Andrea…. I… love…you…so much." The next moment he was gone, hurriedly burying his head once more in his pillows, the moment had been too much for him to bear and I recognized how fragile Derek really was. He was truly damaged and very vunerable.

I picked myself up and leaning over the bed I gently pulled his head up, at the same time straightening the pillows around him. He lay back wanting me to believe he was asleep but knowing that he was not I sat talking quietly to him, encouraging him not to give up and reminding him that all things would be taken care of in their own time.

Suddenly I felt his hand grip mine. "This mountain…. too high…..far…too high…….can't…make…it……sorry…will…never….make…it."

"No you will not," I stated, shocking myself with the sharpness of my voice and the speedy response with which I jumped up so that I could look directly at him, "Derek with that attitude you never will", then realizing how harsh my words must sound I quickly softened my tone and added, "My darling, you cannot ever hope to climb your mountain from the position you find yourself in at this moment in time," I stressed, "how can you when you are lying flat on your back with no strength or energy, right now you are much too weak and confused, of course this mountain is far too high, but let me tell you this……,"

"No, no….can't," he interrupted.

"Derek, please my poor, poor darling, I know this mountain appears too high right now and that's because it is, far too high, but gradually you are going to learn how to pull yourself up. Then you are going to learn how to take one step at a time and slowly but surely you and I will learn how to walk our way through the foothills of that seemingly impossible mountain. When the time is right and you feel stronger than you do right now, we will together, without looking up to the top, keep ourselves focused on only that which stands in-front of us. We will deal with each and every hurdle as it presents itself along the way. Who knows how far up that mountain we will eventually climb."

"I know ….. I will…..never…make….it," he whispered.

"Derek," my voice sounding a little more forceful, "your choices I am afraid to say are quite limited. You can lie here in this bed and give up or you can start on our new journey together, it's as simple as that."

"I can't," he cried pitifully, "I….can't…do……. anything….. can't move".

"Not physically you can't but you can take that first step, that first step of wanting to." He closed his eyes and was lost to me once more. Had I said too much, I sat back praying that I had not been too harsh with him, but at the same time I was strangely excited as this had been the only definite dialogue and understanding which had passed between us. No matter how slow and faltering, Derek had expressed himself clearly for the first time.

CHAPTER FOUR

Sarah had returned to work by this time. There was very little she could do at home during the day but every evening straight from the office she would appear at Derek's bedside just in time to feed him his evening meal of liquid food, she would then spend time caring for him in any way she could, she might have clipped and filed his nails or rubbed cream into his dry and peeling skin as she continually updated him on all that was happening in her daily world.

I was usually exhausted by the end of each day and was so grateful for Sarah's support. Never once did she allow me to carry the bag of washing that had to be taken home each night, it was as though she were trying to carry my load for me in any way she could. Every evening I was driven home, never being allowed into the kitchen except to sort through the nightly bundle of dirty linen and whilst I filled the washing machine, Sarah would prepare a meal for us both.

I would sit and open the day's mail which always included cards from family and friends, each one offering prayers and support. It was greatly uplifting to know that so many people cared so deeply and were holding us in their thoughts. But what I found impossible to deal with were the many telephone calls enquiring after Derek, all understandably wanting to know how he was and how he was progressing, I was simply too exhausted and often too upset to cope. It really felt very strange to me at that time as though in my talking about him I would be betraying him in some way for it felt a very private and personally intimate period we were living through. By the time I had eaten and sorted out clean clothes for Derek which were needed the following day and had my bath I would most evenings be ready for my bed. I would be asleep almost as soon as my head touched the pillow which was unusual as I am normally a poor sleeper.

My mornings were spent in a frantic dash of shopping, ironing and a general housework regime before I set off once again for the hospital. I found it impossible to take on board anything outside of what had shaped itself into my daily routine, this time was Derek's and I could not spend what little time I had in answering each and every call and discussing him repeatedly even though I knew that people were deeply concerned. I had shed no tears, being either too shocked, busy or too exhausted but I had begun to experience a strange new feeling, just every now and then to begin with, but a feeling that was to grow in its intensity as time passed by. I began to feel alone and isolated and in spite of Sarah's constant love and support and the love and well wishes of everyone else, I could do nothing to dispel it.

With the recent forecasted probability that Derek was going to need constant twenty-four hour nursing care I was forced to consider selling our home as he would never be able to manage the twenty five steps leading up to our front door. I found myself faced with the possibility of Derek one day being discharged from hospital but remaining unable to do anything for himself. I never allowed myself to believe that Derek would not be coming home but I had to face the financial implications of such intense nursing care and the probability of moving to more suitable accommodation. I found myself considering all possibilities, a bungalow would be more suitable, somewhere much smaller and more easily managed. To be ready to face such an eventuality I began clearing out cupboards and wardrobes, discarding all that proved surplus to future requirements, I became quite manic in the process.

I experienced the strongest, and admittedly the strangest, feeling of having to do it for Derek but no sooner had I begun than I realized I could not continue with any such plan, how could I ever bring Derek out to a strange new environment he would never, ever recognize as home. I could not do it he must and had to come back to his own home which he loved, a place he would be familiar with. He needed that, and more importantly he deserved it, and I was going to make sure that it happened. We would take care of his future needs as and when necessary. At the same time I was mindful that where we lived was Sarah's home also and this was a fact which needed to be taken into serious consideration, although I knew Sarah would have been the first to understand and would have fully supported any move that I had considered necessary.

What took up a lot of my time during those first few weeks in between the mundane tasks of daily life was the picking up the reigns of the household budgeting, something which Derek had always carried out on computer. This was not for me, I liked to see everything written down in-front of me, had I been doing it previously instead of Derek it would have been the old fashioned book-keeping method and so that is exactly what I did. I purchased a ledger and began my own budget account, it was important to me that I should be able to account for all expenditure and be able to keep control of the family finances, in doing so I exposed a fraud which had been draining our bank balance for some time. It transpired that Derek's bank card had been successfully copied in the past enabling forgers to withdraw small amounts on a regular basis, a matter which had gone unnoticed on his computer system in his belief that I had been making small purchases. I was told this practice can go on for years before anyone ever detects the fault, dribbling away small amounts out of many accounts affords someone a very lucrative living.

I longed to tell Derek all about it, I actually got myself into quite a state one evening incase I never got the opportunity to explain to him what had happened and that he might die believing that I had been spending without his knowing. How ridiculous is that? And yet it really did seem to be important to me at the time; little things I might never be able to explain to him again. It was times such as that which added to the feeling of loneliness and isolation I had begun to experience.

By 31st May, Derek was a lot more settled in himself than he had been the previously and his speech was improving rapidly. The other men on the ward informed me that he had been relating to them something regarding air-conditioning units and huge sums of money, "Been going on about it all morning," they chorused.

"That's good," I replied, "you see Derek once dealt in air-conditioning and the large sums of money he talks about would all be related."

I went onto explain to them that Derek had run a Building Design Co. which covered the design and installation of industrial build.

"That explains it all," they cried, "now we can understand him more."

During the days that followed Derek was to nearly drive everyone mad with his repeated and deeply frustrating talk of air-conditioning. He talked of air-conditioning unit no1 and of air-conditioning unit no 2.

He would cry as he kept repeating his story over and over again. He kept telling me... "important......important....you...must... listen.......air-conditioning unit no1....and.... air-conditioning....unit no2.....unit no1....went bang.......loud bang.... help.....needs help."

I tried to soothe him and the men told him that they understood but Derek grew more and more agitated and continued, "no amount........ of.....money.....not one thousand......not one... hundred thousand......will put it.....right.....unit had it....blown up."

"Must have been a hell of a job that one," said John, "to be playing on his mind like that." I could not recall such an explosion but then again so many things did go wrong on site which I never got to hear of. No-one could have been injured or I felt certain I would have known of it, but I did think it rather strange that Derek should be so disturbed by this incident.

No-one could explain the logic lying behind Derek's words and I was reminded that he had suffered severe brain damage therefore there would be no logic. I tried hard to convince him that I did indeed understand and that those air-conditioning days were long gone and so there really was no cause for him to get so worked up. Once again he became agitated and leaned back onto his pillows as though totally exhausted, shaking his head from side to side and unwilling to talk he closed his eyes leaving me to watch as the tears ran down his cheeks. I gently massaged his limbs for the rest of the afternoon and mentioned to one of his nurses my concern over his peeling skin.

"Not a problem," I was told, "it's good what you're doing, it can only help, it's only dry skin."

I also noted that same day that the Peg tube site was looking sore and infectious and I was informed that a close eye was being kept on it. During the drive home that evening I mentioned my concern over Derek's dry and peeling skin to Sarah.

"Did you mention it to anyone?" she asked.

"Yes I did."

"Well if they say it's only dry skin then it must be alright."

"Yes that's exactly what they said, that it's dry skin and simply needs moisturizing but I don't like it, something feels wrong and I feel a little concerned."

"Why?"

"I'll tell you why," I stated, "because the last time I saw skin peeling like that was when your Nanny contracted MRSA during her last stay in hospital and she sadly died from it."

"But Derek hasn't got MRSA, has he?" questioned Sarah.

"I can't be sure, but I have a very strong feeling that he has," I told her.

The following day on the ward I voiced my concern regarding Derek's now obvious infection and was told that swabs had been taken and that the ward was now awaiting the results which would be due back sometime during the next few days.

Apart from Derek being given continued doses of laxatives and the ongoing distress this caused him he maintained making good progress. He was showing less tremor in his limbs, much greater recognition in what was going on around him and was now trying his best to converse. He was still persistently repeating his story of the two air-conditioning units and would not be persuaded away from the subject.

On 31st May it was noted that the Peg site was showing signs of soreness and oozing of puss. The Peg nurse was asked to check the site and advised that it should be swabbed and monitored.

During the first week in June Derek was to experience his first attempt at sitting out of bed. This proved to be extremely difficult for the physiotherapists to carry out as Derek could not respond to their instruction and sadly proved far too much for Derek himself to bear. It was decided a hoist would be necessary and so a short time later the procedure began again with the aid of a hoist. Derek was fastened into this contraption and as he sat hunched and curled up in a foetal position he was hoisted up, over and away from the bed and deposited into the adjacent chair.

The ordeal was too exhausting for him and during the manoeuvre he unfortunately lost control of his bowels causing Derek to suffer extreme embarrassment despite his inability to be fully aware of what was going on. He became limp and seemingly lifeless. All natural colour drained from his face and I quickly voiced my concern to the girls about his grey complexion. However they seemed rather unconcerned and more annoyed that Derek was unable to follow their instruction. After stating he was not ready for physiotherapy treatment, they quickly swung him back onto the bed and walked abruptly off the ward leaving Derek lying in a crumpled up position and very messy state.

I quickly summoned help and as always the ward nurses were at his side immediately. Efficiently and yet very gently they washed and changed him, quickly stripped and remade his bed making him comfortable once more before checking his blood pressure. I was told there was no harm done and no reason for concern, it had simply been a little too much for Derek's first time experience out of bed and all that was needed was a little rest. Perhaps so, but I thought a little more understanding from the two physiotherapists would have been appropriate and certainly would have been much more appreciated.

It was confirmed on June 5th that Derek had in fact contracted MRSA. I had known the infection was on the ward because I had overheard two nurses discussing the subject at their station just opposite Derek's bed. When the nurses became aware they were being overheard they discreetly and very quickly brought the conversation to a close, but I had heard enough to understand that it had been Derek to whom they had been referring.

I had known that swabs had been taken from his tracheotomy site and sent off for analysis and had repeatedly asked if any results had come back.

Later that same day and again before leaving the ward that evening I asked if any results had come back and was told on both occasions that none had.

Alone in my bed that night I was upset and felt that the results were being withheld from me. Not being able to do anything about it I tried to hold onto the positive happenings of the day, which had seen Derek able to drink small amounts of fluid, in spite of me almost choking him on one occasion. (I had not thought to bring his bed into a more upright position before placing the straw into his mouth.) His drinking along with his improving conversation had proved extremely encouraging.

I did not sleep well that night, after tossing and turning for what felt like forever I finally fell into a fitful sleep in which I relived the suffering my mother-in-law had found herself having had to endure during her last and final stay in hospital. On being admitted into hospital after a serious fall she had been left twelve hours alone on a trolley in the A&E department. (Not in Arrowe Park Hospital I hasten to add.) Eventually she underwent an emergency operation to correct a fractured hip before being subject to the worst hospital care that I had ever experienced. Both the medical and nursing staff should have hung their heads in shame as they must have witnessed on a daily basis the filth and lack of care which this elderly lady was left subject to.

· I lay awake throughout part of the night remembering the effort that had to be applied in simply trying to rectify those appalling conditions. Conditions one would never have believed possible in this country during the twenty-first century but alas conditions we hear of so often today.

Members of Parliament became involved, the Minister of Health became involved and it became feared that I was going to sue the involved Hospital Trust but I held no such intentions. That was not my way, I had no interest in financial gain, my only interest lay with the health and well being of my mother-in-law and the immediate improvement in the care and cleanliness being administered to and surrounding her and all other patients in that hospital.

I had also wished to see a little more understanding from the nursing staff towards their patients and asked that they might remember that they were tending human beings who were, when at their most vunerable especially in need of respect and a little compassion. I did have one other interest and it was that whoever was held responsible should also be held accountable for the gross negligence witnessed during that period.

Today we hear almost on a daily basis about the poor state of our hospitals and of the strides which are being taken to bring about much needed improvement. But when my mother-in-law was in hospital these conditions were only just becoming apparent along with the recognition of how far our hospitals had been allowed to sink into the appalling political mire of bad management and care.

I also witnessed on many occasions in that same hospital food being placed in-front of patients who were too ill to feed themselves, how cruel can that can be? Patients were left unwashed for days and some were left to lie in their own urine and excreta. There is no need for me to continue with the ongoing lists of deplorable incidents which took place on that particular ward because almost every person in this country will have or will know of someone who has experienced the same raw indignities we face and suffer in most hospitals today.

My mother-in-law was transferred from a six-bedded bay ward where she had been left on a bed with no sheet or blanket and she had somehow managed to pull away her medical dressing, leaving a raw wound open to the dust and fluff, which fell like snow all over her naked body. This was caused by a cleaner standing on a chair dusting the curtain rail around her bed. Dirty bloodied dressings were found left on her bed, used syringes were found discarded on the chair next to her bed and heavily soiled bed-sheets were left lying about uncollected.

She was moved into isolation for the treatment of MRSA and the conditions found in that room would have shocked the hardiest of people. The room was splattered with dried blood, urine and excreta and had been used as a filthy store room for some considerable time. Regrettably it had not been cleaned down before the patient had been wheeled into it.

When I first entered her room on the day she had been moved into it I gagged on the smell and was shocked at the sight before me, but what I saw splattered and smeared over the walls was nothing in comparison to what lay behind the door of the en-suite toilet. After opening the door and witnessing the filth which greeted me I demanded that my mother-in-law be moved out immediately. The toilet was full and overflowing onto the floor with excreta that was stale and set solid, indicating that it had been that way for some time.

The immediate excuse was that the room had not been in use for some time except as a store-room. People using that same store-room must have had no sense of smell or eyesight to see what was right in-front of them, I found it hard to believe that they simply did not care enough to do something about it.

Why would I have been interested in suing for personal gain, what would that have achieved? All I wanted was explanations as to how this state had been allowed to occur in the first place. Why had it been allowed to go unattended for so long and how in heavens name could anyone have ever considered placing an extremely vunerable patient into it? How could anyone have ever justified placing another human being into such filth? There are jails in far flung places of this world where we might expect to find such filth and squalor, which are kept in more hygienic conditions than those found inside that room. Under conditions such as these, it should be no surprise to find infections such as MRSA rife on our wards and difficult to treat due to poor hygiene.

The Trust was held accountable and took full responsibility, going to great lengths to put right their wrongs, but sadly it meant nothing to my mother-in-law who died of her infection leaving her family with a sense of not only heartfelt sadness but also a lack of trust and a deep sense of shame in our hospitals.

For goodness sake we need them, how I wish our respect could be brought back for this giant of institutions, for we all, will one day be in need of their care, attention and great expertise.

Each time I awoke that night I found myself thanking God that Derek was not lying in a bed in that particular hospital but nevertheless I was extremely worried. The health authorities need to know that we the general public are, whether naively or justifiably, seriously concerned about these infections. We do not like to be fobbed off with excuses blaming the visitors as being the carriers when it is their own conditions of care and general lack of hygiene that are in need of more serious consideration. I personally will stand and be corrected at any time in my lack of hygienic standards but only when the ward or hospital I stand within has first put its own house in order.

Since Derek had been admitted into Arrowe Park hospital I had been given no reason for complaint. The I.T.U. department had been visibly immaculate and the room we had been allocated for sleeping in, although uncomfortable, was cleaned daily with a constant change of bed linen.

Ward 37 was well staffed with a nursing care quite rare these days and a team of domestic staff who not only cleaned and served the patients their drinks but who also took a little time in helping to boost patient moral. Never once did I see a patient left unable to feed themselves. Those busy nurses always found the time to feed anyone in need of assistance.

During those first three weeks I had come to know the team on the ward quite well, with the exception of his special nurses, who sat constantly with Derek, but changed every shift and were brought in from the agencies, or bank as it was called. It took many more weeks before I got to know them but the regular team were brilliant and I built up a high respect for them as I witnessed the way in which they handled and genuinely cared for their patients and Derek, who needed so much more individual attention than their usual patient.

Sadly on June 6th it seemed I was to cause one of the nurses of whom I had grown very fond of to flee the ward extremely upset. The day began with me ringing the ward (as usual) to check on what kind of night Derek had had and to enquire as to whether any results had been returned. I was informed that he had spent a very restless night and had been given sedation during the early morning to settle him and no, there had been no results through.

I arrived on the ward mid-morning and relieved his special nurse. Derek was still sedated so I gently rubbed cream into his limbs and then sat quietly watching over him as he slept, for even in sleep he would seek to pull his tubes out. Dr. Pinder his consultant neurologist arrived and was once again unable to assess Derek's condition due to him being sedated. But as unfortunate as this was it turned out to be a turning point for myself as the doctor gave me his time and the benefit of some very valuable advice.

On being informed that the doctor wished to speak to me I followed the nurse into the ward office where we were both asked to sit down. Dr Pinder spoke to nurse first, instructing her on procedure he wanted commencing immediately. Firstly Derek should be moved into a side room to avoid sensory overload. Nurse stated that no room was available at that time. Secondly an orientation board was to be placed in-front of Derek's bed which showed the date and where he was, adding that all staff, including myself, should draw his attention to it as often as possible to develop his attention span and help his orientation.

Continuing, the doctor stated that a bowel management program was to be introduced straight away and also recommended that a short acting sedative be given at night to ensure that Derek returned to a good nights' sleep cycle. I felt a flood of relief as I had been very concerned regarding the amount of laxatives which Derek had been frequently given. They caused a lack of bowel control and I knew had caused a great deal of the agitation and embarrassment he had experienced since regaining consciousness. This program had not come a moment too soon and I was so thankful that it was to begin at once.

Dr. Pinder went to great length in explaining as much of Derek's condition to me as he could but felt unable to confirm any true diagnosis as he needed to assess Derek properly.

What was to be the great turning point for me, although I was not to realize it until several days later, was when Dr. Pinder stated how we would have to learn how to break down the code in which Derek may talk. I understood fully, or thought I did, the content of what was being explained but have to admit I could not relate it to Derek, who was not able to string together more than a few words at any one time. However at the time, I naively believed that I understood what he was trying to explain.

The meeting over, I followed Dr. Pinder out of the office feeling more uplifted than I had felt in weeks. At last we could start doing something positive to help Derek but the last words spoken by the doctor were still ringing in my ears, the words which had offered the future promise of a bed in the Neuro-Rehabilitation Unit and the possibility that this patient may make a full recovery. I could hardly contain myself, I literally felt as though I were floating out of that office three feet above the ground but I was soon to be brought right back down to earth again.

Nurse walking out directly behind me asked very quietly if she might have a private word back in the office. She closed the door and nervously explained to me that Derek's test results had come back confirming that he had MRSA. I asked how long this had been known and was told a couple of days.

"Why on earth has this information been withheld from me?" I demanded.

"I don't know," nurse answered timidly.

"Will this make a difference to Derek being accepted into rehab? Did Dr. Pinder know of this whilst we were sat at the meeting just now, did everyone know but me?" I asked.

"It was written in Derek's notes," she stated, "so he probably will have seen it."

"But I have rung each morning and enquired each day for the past two days as soon as I came onto the ward asking if these results had come back, only to be told each time that they had not. I enquired only this morning to be told there were no results through yet, what on earth's going on and how did Derek contract this?"

At that moment I needed answers.

"I'm so sorry, I don't know anything about this but I know how you must be feeling." Sadly the nurse could have no conception of how I was feeling and at that particular moment I could not even rationalize the sense of injustice that was building up inside of me. Of one thing I now felt certain, Derek would not be going to the Neuro-Rehabilitation Unit in the near future.

I went on to inform her that if she were unable to give me answers to my questions then I would like to speak to someone who could. I was told that no-one was available and I went on to explain if that was the case then perhaps my solicitor or the hospital's Chief Executive could look into the matter for me. I left the office far from happy and went back to sit beside Derek's bed. As the afternoon wore on I became more and more aware of the heavy atmosphere which had descended upon the ward. The bay I sat in seemed unusually quiet after the afternoon visitors had left and the nursing station remained deserted except for a couple of occasions when nurse had out of necessity needed to use it, she had not lingered and we did not speak.

Sarah came onto the ward that evening to find me very upset by the afternoon's events and went to have a word with the nurse to find out why we had not been informed of the latest developments sooner. Nurse explained how she thought that I had been too fierce and aggressive in my attitude towards her and after speaking with Sarah left the ward extremely upset. Obviously the rest of the staff were feeling very concerned regarding their colleague but did anyone stop to consider how we were left feeling?

I had not considered myself rude or aggressive towards this lovely nurse, I am not that type of person but I had demanded an explanation I felt I was owed, one she was unable to give me. Being informed later that I might well have passed this infection onto Derek I find it too easy to place the blame on the visitors when hospitals need to put their own houses in order. I was not looking to blame, merely to deal with how it had occurred.

It had been a long day of very mixed emotions and I was pleased to be back at home. The evening routine of washing had, because of MRSA, been changed as all clothes now had to be first soaked and then washed at a very high temperature but by the time I had sorted and soaked the washing Sarah had prepared and cooked and was serving our evening meal. I ate it with no appetite and told Sarah I could not settle until I had rung the ward to speak to the nurse who I knew would be feeling as upset as I was. I wanted to apologize, not for what I had said but because I knew I would not be able to go to sleep that night knowing that the sharpness of my tone had upset her. Unfortunately on ringing the ward I was politely told that she had gone off duty.

CHAPTER FIVE

I was aware during that first week in June of the very sudden and drastic changes taking place in Sarah's personal life but did not have the energy to deal with it in the way that I perhaps should have. At the end of each day I felt too emotionally drained and physically exhausted to cope, I did what was required of me and somehow managed to keep going but there was nothing left, no energy to spare, not for me, not for Sarah, not for anyone, everyone had to manage and cope for themselves.

After dinner each evening I would soak in my bath and be ready to collapse straight into bed, whereas Sarah would be getting ready to go out with the new man who had recently come back into her life. That man was Max, a person who had left her life eight years earlier but had never left her heart and although Sarah had enjoyed other relationships with other men they had never matched up to Max.

Andrea Craig

How I felt for her, for the happiness she had waited so long to find was now marred by all that was taking place around her, events which had cut so deeply into her heart causing a hurt which prevented her from experiencing the joy she should have been feeling. Max was also affected because in being so closely connected to our family, he was painfully reminded of the recent experience lived through with his own dear father.

Nothing would ever please me more than Sarah and Max finally coming back together again and I felt for them and all that they were going through. Derek's devastating collapse had not affected my life alone, it had cut right into the hearts of others and my love reached out embracing them both as one but I could not cope with the changes their relationship began to put upon me.

Everything suddenly felt as though it were happening too quickly, I was already having to deal with as much change as I could cope with and the events of that day and the confirmation of Derek having MRSA proved to be too much.

That evening instead of getting straight into bed after my bath I thought I would try a little television to help me unwind. Sarah had already gone out having first solicited a promise from me that I would ring her if I were to need anything and giving her assurance that she would not be late.

I found I could not concentrate on the television and although the evening was very warm, I felt strangely cold and needed my bed.

I can remember clearly switching the television off, but I cannot remember the exact moment in which I first became aware of a sound which made me feel as though I were drowning in it. It grew increasingly louder, rooting me to the spot where I stood until suddenly I recognised the sound of great heart rendering sobs, crying as I had never heard before. Not even when my father had died and I had cried long and hard into my pillow throughout each night for several weeks afterwards had I heard a sound such as this.

The sound seemed to be coming from deep within myself creating the feeling of a damn having burst and there was now no stopping the massive surge of waters from flooding the very room I occupied. For a short while I became detached from the experience, and found myself wondering and somewhat puzzled as to what was happening. Then suddenly I could stand no longer, I became overpowered and unable to breathe as I felt myself sinking into the waters which were threatening to engulf me. It was all too much, I was no longer strong enough to stand, swim or even care what was happening, I simply gave in. The tightness felt in my heart had vanished and all thoughts had ceased.

Gradually out of the darkness I once again heard the sobbing, some poor soul sounding lost and wretched I thought and at the exact moment of thinking it came the realization that the sobs were escaping from me. I felt totally exhausted and remember thinking and questioning at that point if to feel lost, as I had first imagined that other person to be, could be borne of my own sense of feeling alone and isolated? I supposed it might have been.

I was surprised to discover that I had not been sitting in darkness, in fact the summer sun was still pouring in through the large windows of our sitting room but in spite of the warmth this created, I still felt very cold. Feeling stiff and numb from having found myself lying on the floor I picked myself up and drew the curtains over before heavily climbing the stairs to my bed feeling as though I had shed my last tear. But instead of sleep came more tears, they flowed until I believed they would never stop. They eventually stopped and as sleep drew me into itself, I willingly surrendered to its calming embrace.

I did not hear Sarah come home and thankfully I awoke the following morning feeling surprisingly rested, this was the first time I had cried since Derek had collapsed and instead of feeling weary and exhausted as I had the previous evening I felt strangely rejuvenated.

I awoke remembering the words which someone had spoken to me many years previously, "Andrea never be afraid to shed your tears, for the growth of your inner being shall depend on them." Words I had often recalled when needed and repeated to many people over the years. I could not help wondering if that was the reason for my feeling as refreshed as I did.

Still obviously very concerned about Derek and extremely upset at the handling of the situation by the hospital staff, I felt that I faced the beginning of a new day in which we could hopefully put into place many of the suggestions put forward by Dr. Pinder. Before leaving home to visit Derek I received a telephone call from the hospital wishing to arrange a meeting at 2.15p.m regarding my outburst which had upset one of their nurses. I welcomed this opportunity and said that I would certainly be present that afternoon.

The meeting was chaired by Dr. Oates and in attendance were the chief nursing officer, infection control officer, duty staff-nurse and myself. It proved a very positive meeting with an apology given on the hospitals behalf for the delay in informing me. The reason was that Dr. Oates had been in London and not herself been informed. I also expressed my sincerest regret for having upset a nurse and stated how I would very much like the opportunity to speak to her and apologize personally as I was very fond of her and considered her nursing of Derek and her other patients to be excellent.

It was also stated at this meeting how regrettable it was that there were no available side-rooms to place Derek in but as soon as one came empty then he would go straight into it.

I went on to ask why, when Derek was on twenty-four hour watch had he been allowed to pull out his tubes? I was not exactly satisfied with their response, which explained that Derek could be very quick at doing this to which I replied,

"Yes indeed he can but that is precisely why he is on twenty-four-hour watch so that he can be watched and supervised very carefully."

I went on to further explain that during the times when I sat with him he would often attempt the same thing but I always managed to prevent him from doing so.

This took constant alertness and effort on my behalf and should have been something his special nurses were meant to be doing.

However, once again I must make it quite clear that I held both the entire resident nursing staff on ward 37 and its domestic team, not forgetting many of the H.C.A's who attended Derek, in the highest respect, I cannot state that strongly enough. They carried out their duties and were superb in every way. Nothing was ever too much trouble and a genuine caring and gentle attitude was administered each day. This went a long way in helping the patient's relatives as well as the patients' themselves. Both Derek and I will remember that wonderful team for the rest of our lives.

The following day nurse graciously accepted my apology in the presence of the chief nursing officer and I was truly sorry for having upset her so much, it was never my intention to do so. We spent a little time chatting to each other and parted warmly after sharing what I believed to be a truly genuine hug. I was therefore saddened to hear a little later that she had requested to be moved from nursing in Derek's bay because of the upset.

It was then I began to realize that reactions were running too high, all because I had demanded an explanation I felt entitled to. I had not been aggressive nor had I behaved in a rude manner towards that particular nurse but yes it was true that I was upset (justifiably so in my opinion) and yes, when she told me no explanation could be given, I did state that I would be talking to my solicitor who might be more successful in obtaining one than myself. That was a direct statement of fact, not the firing of bullets with the intention of harming anyone. I do hope that our shared experience will prove to make us both stronger and wiser in dealing with future circumstances.

It had been an exhausting two days but what had helped to uplift me during that time was the fact that a date board had been placed at the side of Derek's bed. This began his daily practice of having to focus on the date, day, year and where he was. At the beginning he could not see the board let alone recognize writings on it, but nevertheless the staff and myself continued to draw his attention to it on a daily basis.

The second thing to uplift me that day was the fact that I had been out and bought books to write in, these became known as Derek's daily diaries. I was never quite sure why the doctor had recommended that I keep one but keen to follow his advice I had decided that a diary would be kept and today was the day I had placed it on his table, open for all staff who wished to pass comment to be able to do so.

At first we were not sure what we were expected to write and the initial daily comments were brief and entered only by myself, but after the first week had passed the nursing staff and therapists began to enter their own comments and as the days turned into weeks and the weeks turned into months the daily entries turned into quite extensive writings.

They record an enormous struggle of one man's climb up a mountain he once felt too high. In the beginning he was overpowered by the very thought of it and had believed he would never have the energy which he knew would be demanded of him. But with the expertise of a magnificent medical team, the day by day determination and commitment from Derek himself and what I consider to be the greatest power of all, Love, he has after many set-backs, learned to overcome his fears and is well on his way to conquering this formidable peak.

Has he reached the summit? ---- Definitely not. Will he ever reach the summit? I cannot say. I believe he stands half-way to the top and is still climbing as I write

CHAPTER SIX

Many of the hospital staff found Derek's diaries fascinating and at times quite moving, Derek himself finds them priceless as they bring back and place before him a part of his life he would otherwise have lost. In the later reading of them he found a form of healing which helped him to move on and also enabled him to find the impetus needed in continuing his daily climb. The following pages are the daily entries recorded just as they were written, along with some of the letters I wrote to Derek during his many months in hospital.

Ward 37 Friday 8th June 2007.

Derek was constantly requesting information, still flaying his arms about but not as much. Was very alert to the mentioning of the year 2007 and was able to repeat to me, "Friday 8th June 2007" and again in-front of nurse.

He was a little emotional this afternoon.

Derek requested bed-pan for the second consecutive day.

Mrs. Lamb passed comment on the ward being rather warm and Derek responded unbelievably with, "Yes it certainly was."

I asked Derek if he could try and count to ten with me, he did so and continued on to fourteen, without being asked he repeated from one to ten.

Asked Derek if he could sing, he sang Elvis Presley's "Blue Suede Shoes" and went on to sing two more songs. He remembers all of the words and sings very well. He seemed to have enjoyed himself.

5 15 p.m. *Derek is now completely exhausted and is resting.*

Entered by Andrea Craig.

Saturday 9th June   2007

Derek was very emotional after lunch because he recognizes he can not find or use the correct words and feels his head is hazy and muddled all the time.

He was asked to count to ten and did so readily but jumbled.

He was a lot more relaxed and cheerful throughout this afternoon.

Derek continues to be able to count to ten, albeit still somewhat jumbled, and was able to repeat the date after me.

Entered by Andrea Craig.

Sunday 10th June   2007

Derek was very emotional when he woke up this morning but was o.k. later on when he became quite chatty.

Entered by unknown person.

Derek responded well to having his hair and beard trimmed by myself.

Was very relaxed today but rather quiet.

He counted to ten on request and again up to twenty, still mixes his numbers.

Could not repeat the day or date but he did know which year it was.

Entered by Andrea Craig.

Monday 11th June   2007

Happy day, I asked Derek to count to ten and he did so although still unable to follow instruction very well.

Derek focused well on date board today for the first time.

Talking again of air-conditioning units and got quite agitated saying I did not understand.

Entered by Andrea Craig.

Tuesday 12*th* June   2007

Derek agitated today.

He could see date board although he could not hold his concentration for more than a few seconds.

He also managed to explain to me why he had refused to eat his lunch, stating that he simply did not like it.

Derek's physiotherapy really exhausted him and left the physiotherapists very unhappy once again but at least he managed to put both his feet to the floor which made it a little easier transferring him into his chair.

Nurses called to help clean Derek and put him back into bed.

Entered by Andrea Craig.

I had left the hospital that evening feeling very upset and despondent. I could not get it out of my mind how uncaring those physiotherapists had been with Derek, no man deserved that sort of treatment.

It had been myself who had kept insisting upon physiotherapy for him, believing that the longer he lay in bed the more unlikely his chances would be of his ever being able to walk again. I had felt it was vital his limbs should be exercised, I had from the very beginning tried to do what I could to keep moving and massaging them but knew this was not enough, so yes I had persisted in requesting that he had physiotherapy and felt badly in having let him down in their mishandling of him.

I had expected the girls to have had a way of exercising his limbs, to perhaps show me how I could be of more use to him myself, but I had not expected them to hoist him out of bed for the second time in the brusque manner in which they did, sit him in a chair and then leave me to hold him up for the following half-hour. On their return the girls apologized for being so long and said they had been detained and felt things would be better in future if a larger chair were to be brought in for Derek to sit on. Derek was completely exhausted by this time and should not have been left out of bed for so long. The ordeal had proved far too much for him during his first attempt and the girls in my opinion should have known better.

I went to bed that evening knowing I must put it out of my mind and as always I had no difficulty in dropping off to sleep. I have no recollection of the exact time I awoke except that it was still dark and must have been during the early hours of the following morning. I sat bolt upright as though a light had been switched on flooding my mind with a knowing that made me want to get up and rush to the hospital immediately.

How or why the realization came to me during sleep seems unimportant but the fact that it had was to prove very important to Derek. No way could I go back to sleep, I needed to clear my thoughts and so slipping into my dressing gown I went downstairs and made myself a drink whilst

Andrea Craig

I went over once again the realization I had just woken up with.

It was now so clear I could not believe I had not known it sooner. I knew with absolute certainty that air-conditioning unit no.1 was Derek himself and unit no.2 was me. The code which Dr. Pinder had talked of had been broken and I at last knew that Derek had been trying his best to tell us how he had "blown up" and that no amount of money would ever be able to put him right again. He had been so correct in his repeated telling me that no one understood him. I could not wait to tell him that I now did.

Much too excited to go back to bed I decided I would write a letter to Derek, which I could read to him in an attempt at cheering him up after his unpleasant experience yesterday, this is the letter I wrote.

To my dear, darling boy, my wonderful, wonderful Blue,

I find I cannot sleep. The excitement of finally understanding what it is you have been struggling to say to me over the past few days is so great. So here sitting with a nice hot drink in the peace and silence of the night I thought I would write and tell you some of the things I would like you to know.

I want you to know that Saturday April 28th was both the most beautiful and the most dreadful day of my entire life. It was the day you collapsed without my being at your side, but at that moment

108

when your world stopped I want you to know that my world stopped also.

I have been at your side ever since and knowing how shocked and damaged you were I knew I had to be strong. I needed to be strong for you, for both of us.

The doctors and nurses have been wonderful, their expertise truly remarkable, I feel we owe them so much but most of all, my darling, I want you to know of the love, respect and admiration that I have for you which has deepened beyond words over the past two weeks as I have sat at your side.

You have at times throughout our marriage been a pain in the backside, your expression I believe not mine, you have been both obstinate and stubborn on the odd occasions but you have always been true, open and honest with me and I have admired and respected you more than you could possibly imagine.

There are so many things I long to tell you and be able to share with you still and I believe that God in His Grace will grant us just the right amount of time needed to do so, for all things are taken care of in their rightful time.

It was not your time to go my darling, and we must take this time and trust that we will be allowed to share an even deeper love than we shared before. I have never, except by Sarah, ever been loved by anyone as much as the love you hold in your heart for me.

I want you to love me always as I love you, until all the little pieces are gathered in, once again making one entire whole, when the world will be united in our love, God's Love. We are you and I and all who share in His love united as one.

The time to come is our journey together, of letting go of all things which do not matter and focusing only on those that are important. Although I realize that this must be a very frightening time for you, please try if you can, sweetheart, not to be too afraid of feeling lost for God knows exactly where you are, He will never lose sight of you, not ever and I will be at your side always, sometimes gently persuading you to do something you feel you cannot do, sometimes pushing you forward perhaps too harshly but please always remember how much I love you and that I would never mean to hurt you, I love you so much it actually hurts me at times deep down within my heart.

I ask that you do not worry or concern yourself about me for I am, with Sarah's help, managing to take care of everything. Know my darling "Blue", that we will face our journey together as we have faced all which came before, with truth, love and the help of God and heaven's armies. Love is the greatest and strongest healing there is. You have my entirety in body, mind and spirit for as long as you should love me, you are the completeness of my soul, you are me and I am yours eternally.

So you can understand why the 28th was the most dreadful day but the most beautiful part of it was shared before you collapsed as we walked hand in hand around the Marina and you told me how happy you felt and of how you had found your inner peace at long last. That made my heart almost burst with joy, I had waited so long for you to feel that and now at last we will, God willing, go on to share that inner peace and If, when God does decide that it is time for one of us to leave the other, we will have come to know and understand, that in the sharing of love and such peace, there can never be separation. I truly believe this truth will help us, each in our turn, find the strength needed to somehow complete the final stage of our journey My wonderful, great big fellow, I want to thank-you, for your never ending patience with me. I often acted harshly towards you, when all I ever intended to be was kind and gentle and a lot wiser than I ever was. I often gave the impression of being aloof with you when all I ever wanted was to be held safe and secure within those arms of yours, so many people have been comforted when held within that huge and warm embrace of yours, I know exactly how they felt and the strength each of them received.

I want you to know how much and how often my heart would swell with pride when we were out together, I loved dining-out with you, I loved so much the holidays we shared, and I loved especially our dancing, how we loved to dance together feeling that special closeness with my Mr. Wonderful. I loved visiting the cinema with you for you would always willingly sit and watch through the silly films that I so loved to see but most of all I loved simply to be with you, talking to you, you are my best friend and lover and I must tell you once again that I shall love you always with all of my heart.

We stand now my darling at a time when we are able to let all the stress and strain of the past fall away and allow the gentleness of our love and the strength of God to take us forward. Remember that I am a Capricorn, the mountain goat and as such I will help you find your way up this mountain which looms so high before you. Rest in my love and the peace you have discovered and all will be well, remember that all things are taken care of.

My love forever and always until the end of time and beyond

Andrea   xxx

However it would be another seven days before I was able to read this letter to Derek or be able to tell him of my realization regarding the air-conditioning units. Circumstances took over as I was to discover the following day.

CHAPTER SEVEN

I set off the following morning, arriving at the hospital much earlier than usual to share excitedly with Derek what I believed was the truth behind his talk of air-conditioning units and that I might be able to read, or make a start in reading my letter to him. I say, a start to read, because Derek did not have a very long attention span and my letter being rather lengthy made me realize that it may have to be read and re-read over and over again in small sections at a time. What I did not expect but was delighted to be informed on entering the ward was that Derek no longer occupied the first bed in bay one for he had been moved into an isolation room at the far end of the ward.

As I walked down the ward I felt sorry that Derek would no longer have the company of the other men, they had taken to him and looked out for him and I felt sure he would miss them but at the same time I felt very pleased that at last he would have some privacy. Nearing the three isolation rooms which where sited adjacent to each other across the furthest end of the ward, I began to feel a nervousness about what I might find when I opened the door of Derek's room.

I felt the eyes of the other patients upon me as I walked past each bay, I was someone new to them and what else had they to do, of course many of them were far too poorly to take notice of anything but the nurses called out good-morning and some asked if I was pleased to hear of the transfer. I answered that I was and hoped that I was not showing the nervousness I felt.

Derek's room was the end one of the three, the first opened straight off the main ward but the other two were reached by walking first into a small anti-type room a little further down the corridor. This room separated the two isolation rooms from the rest of the ward and housed a shower room and toilet which was to be shared by the patients in either of these two rooms.

"Are you looking for Derek Craig," asked the duty staff-nurse as I passed her desk. I said that I was and indicating which direction I should take she added, "Last door opposite the store-cupboards, room 23, I believe his special nurse is in with him and that he is quite settled."

I opened the door and was immediately taken back by the huge expanse of window stretching the full width of the opposite wall, which took my gaze out over open countryside, across the River Dee and as far as the Welsh hills. Sadly Derek was unable to see the beautiful expanse of clear blue sky or the view outside of his window, he could not even focus on anything inside of his new room and had no knowledge or memory of being transferred only two hours previously.

To say that the room was bright would be stating the obvious, being situated on the third floor of the hospital and having such a large window how could it be otherwise but as I stood in the doorway I was able to see that not only was this room bright and spacious it was also clean which was an immense relief to me. I had a brief chat with his nurse as she explained that Derek was not too high in spirits and would probably need a little time to settle after the disturbance of being moved. As she gathered together her belongings and bid farewell to Derek I began putting Derek's clean change of clothes into his new locker.

Taking over from his morning special-nurse became the daily routine for the following five long months. Here is the entry into Derek's diary which marks his first day in room 23.

Wed. 13th June 3, 2008

Derek now in room 23 (side room)
Off his food, appears to be a little down today.

1.30p.m *Derek helped out of bed by physios and sat propped up in his chair.*
Could not take in outside view, unable to sit up properly I had to hold him in his chair. (A little worried at times that he was going to slip)

4p.m Derek very tired but as he was being put back to bed he asked for a bed-pan (excellent)

A few more open windows today into his recent memory which I feel is good,

Also turned towards the notice board when I asked him what day it was.

(But not every time)

Derek remembered how old he was today for the first time (He has always stated 25 before when asked)

He also recognized that his brain is not functioning correctly and feels he has lost part of his memory. This worried him.

As the day wore on Derek lifted in spirit and seemed quite happy once more.

He stated that it worried him because he could not find or use the correct words to express how he feels.

Derek still feels the mountain is too high to climb and is frightened that he has lost all control.

His expression much clearer to-day in spite of how he feels, even if only now and again. (Brilliant)

Able to remember that Paul (Derek's son) had been into see him last night and as we continued to talk of Paul, Derek's face literally lit up.

Entered by Andrea Craig.

Thursday 14th June 2007

Derek a bit upset this morning that we are not giving him any information.

Being very responsive and trying to be chatty while being washed

Entered by M. Clark (H.C.A)

Told us that his wife's name is Andrea.

Derek very quiet and thoughtful

Entered by G.C. Duffy (H.C.A)

Derek was asking for a drink of water.

He has been very upset and tearful.

He has eaten a small amount of his dinner but most of his ice-cream.

Derek was quite talkative a little later.

Entered by M. Clark.

Derek was a little better with his physio today, he sat out and said he felt better for it. He asked to use toilet, said he no longer wished to use bed-pans. Nurses sat him on the commode and he was very much happier. He managed to explain how embarrassed he feels and longs to be able to take care of himself.

Sat back on chair after using commode until 3.45p.m saying how tired he felt.(colour drains from him with any exertion).

Nurses put Derek back into bed and he quickly fell into a relaxed sleep.

Derek stated today that he did not like baby-mush (liquidised food) and wanted no more of it, also asked me how long did I think it would be before he was better. He knew who I was and that I was his wife.

Not as emotional as yesterday.

Has kept repeating that water has always been very important and that he has always drunk it all of his life. (This is true.)

Derek not been talking as rapidly as he has been and seems to be thinking more before he tries to say something.

Was looking out of window more and said he thought he could see some trees.

Derek again concerned that he is not able to use the correct words.

Derek managed to drink a whole beaker of water late afternoon.

Entered by Andrea Craig.

Derek was quite coherent this evening was discussing how he did not feel as much pain as he had previously.

He talked of how bored he feels at times and of how determined he is to get back to "something like his old self."

Was able to state how long he has been in hospital, he feels like it five years and I had to explain to him that it had been five weeks.

Talked about his tracheotomy tube and how disgusting it had made his mouth feel.

Says he feels much better now and enjoys drinking water and milk.

Was able to take his drink unaided.

Entered by E. Leatherbarrow (Derek's sister)

Friday 15th June. 2008

Derek was in a lovely mood this morning, very chatty and smiling as well as talking about going to B&Q to spend some money. He was asking for information between mouthfuls of breakfast.

He has been washed and changed and had his bowels opened.

Speech therapist came to see Derek this morning regarding his speaking, eating and drinking.

Therapist's report below.

Entered by Karl McCavish (Bank HCA)

9.45 a.m. *Engaged Derek for twenty-five minutes.*

He was able to recall therapist's name after a short delay.

Also able to follow some basic instructions within context i.e. to sit up, not to pull at catheter tube etc.

Difficulty in responding to questions but was able to tell me his wife's name and that he likes to be called Derek.

Would suggest: Keep topics of conversation with Derek

simple and relevant.
Give clear and simple instructions with
Visual clues.
Do not give too much information at once.
Entered by Rebecca Smith
Senior specialist SCT.

As the morning progressed Derek became settled, he had a little sleep, he chatted at times. He has taken all of his salmon with cheese sauce for lunch but left some of the mashed potatoes. Has taken half a pot of HIP (high intensified protein) whip but refused the rice pudding.

Derek remains in pleasant and chatty mood, is always asking for information.

Feel I must add that Derek was able to explain for himself with no prompting at all, that he refused his rice pudding because he does not like it.

His wife has confirmed this to be true. Well done Derek.

Entered by Karl McCavish (HCA)

1p.m 15ᵗʰ June *Derek asked me why he should keep thinking of B&Q and shopping there. I explained simply that that was where he had been when he had experienced his heart attack.*

Managed into his chair a lot more easily today.

Asked for and used the commode again.

Physio's arrived and successfully got him to walk a few steps with assistance, Physio's stated enough but Derek wanted to try and do a few more, he managed two and then proceeded to show us how he used to dance by moving his hips, he thought this very funny. I thought he was brilliant.

He also managed on their instruction to stand-up from his chair but was not able to sit himself back in it.

Derek rested after his physiotherapy session. A little later we used the coloured building blocks. He was able to recognize several colours and managed to be able to count them into groups of three. Had difficulty repeating and got confused after approx. ten minutes.

I read the daily paper to him but after five minutes I had lost his attention and he stated he was tired and wished to get back into bed.

He drifted off to sleep after telling me he felt so happy today.

4.45p.m. *Upon waking-up Derek claimed that his toiletry is so embarrassing for him and he loathes it all so much he cries about it in the night.*

He informed me of three things he considers very important to him:

1. *To be able to go to the toilet on his own whenever he wants to go.*
2. *To be able to go to the tap and pour his own drink of water and not have to ask other people all the time.*

3. Not to have to eat any more "baby mush."

Derek did well today, I felt so pleased, he ate all of his dinner and he enjoyed it.
Entered by Andrea Craig.

Saturday 16th June 2008

Derek had a comfortable night, sleeping for six hours. Derek enjoyed spelling out his name using the bricks. He spoke a lot about Andrea and his children and has been in a very pleasant mood since waking up. We have been doing some spelling of his name and his wife's.
Entered by duty nurse.

12.45p.m. *Derek was very emotional when I first arrived today and he begged me never to leave him. Said he was very afraid and asked if I would explain about B&Q.*

He stated that he was too tired to concentrate today but would work tomorrow.

I personally believe that yesterday, which was by far his best day to date, tired him out completely and left him exhausted and low in spirit.

I tried him with his reading specs. But alas with no success, he was not able to focus at all. He got confused with colours and numbers he said, and when I tried to explain that numbers did not go together with colours, he surprised me by stating that in B&Q, numbers and colours did go together because they mixed the colour of their paint by numbers, which of course is quite true, and that some people also painted by numbers.

Derek was not able to focus today but he was able to think and express himself a lot more clearly.

I was told that Derek had used the commode again this morning which he said made him so happy that he could do this. He also asked if I would take him in a decent, proper cup, instead of the feeder-cup he was now having to use because he did not like 'baby-cups'.

3.15p.m. *Derek asked to go back to bed claiming he was so tired. Whilst sitting with him, he told me that he was so frightened that everyone will now believe him to be stupid or daft.*

5.30p.m. *Derek had a good rest and is now a lot more settled but kept trying to find a certain word to describe "something" he wanted more than anything to be able to go back to again. He asked me to try and guess what he meant when he said it sounded like the word air. It was some time before I guessed at the word "church" and Derek shouted out aloud that that was it, "church" was what he had been trying to say. What a relief. Derek cried and thanked God, saying it had been so important to him that I should understand how much he wanted to go back to church. Derek a lot more cheerful and ate his dinner.*

Entered by Andrea Craig.

Sunday 17ᵗʰ June 2008

6.15a.m. *Derek has had a bit of a restless sleep, he slept all night but seemed to be disturbed. He has had his PEG tube fed during the night which seemed to bother him. He woke up early this morning but remembers falling in and out of sleep all through the night. He's very quiet but did greet me with a pleasant, "good-morning love," which was rather nice.*

I do hope Derek has a good day and continues to make good progress.

Entered by (Bank HCA) Nicki Johnson.

Derek is in a pleasant and thoughtful mood and has chosen the menu for tomorrow's meals. Ten minute later he was able to repeat this back to me. Derek has asked if Sarah has returned from abroad yet, he thinks perhaps she has gone to Spain. (Andrea later told me this was not correct, Sarah had not been out of the country

Entry unknown.

Derek was a little talkative and very responsive for ten minutes or so, however he seemed very tired and restless. Paul Jones (staff-nurse) and I helped Derek back into bed, he remained awake but very tired.

Entered by Sarah Crawford HCA.

18th *June 2008*

7.30a.m.   Derek slept well last night although a little restless and fidgety at times. He awoke at 4.10a.m. quite frightened and upset, I gave a small amount of reassurance and he seemed a lot calmer. Derek drifted back off to sleep at approx. 5.15a.m. woke up again at 7.10a.m.I finished my duty at 7.30a.m.
Entered by Mandy Chapman (HCA)

Derek has been settled but low in mood. Derek remembered correctly who his Father's card was from and stated that Andrea was the love of his life. Derek also talked of a pint of bitter but was somewhat confused as to what he really meant. Derek told staff (nurse) this morning what he would like for breakfast without any help, which was good and also stated what he wished to have for his lunch and dinner tomorrow. During the morning Derek became more chatty and was smiling a lot, he has also been telling me about when he and Andrea got married.
Entered by Karl McCavish (Flexibank)

Physiotherapy a.m.   Derek managed to get himself out of bed on his own this morning. He was able to walk with supervision approx. twenty metres, he seems very much better to-day. He was also able to describe the weather to us.

Entered by Liz. (Physio.)

12.30p.m. *Derek eaten all of his lunch including his desert but did leave mashed potatoes, saying it reminded him of the "baby mush." After lunch Derek and I played with the coloured blocks. We spelt out his name, surname and his wife's name. We also enjoyed a conversation about Liverpool and Everton football club. Derek remained in a pleasant, cheerful and very chatty mood.*

Entered by Karl McCavish HCA.

1p.m. *Derek chatty when I arrived, he asked for information over the last five years of his life. Extremely lucid at times and stated that he was able to remember how he felt during his cardiac arrest at B&Q. He went onto describe how he had found himself in a very, very dark place and of how very frightened he had felt. Knew he could not get home and how he was not so scared now but could be if he thinks he is alone. He needed a lot of reassurance.*

Derek remembered that his son and daughter both came into see him yesterday and that Sarah had broken her arm, but could not remember how.

Mid-afternoon Derek asked for commode.

I am surprised and pleased that Derek appears to be more like his old self today, although he still has a problem focusing. If I move around the room he cannot say where I am, he actually appears to be unable to see at times and this truly worries me.

4p.m. Derek put himself back into bed showing me how well he can now stand unaided, he was able to turn around on his own retaining his balance throughout but needed assistance on sitting down on the bed and swinging his legs onto it, in all the whole procedure was a great success.
Entered by Andrea Craig.

Evening visiting. Derek tells me that sleep is hard to come by and that he is very frightened in case he does not ever wake up again. We spoke for a while about mum and dad and where we thought they might be (both died some years ago). He was in a very pleasant mood and telling me all about the progress he has made and of how I should see him walking now. What an amazing improvement!

He was feeling a bit low and depressed before I left and a little weepy, but we talked and laughed about which one of us was the eldest, "not me that's for sure."
Entered by Elaine (Derek's sister).

Tuesday 19th June 2008

Derek bright and chatty this morning, he was telling me about his "problem" in B&Q, also about his son and daughter. He was able to eat a weetabix for breakfast after which he went for a short walk with the physio's.

9.45a.m. Derek had a swill in his room, changed into clean T-shirt and shorts and sat out while his bed was changed.

Entered by Helen (Bank HCA.)

12.45p.m. Derek has been asking for a bitter-shandy for the past two weeks so today he had his shandy and thought it was heaven, (he actually drank 200ml)

Derek was able to get himself up out of bed and stood by himself for a few minutes, I could see how pleased he was with himself at being able to do this, he needed assistance in finding and sitting in his chair.

Harry, a patient from the main ward who had occupied the bed next to Derek, knocked and said they would not allow him to come in but he would like to say a quick, " hello," to Derek and could I let him know how much he was missed on the ward.

Afterwards it was good to hear that Derek remembered him and of how much he used to enjoy their singing together.

Derek is making really good progress.

4.00p.m. *Derek became extremely cold and shivering, was helped back into bed and nurses brought in extra blankets and said they would keep a constant check on him.*

5.00p.m. *Cardiologist visited Derek and seemed very reluctant to take the matter any further stating that it would not be fair to put a man in a vegetative state on the operating table. I am far from happy and asked how many vegetables he had held a conversation with. Cardiologist returned ten minutes later and apologized stating that Derek's notes had not been in the correct place and that he had since managed to read them. Derek will be referred for angiogram.*
Entered by Andrea Craig.

9.00p.m. *I arrived on duty to find Derek sleeping.*

22.30p.m. *Derek's PEG feed commenced without really waking or disturbing him, although his sleep seems restless with lots of tossing and turning.*

23.50p.m. *Derek awoke and said he needed to use the commode. Paul and myself assisted Derek onto the commode, he managed quite well once out of the bed and proved quite steady on his feet. He did not use the commode, assisted him back to bed. Offered him a drink and he said he would rather have a cold one, I suggested milk but he said no, water please.*

00.15a.m. *Derek tucked up in bed once more and now fast asleep.*

6.30a.m. *We are wide awake saying he has had a good nights' sleep, which he has had, and that he cannot remember anything of the thunderstorm we had during the night and could not even remember having had any dreams.*

I asked Derek what type of music he enjoyed and he replied, "All sorts, I asked him if he had ever played a musical instrument and he laughed and said, "no," but that he could sing.

He thought gardening was hard work but that he and Andrea did lots of hanging baskets together. Says that he used to be a good squash player, and that they have an excellent local squash club. He was not born on the Wirral, (Derek had a good think about where he was born and said that I would best ask either his mum or dad about that one.)

He thought that I would not like black pudding as he thought it to be too hard and rubbery. He stated that he would love fish, chips and mushy peas to eat most of all.

Derek then informed me that his mum and dad had both died a while ago.

He tells me that his wife Andrea is wonderful and the nicest person ever.

Derek asked if I was Spiritual, I answered that I was and he said it was unusual to find people who really were and that it was very important to him.

Derek was helping me to spell the word spiritual and I had to tell him that after a long night I found it difficult to spell, he found this really amusing and we had a good laugh about it.

Derek told me that he used to own and run his own business, and that he and Andrea once worked together. He said that he could never wish for anyone other than Andrea and Sarah, (that made him very emotional.)

Derek says that I am daft and that no-one will ever believe we sang nursery rhymes, (1, 2, 3, 4, 5, once I caught a fish a live, 6, 7, 8, 9, 10 then I let it go again, Why did you let it go, because it bit my finger so, which finger did it bite, the little finger on the right.) Sing it all the time to my kids.......was telling Derek all about them.

Derek asked me if I had ever seen any zebra's but feel it only fair to say that we had been talking about safari parks at the time.

Entered by Barbara (HCA).

Seven whole days had passed since Derek had been transferred into his isolation room. Seven days of extreme struggle and deep frustration, seven days and nights which presented great blanks of nothingness to Derek as he fought to remember and piece together his past life. The moment for reading him the letter I had written or my telling him that I understood his talk of air-conditioning units had not presented itself, moving into his new room had taken over and settling him into his new surroundings had taken priority.

It should be remembered that not only was Derek in isolation on his Neurologists recommendation for complete quiet and absence from distraction but for the treatment of MRSA also. Derek had no idea of the infection he was fighting, I on the other hand took it very seriously and each day as Derek rested I took it upon myself to clean out his entire room as thoroughly as I could. The nurses ensured that I was using the correct mop and bucket and informed me this was very important in not spreading infection from one area to another. I used the special wipes which had been placed in his room to wipe down everything I possible could, nothing was left to chance and the discovery of black dust which lay as a carpet upon the top of the wardrobe, obviously overlooked by the cleaners, seemed to justify what might have been considered by some to be an obsession.

Was this necessary? I have no idea, but it made me feel very much better and proved to be the most wonderful daily therapy, I was applying my effort to something useful. Was I paranoid? Probably but I was very thorough. I intended no slight on the cleaners, or domestic staff as they are now known, room 23 had good domestic staff, better than I had experienced in other hospitals I had attended but I needed to do the best that I could for Derek who was unable to do anything for himself. Also the memory of past experience still being so vivid in my mind, I simply could not afford to take chances.

And so that first week passed by, a period of mixed emotions fluctuating between the dread and fear Derek had been experiencing and the often felt excitement of his remarkable progress, which took place in spite of the infection he was having to fight.

It was during the afternoon of June 20th that I was able to explain to Derek my new revelations regarding the air-conditioning units. We had been going over some family photographs in an attempt to trigger his memory when he stated that since his mind had blown-up he found it very difficult to be able to concentrate on anything at all. I felt this was the opening I had been waiting for and having spent what could be considered to have been a very busy program that afternoon, I lay Derek down for his rest and shared with him my new understanding of what he had been trying to say.

He cried so much I became quite disturbed, perhaps we had overdone things and I had tired him out. This was a constant worry to me, such a fine line between doing just enough to help and doing too much that it may cause harm. I was about to summon help when Derek informed me that he was not upset in any way, it was simply the relief at last of someone understanding what had happened to him. He had felt, literally as though he had blown-up and that was the only way he knew of describing it.

It is perhaps interesting to note that those air-conditioning units were never mentioned again. Perhaps this was not the same "breaking of the code" to which Dr. Pinder referred, nevertheless I felt indebted to him for it was his words of advice given to me a few days before which had helped bring me to this realization.

Derek complained of feeling cold and so I covered him with his extra blankets, he said he would like to feel the soft warmth of his new dressing gown and soon settled down after this was put around him. I then continued to explain that I had written a letter to him and asked if he would like me to read it, my reward came as I finished reading and witnessed the smile on his face as he fell into a deep relaxed sleep.

During his stay in hospital Derek requested the reading of that letter many times stating that it formed a bridge of understanding in what he felt to be a great vast sea of muddled confusion.

As Derek slept I found myself going over the happenings of that week and could not help but marvel at the supreme effort he had exerted in his upward climb. How dare the cardiologist, when he had visited the room earlier that week, ask why I would ever consider putting a man in a vegetative state on the operating table to undergo an angiogram. This doctor had held a conversation, albeit a limited one, with Derek during that visit and I found myself asking him how many vegetables he had ever had a conversation with. I had been cross with him for he seemed not to understand why he had been requested to assess Derek.

I did explain to him that before Derek was discharged from Arrowe Park hospital and placed into 'neuro rehab' I would like further information and medical advice on the very cause that had placed Derek into the poor state of health he now found himself to be in. I tried to explain the confusion I felt caused by my ignorance of the situation and also the fear and lack of understanding that Derek was going through. In the battle to save Derek's life and determine the extent of his brain damage I felt the cause of what had led to this event was being overlooked.

The doctor left the room and returned some ten minutes later apologizing for not having read the latest updated report on Derek's condition. Once again I requested that the angiogram which Derek had been booked in for just a few days after he had collapsed, be carried out, I needed to know exactly what had caused his heart attack and what we were dealing with. Derek was in complete agreement with this and stated that it would help to settle his mind.

At this stage Derek had no recollection of the chest pains he had been experiencing during the weeks before his collapse. Pains which he had kept to himself until one day at the beginning March of that same year when we had been out shopping together and he had dropped everything and clutched his chest. I left our shopping trolley and ran for the car, taking him directly to our doctor's surgery which was two minutes drive away. Regrettably I should have driven him straight to hospital but in my ignorance I drove him to the nearest source of help. He was seen immediately by a doctor and put onto medication of Beta- blockers, GTN spray and Aspirin. An appointment was made and kept at the chest pain clinic on the 12th March which resulted in a further appointment being made for Derek to undergo an Angiogram during the first week in May 2007. An appointment sadly which proved to be too late for Derek to keep.

The doctor was reluctant to request an angiogram and as he left the room for the second time that afternoon I could not believe my ears when I heard a faint voice from the bed saying, "Just call me Derek, Carrot Craig from now on, 'cause that fellow doesn't know his radishes from his onions." I was so thankful that Derek, out of weakness had spoken in no more than a whisper and had not been overheard by anyone other than myself.

As tired as he was we enjoyed a good laugh and it felt good knowing that Derek still had his sense of humour and had just expressed it

CHAPTER EIGHT

20th June 2007

Derek has spent a comfortable morning discussing sailing, beer and local restaurants. His oral intake is satisfactory as per chart and his fluid balance has been recorded. Two areas of confusion on my behalf were the significance of the letters B&T and numbers 5467 (Later explained by Mrs. Craig as past phone no.) and the name of a boat owned by his friend George Hollis. Derek remembered the name of his friend but I unfortunately took this to mean the name of the boat (sorted later).

Derek walked as far as ward 34 and back with two physiotherapists, and was able to stand unaided for 10mins. on two separate occasions whilst holding a conversation.

Later conversations initiated by Derek himself included his desire for independence and of how he understood what was going on around him but could not find the words to help us understand him.

Derek also talked of the disappointing business partnership he had a few years ago.

Entered by B.Jones (H.C.A.)

1p.m. *Derek was settled and calm when I arrived, he asked to use the commode after 45mins. he had a successful bowel movement. Stated how much happier he feels now that he can use the commode but cannot wait until he can go to the toilet in private.*

Looking at photographs he was at last able to recognize me as Andrea, his wife but unable to recognize himself. He remembered Tiger and Tizzy (our two cats) and tried very hard to explain how, since his mind blew up he finds everything so very strange and how nothing seems to be registering or sticking in his mind anymore. So many things no longer make any sense to him because he could not recognise the meaning of anything. He really struggled with this and became upset.

Derek still very confused over his age. (Not as bright or as lucid as he was yesterday).

2.45p.m. *After a rest Derek was able to recognize several more photographs, but still unable to recognise himself then as I was putting them away he suddenly stated that he feels much older now* *than he looked on the pictures of himself. I then asked him how old he was and he answered 5 years old. I explained that he was in fact 65 years of age and he irately stated that he had meant on the photographs of himself. (The snap shots had been taken over the past twenty five years). He is very confused over age and years.*

His movement is improving daily although still very wobbly in standing and somewhat shakey in his hand movements but his legs are definitely becoming very much stronger.

I have been trying to get Derek to take the wooden blocks or picture cards from me but he cannot. I have to still place each of them into his hands but at least he is now allowing me to take them back from him whereas previously he has kept a firm grip on them.

Today he was able to recognize me in the mirror but failed to recognize his own reflection. He could not see it at all, (perhaps it was just not registering in his mind or still not liking what he sees!)

His counting is now reaching into the twenties but he has difficulty counting the objects on the table in front of him. (He sees these objects as either one or five. There are actually five items on the table.)

Derek put back into bed at 4p.m. He becomes very tired about this time each afternoon and turns extremely cold.

Entered by Andrea Craig.

21.00hrs. *Since Mrs. Craig left, Derek has been cheerful and chatty. We have had conversations about fish, chips and mushy peas, his good friend George Hollis and various different colours.*

22.00hrs. *Derek became sleepy but stated that he was too cold to sleep. Two extra blankets and a green top cover have been added to his normal bed clothes.*
Derek has taken 100mls. of water.
Entered by P. Horan (H.C.A.)

21st June 2007

6.45 a.m. *Derek spent a very chatty and pleasant night. He slept for about four to five hours and was wide awake the rest of the time, chatting away happily.*
He used the commode and couldn't stress enough how embarrassing this is for him, I did state that in time he will be able to attend to his own needs and that he just needs to give himself a bit of time and not try to rush into things too quickly. He said he "knows that" and "thank-you".
(He did not open his bowels)
We held conversation about his friend Harry who he knew from Arrowe Park, also about his children and the weather.
Derek claimed he was too cold to sleep, even though he had two blankets, two counterpanes and his cardigan on, so one of the nurses brought

in a heater and he then said he was too hot, I therefore took the two counterpanes off him and also his cardigan, he laughed at this.

He enjoyed looking at the scenery outside his window this morning and said he thought it was going to be a nice day.

Derek and I laughed a lot and he has been a pleasure to look after.

His Peg feed was running throughout the night which did not bother him at all, he also had some "Horlicks" before he went to sleep and also drank a lot of water.

He stated that his wife would be coming in later and does so every day and that she has been right there at his side through all the bad times and that he could never thank her enough as it must have been terrifying and very upsetting for her but he is determined to get himself back to as near as possible to the life he had before all this happened to him.

Entered by M. Jones (H.C.A.)

Occupational Therapy 21st June

Washing and dressing assessment carried out this morning.

Bowl placed by bedside. He required assistance of two to carry out this activity, verbal and physical prompts provided.

Derek demonstrated problems with all following instructions other than sit and stand.

Andrea Craig

Derek was unable to locate his own body parts.

Further assessments and practice will be carried out.

<u>If you would like to discuss the same, or have any questions please contact the ooccupational therapy.</u>.

Entered by Michelle Kozlouski

Derek has been communicating clearly this morning. 11a.m. he returned from a long walk with his Physiotherapists (as far as ward 32 and back) he expressed that he felt very tired afterwards and so a quiet time was instigated.

Conversations have revolved around his age and of how he can now recognize that he is sixty five years old, his inability to differentiate periods of time.

Earlier at breakfast he made it quite clear that porridge was rather dull and he could remember that "Rice Cripies" were advertised as "Snap, Crackle and Pop".

Derek has talked of Venice a great deal and would like some photographs as a reminder. Also the prospect of using an exercise bike with the Physios' was appealing.

Derek has been holding his water glass well. I wonder if he is ready to adapitive cutlery, especially the large handled spoon. (I must query!)

During his conversation with the Physio's he was able to identify the view from his window *as Arrowe Park, but was still unable to identify specific features.*

Derek used fork at lunch time and after being helped to load food onto it he successfully managed to take it to his mouth.

He is now much brighter in spirit and also capability.

Entered by Brandon Jones (H.C.A.)

13.00hrs. *Derek was so happy when I walked into his room today. He has a very good relationship with Brandon and always seems to be much more motivated after his company.*

He asked for the commode at 2 p.m. he used it and managed to take himself off it and asked if I would clean him myself instead of calling the nurse, I was only too happy to do this for him and afterwards Derek stated how much he enjoyed a little more privacy at last.

He then walked over to the basin and following my instruction was able to wash his own hands and then proceeded to dry them after which he walked himself back to his chair and sat himself down. I noted the "cock-a-hoop" expression on his face which clearly stated, "What do you think to that then".

I was so impressed, most successful I have seen to-date, well done Derek.

Derek said how much he would like to speak with his friend Ron. So I rang him immediately and although a little nervous at first, he was soon enjoying a conversation about football and mans talk, as Derek put it. Afterwards Derek stated how much he missed having someone to whom he could discuss sport with.

Totally unprompted and unaided Derek suddenly stood up and took the box of photographs from the window-sill and placed them before us on the table, this amazed me but seconds later shocked me somewhat because he had no recollection of having done it.

He did not really recognize any of the photographs.

Derek was able to focus on me as I walked around his room this afternoon and held it for the longest period to-date.

3.15p.m. Derek stated that he was feeling very cold, I placed extra blankets over him. Five minutes later he complained that he was still cold and that something felt very wrong. I called the nurse who after checking him said she believed that he had perhaps over done things a little.

Derek was settled back down into bed and soon fell asleep.

5p.m. Derek, although previously stating that he was not tired, has slept soundly for the past hour and will soon have to be awakened for his dinner.

5.45p.m. *He ate heartily everything put in front of him.*

Entered by Andrea Craig.

Friday 22nd June 2007.

Occupational therapy advised us to help Derek recognize the different parts of his body when performing tasks i.e. put the toothbrush in your hand, move toothbrush to your mouth etc.

Entered by unknown.

11.30a.m. *Good session today with Derek, I noticed improvement from last week with his attention and more appropriate responses to questions.*

I found it useful to give Derek the first sound of a word (as opposed to the letter name) and giving him choices e.g. "Do you live in Heswall, Greasby or Wallasey" this helped Derek to answer questions he was not sure of without me giving him the answer.

I will provide a word pack for him.

Entered by Rebecca Smith (Speech & Language Therapist)

1.00p.m. *when I arrived the nurse on duty seemed a little concerned regarding the towels in Derek's room, all of his clean clothes and towels had been cleared out of his locker and left in corner of room, when I questioned as to why this was so I was told* *it was ward protocol. Staff nurse was summoned to explain to me "ward protocol". I then tried to explain to her that it was on the hospitals request in the first place that I kept a good supply of clean clothes and towels for Derek as he had so many accidents.*

I assured her that his clothes and towels were changed daily and proceeded to show her the clean towels I had brought in today, but she would have none of it and went onto state that she wanted her staff and everyone else brought up to speed over such matters.

Staff got quite excited and when she began to shout me down Derek ordered her not to speak to his wife in that manner and asked her to leave the room. I held the door open for her and requested that the duty nurse leave also asking that they did not come back until they had calmed down.

Will only use hospital towels from now on but want it noted that Derek's clothes and towels were changed daily by myself.

Derek extremely agitated after incident and requested that I go over it with him as he could not remember what had started it.

__2.30p.m.__ Derek appeared to be in discomfort and claimed there was something terribly wrong. He was flushed and said he felt dreadful, when I checked I discovered his catheter bag was so full it had burst. (This had not been checked for some *considerable time) Nurses called to change it, not very happy.*

Derek had a visitor this afternoon and was so happy to see George, with whom he shared and managed to hold an enjoyable conversation with about boats and sailing and their friends on the Isle-of-Man.

He could not recognize any photographs today but did not seem upset by this, he said that he wanted to get on with some work and enjoy talking.

Entered by Andrea Craig.

20.00p.m. *Derek has been extremely talkative this evening but was showing obvious fatigue by 19.00hrs. (Vocabulary errors, repetition and much reduced clarity of meaning)*

He requested some physical exercise to make him tired. Rather than leave the immediate ward environment, this was too a great a risk with limited staff and no Physio. Involvement. We stood and bent our knees and then walked to outer corridor and back several times.

After fifteen minutes Derek asked for the commode, while sitting he became quite grey in facial colour and weak in limb strength.

Observations taken as per chart, no variance noted.

Result of commode positive, after which Derek was settled into bed.

Topics of conversation: 'Murano' glass, retiring abroad, having a little boat for fun, and the smoking ban in public places. Also noticed improvement in Derek's arm until fatigue overcame him.

Note to all staff.

Please hand over to your replacement the need to read previous day's diary entries as well as adding your own at the end of each shift. Also please note that Derek is subject to the Trust's MRSA procedure, a copy of which can be found at the back of this diary.

20.30hrs. *Derek's colour has returned to normal, mouth-care has been maintained, night bag fitted and P.E.G. feed commenced early to enable longer sleep post feed. Derek is now asleep after last administration.*

Entered by Brandon Jones (H.C.A.)

21.00hrs. *Derek settled and asleep at this time. Awake at 22.00hrs. a little restless, requested drink of water, then getting a bit upset he was saying how they had got the information all wrong and that he was going to die, I calmed him down by reassuring him that he was going to be just fine.*

24.00hrs. *Derek requested commode as he wanted to pee, no luck, he got agitated when I tried to direct him onto and off the commode. I settled him back into bed. Slept on and off throughout the* *rest of the night but was very cheerful when he awoke this morning.*

Derek was talking about going on a plane to Spain and other countries with his wife on holidays.

Entered by K. Gardner (H.C.A.)

Saturday 23rd June 2007

8.00a.m. *Derek is in a good mood this morning, cheerful and chatting about his family, his wife and daughter, his son and was telling me about his friend George who has a sailing boat. We looked over his photo's and he was able to recognize several of them and explained to me who they were.*

Derek enjoyed his breakfast, a bowl of cornflakes, half a glass of water and a full glass of orange juice.

I had to help him wash himself but he managed to clean his teeth with just a little help.

Derek sat in his chair without any help from me.

Later he enjoyed his lunch but stated that he would really love to eat some fish and chips. Perhaps we can order some for tomorrow I told him.

He is concerned about his constipation so I suggested he drinks as much as he can.

I found Derek to be doing well and noticed how much his communication has improved.

Entered by Odette (H.C.A.)

1p.m. Derek is subdued this afternoon and explained it was only because he was thoughtful. We worked on his exercises given by Rebecca, his speech therapist, and I was thrilled with how well he did, much better than yesterday but I feel he is low in spirit.

He stated that he would like to have his own phone so that he could ring me at night-time or perhaps a friend now and again, feel he is lonely.

Derek had no trouble whatsoever rising from his chair and walking around the room. He really thought I was going to take him out today he said, just for a little fresh-air before I go mad altogether. (Wish I could take him)

He walked back to his chair and sat down with instruction, (This was the first time I had witnessed this)

He was given a tablet with a drink of water followed by 220mls. of, "Enlive Plus"

Derek is much improved in his ability to hold his glass.

2.45p.m. Derek lay on his bed, surprising me by being able to do so himself, I was amazed at how he managed to swing both his legs with very little trouble, (This was yet another first for me to witness)

He listened to his "Barber Shop" music and said how very relaxed he felt.

Feel I must note that Derek's colour has been changing from normal to grayish throughout the afternoon.

3.30p.m. *Derek had his catheter-bag changed and then we walked around the room. He stated once again how he longed to go out for a breath of fresh-air. I told him that perhaps Sarah and I would be able to take him tomorrow.*

Derek worked well with his body this afternoon and discovered that sometimes things are the opposite to what he means, eg. if I asked him where his nose was, he would point out into the room away from himself, but at the same time realizing that this was in the opposite direction to where his nose really was.

He claimed this happened only when dealing with himself.

He was able to identify and touch some areas of my face but needed to concentrate extremely hard. His attention wanders very quickly but can be pulled back more easily now than he could before.

We stood at the window and I pointed out various things and several people out walking their dogs down below and although Derek can now recognize the trees and one or two familiar things outside he was unable to recognize the people walking or their dogs.

Derek sat out in his chair for his evening meal and is looking very well and relaxed.

After his dinner Derek held a little conversation over the phone with Sarah and surprised me at how good he handled the phone. When finished he asked if I would read out the prayer card that Harry had passed in to him. (So good he remembers this). Says he would like someone to read this to him before he goes to sleep at night.

Derek now seems fully aware of where he is and why he is here. I feel today has been a very good day.

Entered by Andrea Craig.

Derek asked me if I would take him to the toilet. We walked to the toilet together with the nurse.

He was talking really well and we held a good conversation.

He also told me that he is going out soon in the car. (Marvellous!)

Derek was really clear in his speech for quite long periods. I am so pleased.

Entered by Elaine Leatherbarrow.

21.00hrs. *Derek in a very cheerful mood after his sister and niece left, he said they had cheered him up. I settled him into bed and he listened to some music which he enjoyed a lot.*

23.00hrs. *Derek is fast asleep at this time.*

Derek has been twisting and turning in his bed for most of the night and managed to accidently pull his catheter and unfortunately the bag came undone causing the bed to have to be completely changed at 4.00hrs. Other than this he was fine.

Derek is very calm this morning and is looking forward to going out with his wife and daughter.

Entered by Kath Gardwell (H.C.A.)

Sunday 24th June 2007.

7.45a.m. I introduced myself to Derek who seems to be in a very bright and cheerful mood.

8.30a.m. We talked about tennis, Derek was telling me that he liked to take a bit of time off work when the tennis finals were on. I asked him if the " love of his life" watched it with him and he said she sometimes did but it was he who watched it mostly.

Assisted Derek to wash and brush his teeth, he enjoyed beakfast. I asked him if I could wash his hair but he said he was o.k. for now. I will ask again later. We had a lovely talk about Scotland this morning.

Derek enjoyed his lunch and his ice-cream to follow.

Entered by Jackie Newcombe (H.C.A.)

1p.m. Derek had used the commode successfully and had his catheter bag changed, he is so excited to be going out (as are we). He was easy to change and dress but he is very worried incase he should soil himself while out. Nurse put a pad on him to give him that little bit of security.

While waiting to go out we sat and pointed out body parts and facial features. Derek still has difficulty identifying his own body parts. He is still pointing in the opposite direction but knows he is getting it wrong.

2 p.m. Sarah and Max brought the wheelchair up and we took Derek out into the park. He absolutely loved it. The weather was not brilliant but he said he did not care if it rained, he was so happy to breathe in the fresh-air. His ability to focus seemed so much better. He took in so much of what was going on but when asked to look at something in particular he had difficulty in doing so and would become agitated. (I felt this was because he was afraid of appearing foolish).

He had a very short walk holding my hand before we brought him back in his wheelchair. Derek was very tired but extremely happy.

4 p.m. Derek eager to get back into his bed on arrival back to his room, he listened to sport on the radio until dinner was served.

5.15 p.m. Derek was going to be served an omelette for his dinner and I stated that this was not enough as he was so hungry. Nurse kindly changed it and brought in cottage-pie served with *green beans and carrots, followed by chocolate mousse. Derek has drunk well today and enjoyed his dinner.*

Entered by Andrea Craig.

6.15 p.m. *Derek listening to his radio, football seems to be cheering him.*

6.45 p.m. *Fast asleep and seemingly very relaxed.*

8.30 p.m. *Derek is wide awake, we have been talking about his day out in Arrowe Park earlier today and how much he really enjoyed it, said it gave him hope.*

Entered by duty nurse.

21.00hrs. *I introduced myself to Derek, I asked him if he was warm and comfortable, he smiled and replied yes. We talked about tennis and his trip out.*

Every 15 mins. or so Derek would ask for a sip of water and reposition himself.

23.00hrs. *I assisted Derek to wash his face and hands and then settled him down for the night after first giving him a drink of water. I needed to put extra blankets on him. It is now 12.20a.m. he is sleeping soundly, comfortable and peaceful.*

4.30a.m. *Derek opened his eyes but remained settled and has gone back to sleep.*

6.05a.m. *Derek awoke saying he had had a good sleep and of how happy he felt. Chatted away saying how he wanted so much information about everything all the time. He then listened to the radio.*

Derek was a pleasure to look after and I wish him well and hope that he continues to improve day by day.

Entered by Chris Mepham (Flexibank)

Monday 25th June 2007

8 a.m. *I was introduced to Derek, as we talked he told me all about tennis and how he used to love to play. He went onto tell me about his wife Andrea and about Sarah and Max. We then chatted about other nurses who had sat with him, he said he liked Odette. We also chatted about his work and that he had retired six years ago.*

Derek and I practiced telling the time on the wall clock.

Derek spoke of Germany and of how much he loved the Isle of Capri.

Entered by Nicky Byrne (H.C.A.)

10.10 a.m. *I took over from Nicky and assisted Derek to wash and dress. Derek seems in good* *spirits today also chatting about Andrea's choice of his clothes, said she had good taste.*

Derek has eaten porridge and toast for his breakfast.

We spent some time with the flash cards but he was a little confused with the colours and some letters. We moved onto the lettered blocks and he has just managed to spell out his name with me helping to first find each one. We also spelt out Sarah, Max and Andrea. Derek told me with a great big smile that Andrea was the love of his life. He talked of a dog named "Blue" and a cat called "Tizzy", who have both passed away some time ago. Told me his dad's name was Ron. And that his son Paul lives in Germany.

Entered by Mary Hollig (H.C.A.)

10.50 a.m. Occupational therapy. *We practiced colours and body parts. Appropriate answers were given to questions asked about where he was and what month was it. Derek was able to spell out his name and that of Max when looking at photographs.*

Please continue with body part identification.
Entered by Michelle Kozlouski.

Derek was a little confused trying to hold his drinking cup. He told me he went out for a walk yesterday around the park and how he was able to recognize the golf links and of how much he had enjoyed it.

Derek has just eaten all of his lunch and tells me he can't wait until he has fish and chips, he longs for them.

We had a difficult moment when Derek got confused trying to tell me that his catheter bag need changing and laughed heartily when I finally realized what he had been struggling to say.

Continued entry by Mary Hollig (H.C.A.)

1 p.m. Derek was sitting pleasantly chatting away with his nurse, Mary, when I arrived. He became a little agitated with me when I tried to help him focus his mind as he tried to explain something to me. He seemed quite confused over something. He claimed that he did not want to focus and that he should just be able to do and say what he wanted to, when he wanted to. I went on to say that he had not done too badly just then and he laughed.

1.30 p.m. Practiced pointing to different parts of my body successfully but had trouble once again with his own body. Derek cannot distinquish between mine and his.

Derek asked for the commode and it was agreed that he can now use the toilet next door. (Wipes and gloves have been provided on stool by door to wipe over toilet before and after Derek has used it.)

Derek managed quite well to wash and dry his hands after using the commode but had trouble putting the soap back in its place.

2.30 p.m. Derek was disappointed the Physio's had not been again.

We talked over food intake with the dietition and it was agreed that Derek was eating well and gaining weight nicely.

Derek listened with great interest to the tennis.

3.30 p.m. Physio's arrived to take Derek to practice walking up steps but he was unable to manage them. He was asked to bounce a huge ball and also found this difficult to carry out. I said this was something we could practice ourselves and he said he was very keen to do so. (I will buy a ball tomorrow). Derek was much brighter after his physio.

5 p.m. Derek very tired and sounding very weak in voice. I will feed him his dinner before I put him back to bed.

6.00 p. m. Derek now settled back into bed and wanting to go asleep.

Entered by Andrea Craig.

21.10hrs. Derek was fast asleep when I took over my shift but was awake when medication trolley *came around. I helped him to take his tablets which he took without a problem and went straight back to sleep again.*

Entered by Odette Simpson (H.C.A.)

Tuesday 26th June 2007

Derek very chatty this morning, he was able to sit at his basin for a wash after he had eaten all of his breakfast which was, "Ready Brek", toast and marmalade and then sat in his armchair from 10.20 a.m. he watched tennis for a while.

Entered by duty H.C.A.

11.45 a.m. *Rebecca Smith (Speech & Language therapist).*

I continued with word, orientation and engaging in conversation with Derek.

He did well.

1 p.m. *Derek tells me he had a good Physio. session this morning (but meant Speech session). I brought in a ball to practice bouncing and passing it between us, he enjoys the exercise with the ball very much. His voice is low again (whispering almost), think he is very tired.*

Derek is saying that he is very hungry and that he has had no lunch to-day, have checked sheet and his lunch has not been entered but on checking with Claire (duty staff nurse), discovered that he has been fed.

2.40 p.m. Derek has been taken for his first bath, (stating that he would rather have a shower).

3.10 p.m. Derek was a new man after his shower, stated that he felt wonderful but that his fingers and skin are still very sore and tender to touch.

We spent a pleasant hour with me reading the paper to him.

Karl, his duty nurse arrived at 4 p.m. to say that he was about whenever I wanted to leave, I explained that Derek was eagerly awaiting the arrival of his fish, chips and mushy pea supper at 5.30 p.m. and how he had waited for this opportunity ever since he could remember. Derek and Karl enjoyed a good chat.

Nurses keep popping in, seems they are just as excited as Derek over his fish and chips. Table has been set for four (Sarah and Max will join us as they are bringing in the feast). New glasses have been handed in to us for his first taste of bitter shandy. Poor Derek his mouth is almost watering.

Derek is now having a rest on the bed whilst a waiting supper.

Entered by Andrea Craig.

19.00hrs. Derek washed and settled into bed by his wife, Andrea. He was listening to the tennis. He told me how much he had enjoyed his fish and chips and Sarah and Max's company but what a shame there had been no champagne, he was *laughing about that and said he had enjoyed his taste of shandy all the same.*

20.35 hrs. *Derek has been quiet this evening and is fast asleep now. The staff nurse came in to change the dressing around his Peg feed entry. The site was clean with no problems.*
 Entered by Karl McCavish (H.C.A.)

21.00 hrs. *I came on shift to find Derek fast asleep. He looks a million times better than when I first met him a few weeks ago.*
 Entered by unknown.

27th June 2007

6.25 a.m. *Derek has just woke for the toilet, he is very bright this morning and told me about his fish and chips and that he is going to be watching Wimbledon on the television today.*
 He tells me I sound just like his daughter Sarah.

7.05 a.m. *Derek up sitting in his chair watching his television, he says that he had a good nights sleep.*
 Entered by Angie McCormick (H.C.A.)

Derek has stated his date of birth for the first time. (I checked and found this to be correct).
 Entered by unknown.

10.45 a.m. Occupational Therapy. *We attempted to play "connect-four" with little success. (Unsuccessful because Derek unable to follow instructions or able to identify colours.)*

We practiced body recognition using jigsaw puzzle.

Also attempted a shape jigsaw puzzle, again Derek demonstrated problems following instruction. He tired quickly but remained in good spirits throughout.

I will continue and report on developments.
Entered by Michelle Kozlowski. (O.T)

1 p.m. *Derek stated that he wished to discuss something with me he considered to be very, seriously important. He went on to describe how frightened he is when he wakes in the night. He feels his heart racing and his head hurting and is so frightened he is having a heart attack. He needs to know if this is actually physical or just him being scared, either way it feels very real to him and he feels great pain in his chest and panic sets in.*

3 p.m. *Derek has managed to play bounce the ball and managed to pass the ball very well today, but now tired.*

Derek does seem extremely scared and afraid and I have talked him through this the best I can.

He pulls himself together for a little while but then goes down again.

4 p.m. *Derek requested that we played with the ball again as he enjoys this, but once again he became anxious and troubled. Without prompting or questioning he stated that he was very concerned that he could no longer retain any facts whatsoever. He went on to explain how the staff and myself were feeding him so much information i.e. the day, month and year each day but he could not remember any of it and this worries him*

5.15 p.m. *Dr.Pinder has just left the room having assessed Derek and requested that I make an appointment with Occupational Therapy as soon as possible. He found Derek much improved but states that there are still problems with his attention, memory, perceptual ability and Dyspraxia.*

Dr. Pinder has stressed that still only one person at a time talks to Derek and must be clear and slow.

We must continue to pull Derek's attention back from wandering so that he can focus on what is being said or taking place now.

He recommends that Derek be taken off his catheter.

6 p.m. An E.C.G. has been carried out and Derek feels the day has ended well

I am leaving him happy and settled watching Tennis.

Entered by Andrea Craig.

7 p.m. *Derek very clearly knew who I was and even mentioned Bernie. Told me he was worried about his heart condition and having another heart attack. I tried reassuring him and told him that he was taking a good cocktail of pills to help prevent this and that he was doing exceptionally well. He seemed quite happy with that.*

He asked me how I was going to get home, bless him, then added, "You still can't drive you daft thing." This was more like the Derek I know and love.

I sat beside him until he fell asleep.

Entered by Elaine (Derek's sister).

21.00hrs. *Derek is fast asleep still.*

22.00hrs. *Awakened for his medication and Peg feed, he asked me where was the eggs and bacon.*

Derek soon settled back to sleep.

6.45 a.m. *Derek woke up and I asked if he would like the T.V. on and he said he would to see the news. He asked what I had been doing while he had been asleep and I told him I had been reading*

Andrea Craig

magazines, he laughed at this. He is happy to see the sun shining.

Entered by Angie McCormick (H.C.A.)

28ᵗʰ June 2007

.

Derek is in a chatty mood this morning and has eaten all of his breakfast, we had a lovely chat about his friend George and his boat and all the places he has been to abroad and asked me where I had been to.

Derek had a walk to the shower where I assisted him to wash his hair, he was able to wash his hands for himself, which I said was a great help.

We returned to his room where we played catch with the ball and Derek was keen to show me how he could bounce it, he also managed to kick it once or twice.

10.30 a.m. *Derek had an E.C.G. this morning after which he asked if he could go to the proper toilet and successfully opened his bowels. He was pleased with this.*

Derek has eaten roast turkey, mashed potatoes and veg. and eaten all of his "Manchester tart" for desert.

Derek was able to hold a fork with assistance for the first time today.

Just load the fork for him, then place fork into Derek's hand and Derek will put it to his mouth.

I thought this was brilliant and Derek was rather pleased himself.

Entered by Karl McCavish (H.C.A.)

1p.m. *Derek is in much better spirits today. Michelle came up from Occupational Therapy and we went over games to best awaken and stimulate Derek's instruction and attention abilities.*

Wooden cut-out piece and shape boards, connect-four game recommended for immediate use.

Also asking Derek to go and pick up objects from table i.e. knife, fork, spoon, glass, etc.

Asking him to identify objects that are handed to him i.e. pen, photograph, glasses, key or mobile phone etc. keep it simple and do not overload.

Recommend that we talk even more slowly so that Derek can digest and register it more easily. I welcome this advice.

Derek really does love to play with the ball, passing and bouncing it, I could almost see his old competitive streak returning. His ability is improving daily and it is good to see his excitement and keenness.

Although he was very concerned and upset when we both bent down to retrieve the ball at the same time and his thumb nail caught me between my eyes and made a small cut. I was actually very pleased at how focused he had been in going down to retrieve the ball.

Derek has been talking about the time a lot today and at one time was very focused on the clock counting the numbers around it and was able to describe the little finger position but he was unable to tell the actual time. He stated that he would love to be able to just look at the clock and tell what time it was. I told him how well he was already doing and that he seemed to be well on his way to being able to do just that.

Derek managed to walk to the toilet today unaided but needed directing there. Still need to clean him afterwards but will see tomorrow if we have any success in Derek having a go at cleaning himself. I would so like him to be able to do this for himself so that he may reclaim his dignity back.

Afterwards he was able to wash his own hands and dried them with paper towels which had to be handed to him.

Derek was weighed and found to have gained yet another 2lbs. Ally (dietition)

Was very pleased and is cutting his night feed by half.

We played with various objects i.e. my sunglasses, mobile phone, pen and glass of water. During this period I asked Derek if he could remember where the clock was, after several minutes he suddenly became very agitated and extremely angry. I had pushed too far and had obviously overloaded him. I was so sorry and tried to calm him down but just as quickly as he had become agitated he was calm once more and told me to take no notice of him, that he had just been so frustrated and felt he was getting nowhere.

My heart breaks for him a little more each time he gets upset this way.

I felt Derek needed rest and persuaded him to return to bed where he is now dozing.

Dr.Oates made a visit this afternoon asking if we minded her bringing in two student doctors to see Derek. Derek was only too happy to play a part.

After their visit Derek asked if I minded him watching a little television. I switched on to "Countdown" and was amazed at how it held Derek's attention.

4 p.m. *Physios. arrived and Derek was able to get himself off the bed unaided and followed them willingly with the ball.*

Derek enjoyed his physio. but still worried that he gets most things wrong.

I believe his attempt at steps was slightly better than Monday's attempt.

Derek is feeling very happy and says that it has been a good day. He is tired in a nice relaxed kind of way, (his words).

He states that his hands and fingers are still very sore and hurt him and he finds this very puzzling.

5.45 p.m. *Derek has eaten all of his dinner and is so alert as though a window has been thrown* wide open. He described the colour of his jelly and ice-cream and the blue and green design of the desert dish. I was surprised at his sudden ability to be able to do this.

Entered by Andrea Craig.

6.30 p.m. Derek very relaxed watching T.V. when I took over from his wife. He asked for the T.V. to be switched off at 7 p.m. then fell asleep.

Derek had his catheter removed by Matt. And did not like it one little bit, he was not happy.

Entered by Julie (H.C.A.)

21.00hrs. Derek was awake when I came on and he was not very happy at all but would not tell me why. He watched T.V. for a while, had his tablets and night feed and settled down about 22.45 p.m.

Derek incontinent of urine twice in the night but asked if he could use the bottle when he awoke at 6.30a.m.

Entered by Angie McCormick (H.C.A.)

CHAPTER NINE

Two whole weeks had now passed since Derek had been moved into room 23, and two months to the day since he had first been admitted into A&E.

It felt more like two years, life as we had once lived it was no more, in less than one second one bright and sunny morning, it had been snatched away leaving us both floundering in a deep, cold ocean of dark uncertainty. Our past had disappeared and no future presented itself upon the blurred horizon of doubt and fearfulness.

During the last two weeks, Derek, finding it increasingly difficult to maintain his foothold on the mountain he was climbing, had found himself almost drowning in these dark cold waters. Pain, fear and the panic attacks he was experiencing were naturally taken very seriously by his doctors and all necessary steps were taken to discover the cause.

A further review by his Consulting Cardiologist was requested and arranged, even though his E.C.G. results were showing no change, Derek's chest pains could not be ignored. After further assessment it was arranged for the angiogram to go ahead.

When Derek had told me of the pain and grave anxiety he was suffering it disturbed me deeply and I went to sleep that particular evening with it playing on my mind, only to find myself wide awake again in the small hours of the morning having experienced a dream. Was it a dream, I shall never know but I do know this, after sharing this dream with Derek the following day, he never had a chest pain again or suffered another panic attack.

In my dream I was standing alone feeling very aware of the silence, not a sound to be heard, but there was definitely something tangible present. I could not see anything but knew I was not alone for I could feel a presence. I felt un-afraid, in fact I felt nothing only a tremendous sense of peace growing deeper as each moment passed. Suddenly out of nowhere I heard a voice telling me, 'that all would be well, for the "Angel of Peace" and the "Angel of Calm" would take up their place and remain at Derek's side from that moment on.' I awoke remembering every word and I knew with full conviction that, dream or not, what I had just heard was true.

The following day as I entered Derek's room his nurse told me how he had been looking forward to my visit, a little more than usual she had said, as he had been waiting with great excitement to tell me something.

"Who goes first?" I asked, "Because I also have something to tell you, but do you mind if I put everything away before we start?"

Nurse left the room and after I had sorted out his locker and sat myself down beside him he told me to go first. As I related my dream I could not help noticing the growing excitement in him, I had not expected him to ridicule what I had to say but neither had I expected his drinking in of every word with bated breath, so to speak.

I had no sooner finished when he whispered, "Andrea, I saw them or I think I did. I saw two white birds fly into my room, one flew to either side of my bed. I really didn't know what it meant or what was going on but I liked the feeling they brought with them very much. I've been waiting to tell you about it as it all seemed to be so real. It didn't feel like I was dreaming."

As Derek struggled through his excitement to relate his experience I literally felt the fear leave him, and as I sat watching I saw the strain leave his face and sensed his inner strength returning helping him once again to rise above the dark waters of that unknown sea and place his feet firmly back upon the mountain he was climbing.

These were the ups and downs of Derek's progress, the highs and the lows of his journey. During the low periods, those past two months had felt more like two years but during the highs

I could not help but be amazed at how much progress had been made in such a short period of time. His medical consultant and her team were truly delighted with him, Derek was deemed their miracle boy and they felt sure that Dr. Pinder would be well pleased with him on his next visit.

I felt Derek needed this renewed strength to help him cope with his latest struggle of urine incontinence. Just as he was regaining his dignity of bowel control he had to endure the nightmare of one wet accident after another. I had been told that it is sometimes impossible after long term catheterization to regain normal bladder function and must be prepared for this. I refused to consider this as an option, wishing only to focus on the success of retraining his bladder and helping Derek retain as much dignity as possible.

The nurses had been brilliant in teaching me the correct way to help Derek go to the toilet. They showed me how simple it could be to clean him afterwards with as little embarrassment as possible to him and at the same time being a lot easier on myself in the physical handling of him.

So much had been lived through within the space of time Derek had spent in room 23 but one of the greatest days to-date, not of course forgetting the day he enjoyed his fish and chip supper, was the day we took him into the park for his first trip outside. I only wish we had taken a video camera with us, the expressions upon Derek's face rivaled those of a child when discovering new things for the very first time.

I had been worried as the weather had not been too promising that day and clouds had been gathering on my way into the hospital. No way could we take him out in the rain and my gaze kept going to the window as we waited for Sarah and Max to bring up the wheelchair. As one or two drops hit the window I began preparing Derek for the possibility of not being able to go out not wanting him to be disappointed. I need not have bothered because he simply was not listening to one word I was saying, he was going and that was that.

Max brought in the chair and Derek, as if by magic, had seated himself in it and was rearing to go in a second. He was quickly wheeled out as Sarah and I hurriedly collected the items we felt might be needed. We left the ward with nurses and patients waving farewell and bidding him a good trip, you would have thought we were going on holiday and Derek probably felt he was.

As we arrived at the hospital's side entrance which was situated on the ground floor our faces dropped, it was raining, not heavily but enough to make me hesitant, "Not to worry", said Max taking off his lightweight but most importantly waterproof jacket and wrapping it around Derek, "a little rain never hurt anyone," he added running out through the doors and away towards the park.

The fine rain hit Derek in the face as we ran for cover under the trees where we were sheltered from the wet but found ourselves bombarded by a swarm of mosquito. Derek was delighted and laughed at Sarah and I, who were worried about the rain, saying how good it felt to feel it upon his face. He had begun to believe he would never feel it again. He did add that he could remember what it felt like to be bitten by a mosquito and how poorly it had made him feel at the time.

The rain could not dampen his spirits and as it proved to be only a light shower we were off once again exploring all that the park had to offer. We watched model aircraft flying which greatly surprised us as we witnessed Derek's ability to focus his attention on their flights.

He was able to recognize the golf links and said he could remember that 'Arrowe Park' boasted a golf course. We found a picnic table and wooden benches where we sat and had a drink as we listened to some children shouting with delight as they played a game of tennis with their parents. Derek told us how much he had enjoyed playing himself before he had collapsed. The sun came out and Sarah took photographs of us all. I asked Derek if he felt strong enough to have a little walk and he was out of his wheelchair like a bullet fired from a gun. He willingly took my arm and Max kept one step behind us at all times just incase.

Derek then turned to me and said that although he never wanted to go back he thought that it was time that we did, I knew he was tired. We helped him back into his chair and wheeled him back to his room. What a happy chappie he was that night, our outing had proved to be a huge success.

Yes, Derek was finding it difficult climbing his mountain but at the end of two months he was still applying every ounce of effort he could muster, still being the gentle gentleman he had always been and not wishing to be a trouble to any of the staff whose job it was to nurse him.

Friday 29th June 2007.

Derek awoke, washed at his basin then enjoyed his breakfast, ate all of it. He seems quiet and thoughtful today, he had a little weep. When I asked him what was wrong he said that he was "happy crying" because he loved his wife so much.

Derek went to the toilet to pee before he went down to the eye clinic.

He enjoyed and ate all of his lunch of fish, potatoes and peas followed by high protein whip.

Entry unknown.

12.45 p.m. *Derek was unable to see me as I entered the room not even when I walked right up close to him, but seemed happy on hearing my voice, perhaps this is caused by eye drops.*

Window on vision opened at 1.30 p.m. and Derek was quite chatty, he wished to walk up and down the ward several times.

Since visiting the eye clinic he does seem a little worried about why he cannot see things. He is blaming me for holding up different objects to those I am telling him they are, or for telling him that the television is on when he knows that it is not. (In fact it is on but sadly he cannot focus on it.)

Today Derek was able to remember and recognise what my sun-glasses were. He says he is not concerned in everyone always asking him what day is it, when all he really wishes for is to be able to tell the time himself. He feels lost not knowing what the time is, says no-one could possibly understand what it feels like.

The more we talked the more irritated Derek became today. He asked to go outside but I had to tell him that I was unable to take him on my own.

2.45 p.m. Derek told me that he would like to go to the toilet to pee. Mission successful and then said he would like a walk up the ward and back. We did this several times.

3.15 p.m. Derek said he would like to watch the tennis, and after a very frustrated and angry five minutes of believing that I had not yet switched the television on (I had of course but Derek was looking in the wrong direction and could not focus at all) he finally tuned in and settled back stating that if I had switched it on when he had first asked me we would not have had all this fuss.

Derek then became very remorseful and upset stating that he did understand it was all to do with his brain damage and wished it could all be sorted out very quickly as he did not think he could stand it for much longer.

We had a talk and he did calm down but I cannot truthfully say that he is happy. He seems bored beyond belief, frustrated and extremely emotional to-day.

He says that he feels he is making tremendous headway one moment then falling right back to square one the next.

I have noticed that Derek is reluctant to drink his water and feel this might be for much the same reason as when he did not want to eat when he was on his bowel retraining program, for fear of it would open his bowels more.

He believes that the less he drinks then the less he will pee.

4 p m. *As the afternoon wore on Derek explained that his eyes have been blurred with the drops used in the eye clinic.*

He was able to remember all that has gone on but felt he could not deal with anymore games of any kind today, but did have a game with the ball and is progressing. I felt we should keep it short and Derek is now resting on his bed.

Derek has improved and progressed more than he knows with so much more of his memory returning. He works so hard with a full understanding of all that has happened to him, but sometimes I feel the development of his ability to focus and be able to hold his attention is so very,

very slow, so much so I find myself wondering if it has improved at all.

Derek is slow to take instruction but I can see the gradual improvement here, only fair to say he works so hard, I mean really, really hard believing that at any minute it will all come right. I can only pray that I can find the strength to continue watching him struggle this way because right now I feel it might be very close to breaking my heart.

I know that love is all powerful and pray that God's Love will strengthen us both at the same time asking that He forgive me my moment of weakness.

5 p.m. *Derek seems to be in a deep sleep, he needed this rest as I believe his eye drops have really disorientated him today.*

Derek can assess correctly on some occasions but is not consistent, I feel it may be to do with the windows in his mind or brain being open or shut (the only way I know of describing what I see).

Derek is now able each day to describe the weather, and that he enjoys listening to the news of a morning and evening but he cannot make some of his nurses understand this. I tried to explain that he must tell them the way he has just told me and that I felt sure that they would switch it on for him.

"I know they would," he replied, *"but I forget to ask them".*

Derek has stated once again of how much he is enjoying colours and has asked me if I would buy some soft sponge balls in various colours. He tells me they are similar to tennis balls in size but softer in texture. (To practice hand exercises).

Derek was disappointed that he did not have a shower this morning. (I was rather pleased that he actually remembered this).

6.15 p.m. *He asked if could go the toilet as he wanted to pee. (Again I was delighted with his awareness of his wanting to go and his control until he was able to get there).*

I had an attempt at encouraging Derek to feed himself at dinner this evening. He really struggled, but his first attempt at it was hopeful.

Derek was much more cheerful after his dinner, which he ate all of.

Entered by Andrea Craig.

21.00hrs. *Derek was fast asleep when I first came on duty this evening.*

22.00hrs. *He awoke wanting to pass urine, unfortunately he had already gone and the bed was changed. Changed Derek and settled him back down again.*

He had a fairly settled night, waking at approx. 3.30a.m. We had a chat and he mentioned his right hand had been aching earlier but that it was fine now. I made him comfortable, his night feed has finished and he is settled back to sleep once more.

6.30a.m. *Derek washed and the bedding had to be changed again due to second accident with urine, this is worrying and upsetting Derek, who cannot understand why this is happening.*

7.40a.m. *Derek asked for the commode and had to be assisted on to it.*
Entered by J. Lomax (H.C.A.)

Saturday 30ᵗʰ June 2007.

7.45a.m. *Derek asked to go to the toilet and after helping him onto the commode he successfully opened his bowels.*
Entered by Debbie McKenna (student nurse).

Derek has had a good morning and eaten all his cornflakes and one slice of toast. He has been very bright and alert looking at his photographs, recognising some of the places and people, and telling stories.

Derek has used the building bricks spelling out his name and going over colours. He has enjoyed throwing and catching the ball.

Derek has had his shower. I assisted him in washing his face and afterwards the cleaning of his teeth.

Derek enjoyed his lunch and pudding after.
Entered by Maureen Clark (H.C.A.)

1p.m.   Derek was in a wonderful mood when I came in although he was upset about wetting the bed in the night. I explained that he should not worry too much as it was still early days after the removal of his catheter and that he was doing just fine during the days. He seemed to relax knowing this.

Derek was able to get a grip on the handles of wooden jig-saw and made a very good attempt at trying to place it together, he actually achieved to place two pieces correctly, he got a lot out of this and seemed to thoroughly enjoy it, we also had a good laugh at trying to play "connect-four", after two games he was exhausted and said that he had to go to the toilet. (passed urine and had bowel opened)

3.50 p.m.   George arrived at 3 p.m. he talked and played ball with Derek and then walked with him up and down the ward for twenty minutes, Derek was so pleased and said how much better seeing George made him feel.

He is delighted that his television is working once more as he is keen to watch the tennis this evening. To-day was really wonderful seeing Derek so happy.

He said that he is so looking forward to seeing Sarah and Max to-morrow and the possibility of going into the park once again.

Entered by Andrea Craig.

18.00hrs. *I have just arrived and taken over from Andrea, it took the three of us to get the T.V. working before she left, but finally we managed to find the tennis for Derek.*

19.30hrs. *Derek asked that the T.V. be switched off to give his eyes a rest.*

I asked him if he needed to use the toilet and he said that he thought it might be too late and he was very upset. I explained to him how well he was doing and explained that it always takes time after a catheter is taken out to return to normal. Derek seemed happier after our conversation and being changed and said that he understood.

Entered by Jackie Newcomba (H.C.A.)

21.00hrs. *Derek was asleep at the start of my duty. I checked him and he was dry. I checked him again at 22.00hrs. and found he was wet but he also wished to use the bottle. Bedding was changed.*

It had been discussed with Derek last night that we would use the bottle every three hours with my help, he agreed to this.

We have discussed this again this evening and he is willing to continue trying to set a pattern (Feel this is less disturbing to him than his continual accidents and having to change his bed which is distressing to Derek.)

23.00hrs. *I checked him again to find him still asleep but bed wet. The bedding and Derek were changed and he once again used the bottle.*

Night-time meds. were given and he settled down.

1.30a.m. *Derek extremely restless, his bed wet again and was changed. Derek was made comfortable, he used the bottle and settled down.*

2.45a.m. *Derek woke and asked if he could use the bottle, he successfully passed urine.*

3.30a.m. *Derek once more asked if he could use the bottle, he did so with success and informed me when he had finished. (Derek was so pleased with himself.)*

Entered by ward H.C.A.

4.15a.m. *Derek was very unsettled. I checked him and found him wet. I remade bed and changed Derek.*

5.15a.m. *Derek used bottle and passed urine x 2*

7.00a.m *I helped to wash and change Derek and changed the bed.*

Entered by J.Lomax (H.C.A.)

1st July 2007

8.00a.m *Derek sat on the commode and had a good bowel movement. He was very good this morning at standing and getting back into bed. He had a good drink of water then we had a chat about his family and holidays. Derek appears to have a good memory.*

Derek had cornflakes followed by toast and jam for breakfast. He needed some assistance with his cornflakes but needed no help at all with his toast and jam he also drank a full glass of water unaided.

After breakfast Derek watched the news on T.V. but I soon realized that he was unable to watch it and that he was only listening to it.

10.00a.m. *Derek had a shower and went to the toilet. He was not too bad with his walking just needed a little guidance. He was able to brush his teeth and rinse o.k. His T.V. is not working so is now listening to the radio. He enjoys the news.*

He is sitting up in his chair in very high spirits.

11.00a.m. *Derek ate a "Forticreme" yogurt and had a drink of water then went through some colours on the play board.*

He has been looking at some pictures of his garden and his house. He can remember the names of his cats etc. and we went on to discuss the morning's news.

11.30a.m. *Derek wanted to go the toilet and was able to walk there and back very well. He wanted to doze on his bed before lunch. He slept on and off until 12.10p.m when lunch was served. He ate all of his lunch with Andrea, his wife here to help him with it.*

Entered by H.C.A. (Bank)

1p.m. *Derek is down today because of his incontinence and disturbance through the night. He is suggesting that he be wakened three times nightly but it seems that this was carried out last night and Derek still needed to be changed in between checks. (I am told this is probably due to night feed and the washing through of the Peg tube.)*

After ensuring that Derek ate all of his lunch he went to the toilet and opened his bowels and passed urine. (Seem to be no problems during the day but does feel more secure with a pad in place.)

We practiced Derek going out of the room with him trying to locate the door handle and then opening the door himself and then closing it behind him as he went out. He did need guidance but managed quite well for first attempt.

We continued with Derek trying to focus on his room with the outcome that Derek could see the room but his brain was unable to recognize anything.

I suggested that he pointed to or felt each object and I would state what each one was. This time he did much better, he actually recognized the towel, the towel rail and the basin.

We stood looking out of the window and he was able to recognize a gentleman walking his dog.

2p.m. I changed Derek into warmer pair of trousers and put on his socks and shoes as Sarah and Max are coming in and we are going for a walk. (Hopefully that is, for as soon as I had finished dressing him he was tired and is now lying down fast asleep.)

As I was changing him, Derek told me that he is so fed up with it all and felt he could no longer cope with the frequent accidents he was having. I explained that I had been pre-warned that it would take time and asked that he did not upset himself too much over it. He did not seem to be listening and went on to say that he could do no more brain games today as they hurt his head physically.

3.pm. Sarah and Max arrived, Derek heard them enter the room and was very pleased to see them both.

The rain had gone off so a trip around the park took place which Derek so enjoyed. He managed to walk all the way from the ground floor (coming up in the lift of course) along the corridor, down the length of the ward and back into his room having first found the door handle and opening it himself at 4p.m.

Derek paid a visit to the toilet but passed nothing. Stated that he would like to lie down and rest which he did.

He enjoyed watching a little television and was able to focus quite well.

(Derek's focus has held well over the last two days, the best to date.)

5.15p.m. Derek stated that he felt very sick and must sit up. I sat him up and called for the nurse. Derek was shaking and his hands were trembling, he was sitting in his chair. His blood pressure was taken and proved to be normal.

Derek tried to eat his dinner but could not touch any of it saying it would make him vomit. He drank 400mls. of water and suddenly wanted to pass urine. I quickly assisted him to use the bottle when he began shaking again and stated that he was in serious trouble. He managed to tell me that it was very sore and painful passing urine but managed to pass 50mls.

He wanted to be put back into bed immediately afterwards and then began to panic incase he wet the bed. He was given a little talk of reassurance and fell into a deep sleep at 6 p.m.

(Thought I should mention the fact that Derek has had a runny nose this afternoon.)

Entered by Andrea Craig.

21.00hrs. Derek was watching T.V. and appeared to be fully absorbed in the program about Princess Diana.

22.00hrs. Derek asked for and used the commode, he managed to pass urine but sheet was still found to be wet and had to be changed. He settled afterwards and went to sleep.

Derek again used the commode (passed urine) then fell back to sleep and appears to have had a restful sleep for several hours.

5.00a.m. Derek had to be changed once again and sat out while the bed was changed. I made him comfortable and he went back to sleep.

7.00a.m. Derek awoke very upset about the bed wetting throughout the night but I reassured him that he had in actual fact improved from the previous night which he should be pleased about. He complained once in the night of it hurting him as he passed urine but I *was* informed that a sample had been taken.

Another morning sample *needs* to be taken when he is ready.

Entered by Joan Lomax (H.C.A.)

Monday 2nd July 2007

8a.m. I was introduced to Derek this morning and the first thing he told me was that he had to give a urine sample. After passing his sample he ate breakfast of 2 Weet-a-bix with milk followed by toast and jam.

We were then looking at the clock and I asked if he could tell me the time, Derek knew that it was on the eight but could not recognize the half past. We practiced with the time for a while and then began talking about his wife Andrea and what time she would be coming in to see him, he said she normally came in at lunch time.

Derek then stated that he was tired and would like to rest. He is drifting in and out of sleep. A cough seems to be disturbing him. He finally woke up at 10.45a.m.

Entered by Diane Pegg (H.C.A.)

11.20a.m. Occupational Therapy.

We played Connect 4 and did a shape jig-saw. Derek concentrated well on the game. He informed me that his catheter had been taken out.

Andrea Craig

We practiced following instructions when playing a game.
Orientated him today with date and month.
Entered by Michelle Kozlowski.

11.45a.m. *have been playing ball with Derek and have had a good talk about his family. He has been telling me about Sarah and Max, Andrea his wife and his interest in football. I put the television on for him but he became very upset because he was unable to focus upon it. He has said that he just wants to sit quietly and rest his eyes.*

Derek has eaten his lunch of lamb, mashed potatoes and carrots followed by cheesecake for desert and then he drank a full glass of water.
Entered by Diane (H.C.A.)

12.45p.m. *Derek had just finished his lunch when I arrived today. He had been given a suppository and had to remain lying on his bed for a rest. He fell into a deep sleep. He appears to be very washed out and extremely tired.*

2.30p.m. *Derek woke up and asked for the commode. He opened his bowels and passed urine. He wished to go back to bed stating that he felt happy but would feel even better if he could just have another sleep.*

3p.m *Physio's arrived and decided that he should do his therapy, he went off disorientated but did manage to walk unaided.*

(Derek was confused as to the correct doors.)

Derek has informed me of two things today;

1) *He does not like the days and date notice board as he is very fed up with it now, and*
2) *He believes that he is almost ready to come home.*

I did not dwell on either point as I thought he was too tired to deal with it. I will try to explain as simply as I can when it next arises.

Dr. Oates was here when Derek arrived back from his physiotherapy. We talked about Derek's night feed being discontinued and all being well the Peg tube would be coming out soon.

3.30p.m. *as soon as Dr. Oates had left, Derek requested the commode and opened his bowels and passed urine. He then asked to lie on his bed as he felt exhausted, he was soon fast asleep.*

4.45p.m. *Derek awoke and asked to go to the toilet. He passed blood and a lot of mucous from the bowel.*

Derek is once again refusing to eat believing that the less he eats then the less he will go to the toilet. He is extremely low in spirit and my heart aches for him.

Entered by Andrea Craig.

21.00hrs. *I sat with Derek when his wife and daughter had left at 6.15p.m. He had been washed and put to bed comfortably watching tennis on the T.V. with his head phones on.*

He seems very tired, dozing in and out of sleep until 7.30p.m when he asked if I would change the station for him, he fell back to sleep waking again at 8.15p.m. asking to use the toilet. He opened his bowels and passed urine.

After returning to his room we chatted about Venice, Max, and how he would like to learn a foreign language amongst many other topics.

Derek was very chatty this evening describing how fortunate he feels after having had the heart attack.

9.00hrs. *Derek needed to use the toilet again to pass urine.*

Derek's mood seemed good and we enjoyed our conversation.

Entered by Elaine Brocker (H.C.A.)

21.00hrs. *I introduced myself to Derek. He had just used the toilet and was sitting on his bed when I came on duty. I asked him what he would like to do and he replied that he wished to go back* to bed and get as much information as he could from the radio.

I switched onto Radio 5 and Derek promptly fell asleep.

23.00hrs. Derek woke up asking for Andrea then said he needed to use the toilet, he used the bottle instead then had a drink of water with his medication and was soon back to sleep.

2.30a.m. Derek woke needing the toilet I gave him the bottle but had difficulty using it and wet the bed. I changed the bed and he went straight back to sleep again.

4.00a.m. Derek asking for toilet and I gave him the bottle, he went back to sleep.

6.00a.m. once again Derek asked for toilet and I gave him the bottle, he went straight back to sleep.

7.00a.m. Derek awake and is very quiet and subdued. He said he was thinking lots of things which were going through his mind, like the weather, it was raining very heavily at the time and he was looking out of the window, and of how much he longed to go home.

Derek seems to be very sad and thoughtful this morning.

Entered by C. Mepham (H.C.A.)

Tuesday 3rd July 2007

Derek was in a pleasant mood this morning but was tearful when listening to some music. He enjoyed his breakfast.

Derek had a shower and was assisted in washing his face and brushing his teeth.

We later played Connect Four and Derek found it very difficult to co-ordinate the counters into the frame. We played ball and his co-ordination with this was very good.

Derek's sister and niece came in for a short visit and left Derek in good spirits.

Derek enjoyed his lunch.

Entered by Maureen Clark (H.C.A.)

1.00p.m. Derek was very thoughtful when I first came in. I feel he is low in spirit and subdued. Derek asked if I would take him to the toilet. He walked unaided but I was unable to sit him quickly enough and he wet on the floor. Derek broke down and sobbed like a baby. I tried to make light of it as I washed and changed him, nurse mopped out the toilet area.

1.30p.m. I had brought in some new up to date photographs of family members and Derek was able to recognize every one of them, especially those that Sarah had taken the previous week in the park. He had needed no prompting.

I read him a letter of news from a personal friend which pleased him enormously. He stated how much he keeps wishing he could come home and that he hopes it will be soon. I promised him that he will definitely be coming home but again reminded him that we must be patient.

2.00p.m. *I played him music from his "Barber Shop Choir" which he sang and cried along with. I laughed at one point believing I was keeping the occasion light and fun only to be accused by Derek of being devoid of emotion and could I take it a little more seriously. I promised that I would after he had assured me that his tears were of sheer joy and not of sadness.*

2.30p.m. *Derek and I played ball. He is now good at throwing but still finds it difficult bouncing the ball onto the floor or throwing it up in the air.*

We played with the board and fitting the pieced into it. Derek hates this exercise as he maintains it causes his head to actually hurt. (But he is better at it now than he was.) He can grip the pieces firmly and lift them onto the board but has great difficulty placing them in the correct spaces.

Derek said he would like a walk down the ward and back for a little exercise.

He started sneezing a little earlier and it would now seem that Derek may have the beginning of a cold or chill.

We walked down the ward, along the corridor, around the lift area and back again to his room where he asked to go the toilet, Derek did not pass anything but said that he felt so much better for having tried and managed to take himself there.

Derek stated that he felt he would like to lie down as he felt tired and needed to rest and hoped that the Physio's did not come for him as he had no energy at the moment.

4.00p.m. *Julie topped up his T.V. card so that he could watch the tennis. (She had more luck with the machine than I had.)*

5.15p.m. *Derek ate all of his dinner and desert and drank 200mls. water. He requested a visit to the toilet but once again passed nothing.*

He washed his face with help but managed to dry himself successfully.

Derek asked to go back to bed so that he may finish watching the tennis but he was very tired and was unable to focus on the screen. This disturbs Derek very much. I did try to explain that it was because he was so tired and reminded him of how well he had done earlier on focusing on the date board. He came back and claimed that it was much easier for him now that it was being underlined.

Entered by Andrea Craig.

8.00p.m. *Derek watched tennis most of the time from my coming on duty and fell asleep waking up at 8.30p.m. asking for the toilet. He was able to wash his hands before going back to bed and falling straight back to sleep. All was well until I changed over.*

Entered by unknown.

21.00hrs. *Derek asleep when I took over shift but still had his head phones on.*

21.50hrs. *Derek awakened and used the bottle and went straight back to sleep.*

7.30a.m. *Derek woke several times in the night to use the bottle but apart from that he has had a good nights' sleep.*

Entered by Angie McCormick (H.C.A.)

4ᵗʰ July 2007

10.20a.m. *Derek was still asleep when I came into his room at 8.30a.m. he asked to go to the toilet, he went and passed urine.*

Derek ate all of his breakfast and said that he had enjoyed it.

After breakfast I assisted Derek in the shower and with washing his hair. Derek did manage to brush his teeth with minimal assistance.

We discussed how he felt that showers were so much better than having a bath and he related to me the history of his beard.

Entered by Elaine Brocker (H.C.A.)

10.50a.m. Occupational Therapy.

We practiced object recognition (i.e. comb, cup and glasses etc.) colours and body parts.

We lifted shapes out of the jig-saw.

Entered by Michelle Kozlowski (O.T)

11.00a.m. Derek enjoyed listening to Radio 2 and has been singing along to the songs.

Entered by Elaine Brocker (H.C.A.)

1p.m. Derek looked and sounded very bright when I came in today. We had a little chat and then asked to go the toilet for a "pee".

1.45p.m. We practiced placing the pieces on the board. Derek managed to take them all out successfully but then suddenly threw one piece across the room when I asked him to place it back into its correct position. I quickly moved onto playing Connect 4.

Derek said he would have a go at this but wanted me to know how much he hated this game. I tried to explain to him why he needed to practice but he became even more angry, I put it away and asked what he would enjoy doing.

He then broke down and between the sobs told me anything normal, just something which would help him to feel normal once more. I tried to hold him but he would not be held, so I simply waited until he was all cried out. He said how very sorry he was and went on to explain how exasperated and frustrated he felt and that no-one could possibly realize just how extremely bored he was.

He claimed that no-one understood how hard he was trying and that he seemed to be getting nowhere what-so-ever in his recovery. He began to cry once again and held onto his head murmuring how much it hurt him all the time and that his hands were so sore whenever he touched anything.

For a moment my heart felt it was about to break and I nearly broke down with him but I quickly felt that this would not help Derek and so I bathed his face and rubbed his shoulders and gently massaged his head for a little while. Neither of us spoke. A few minutes later I switched on his music for him to listen to and he began to softly sing along with it, ten minutes later he was returned to a much calmer state and I asked him if he would like to have a walk. Suddenly he was out of his chair, high in spirit and demonstrating a sudden remembered step from "Tai-Chi" stating that he could give me a demonstration if I so wished when Liz and Peter (Physio's) came in and whisked him away to the gym at 3p.m.

Derek returned at 3.20p.m. very happy and animated once more.

Liz stated that Derek had been unable to focus very well today. He was unable to manage any steps at all.

Derek went to the toilet but did not pass anything. He lay down on his bed at 3.45p.m.

Entered by Andrea Craig.

21.00hrs.   Derek was asleep when I came on duty. He woke and asked to use the toilet. I walked him through and he managed to successfully pass urine. He was a little confused in washing his hands as he could not locate the soap even with my prompting him. He kept using the plug thinking it was the soap but he did manage to dry his hands with no problems at all.

I made Derek a cup of 'Horlicks' to drink which he declined saying that he was more a water man.

Derek watched Cherie Blair's interview on T.V. in between nodding off to sleep.

Derek was able to remember me from last time which was the 20th June, he kept saying that he remembered that I had a strange name. (I believe it is my accent he remembers.)

00.10a.m.   Derek woke and asked to use the toilet, but when I went to help him out of bed it was too late. He was very disturbed and agitated and kept claiming that he could not understand *why this was happening to him. I explained it was because he had been in a very deep sleep and was nothing to worry about.*

Gave Derek a wash and changed him and the bed linen and he was soon re-settled and back to sleep.

6.45a.m. *Derek had slept through the night and asked to go the toilet on awakening, I walked him through where he managed to have a pee with no problems.*

He claimed he was able to recognize himself in the mirror today and was able to recall that I came from South Africa.

Derek has been watching the news on T.V.

He asked me if I liked strawberries and cream and I told him that he should go to Wimbledon because they have lots of them there.

Entered by Barbara (H.C.A.)

Thursday 5th July 2007

Derek has been in a cheerful mood this morning. He ate all of his breakfast with him managing to eat his toast himself. I help him shower trying to encourage and guide him in washing his hair, he managed to wash his genital area himself. We had a good laugh when I stupidly called him Peter and joked about him changing name.

Derek remembered that his bacon was fatty and a bit chewy yesterday but that he had enjoyed the scrambled egg. I read out the menu for tomorrows meals to him and he chose for himself what he would like to eat.

I read out the spiritual card which he enjoyed, he remembered that Harry had sent it to him and we chatted and laughed about the singing they used to do.

We chatted about sailing and of how I suffer from sea sickness. Derek told me all about George and how he enjoyed sailing with him on his boat. In all we have enjoyed a good laugh this morning since I came on at 8.00a.m.

Entered by Elaine Brocker (H.C.A.)

1p.m. *Derek very cheerful when I came in which was so lovely to see. I read him a letter and cards sent to him sent from friends in the Isle-of-Man.*

We practiced with pen and paper and Derek surprised me by drawing a circle and being able to recognize the difference between that and a straight line (which I drew.) This made him very happy and said that he wanted to practice this every day.

2p.m. *John (friend) arrived to visit with him. They chatted about football and lots of interesting topics. John left at 4p.m.*

Derek was able to walk unaided to the toilet where he managed, with a little help in sitting, to go successfully.

We then went for a walk around the third floor and back after which I cut Derek's hair and trimmed his beard.

4.30p.m. Sarah and Max arrived and played ball with Derek. They left at 5p.m.

5.15p.m. Derek ate all of his evening meal but was telling me how much he longs to come home and did I think he ever would.

5.45p.m. Derek was feeling sore from sitting down, I told him we could have a little walk but he said that he felt tired and that he thought that his dinner should be allowed to digest first. He said he wished to listen to his music.

6.30p.m. I am waiting for nurse to come and relieve me, she is occupied on ward at the moment.
Derek has used the toilet, washed his hands, face and body and cleaned his teeth. I found him much improved with these tasks but he still needs a lot of assistance. I put Derek into bed where he is now watching tennis and feeling very relaxed.
Entered by Andrea Craig.

6.35p.m. when I walked into Derek's room I found that Andrea, his wife had already prepared and put Derek to bed where he lay comfortably. A little later he complained of some pain in his left hand, *like sharp needles pricking into his fingers. This was coming and going it was not continual.*

I took over from his wife and after a short while he had fallen asleep.

20.30hrs. *Derek woke up and asked to use the toilet. I walked him through and he successfully passed urine. He washed his hands under supervision as he is unable to do so for himself. Found that Derek needs assistance in all things.*

We walked back to his room I helped Derek back into his bed where he is now asleep but restless.

A little later I asked him if he was alright and was there anything which he needed such as an extra blanket, he said that he was alright but felt very tired.

Entered by Odette Simpson (H.C.A.)

Derek had an unsettled night, he was moving around the bed a lot. He asked for and used the bottle but missed a few times, (he is unable to use it for himself)

This really upsets Derek and he says that he finds it so strange that he manages to go alright during the day but cannot seem to manage during the night and said that he preferred to use the toilet and not the bottle. I walked him through to the toilet but he found he could not go but felt happier. He went back to bed and fell asleep.

Entered by Linda Kearns (H.C.A.)

Friday 6th July 2007

11.30a.m *(Speech and Language Therapy)*
We did orientation work.
We looked at photographs.
We talked about cats.
Derek is tired and was talking in whispers at times but was able to raise his volume on request.
Entered by Rebecca Smith (Speech and Language Therapist)

12.15p.m. *Derek has had a very busy morning. He awoke in a chatty mood and we engaged in good conversation. He was talking about his progress so far and of his frustration in not being able to do certain things yet. He is in a bright mood and has enjoyed his breakfast and a shower.*
Dr. Newall visited Derek and requested that I ring Derek's wife to arrange a meeting with her to-day.
I would like to note that it has been a pleasure helping to care for Derek and I hope that he makes a speedy return home.
Entered by Elaine Brocker (H.C.A.)

12 noon. *I received a phone call asking if I could be on the ward to meet Dr. Newall, who has proven to be extremely helpful with his detailed explanation of Derek's heart and arterial condition. He was also very helpful in explaining the nerve damage* *to Derek's hand, arm and leg (left hand side.) He recommends that Physios guide me in daily therapy to help reinstate normality (hopefully.)*

Dr. Newall introduced himself as taking over in this instance from Dr. Silas, senior consulting cardiologist, to whom Derek had first been referred several weeks before he had suffered his cardiac arrest.

I liked Dr. Newall and took to him immediately, he explained that he could, if we so wished, perform an Angiogram on Derek immediately but he would in actual fact sooner wait two more weeks when he could take Derek into a new theatre and spend a little more time with him than would be possible if we chose to have it carried out now.

His angiogram has been scheduled for the 20th July. Derek seems highly delighted with this in spite of the risks which have been outlined to us.

Derek drained very suddenly after eating his lunch and his nurse quickly checked his blood pressure which was found to read normal.

Derek seemed happy enough in himself and sat listening to Elaine (H.C.A.) and I catching up on his morning therapy sessions.

1.20p.m. *His nurse went off duty and Derek and I had a walk up the ward, we paid several visits to the toilet trying to obtain urine samples with no success (how typical is that, Derek could* *normally pee at the drop of a hat but obviously not on request.)*

We proceeded to practice picking up coloured counters and placing them into their correct box (he managed quite well with this but complained that it hurt his fingers causing little shocks every time he touched something.) I told him of someone I once knew who had suffered severe nerve damage to their hand after an operation and of how his consultant had advised him to gently tap the sore area as often as he could. He was told that it would take time and that he must persevere if he was to succeed, I went on to explain that this person had persevered and it did indeed work, his hand eventually returned to normal but it had taken approx. six months.

We tried it with Derek's fingers but it was too painful so I gave him a soft ball to keep squeezing with his fingers and he seems able to manage this without too much discomfort.

Later he stated that he enjoys exercising with the soft ball and feels he is doing something useful.

Derek has been practicing drawing circles and squares, he is quite excited with this exercise.

He has said that he would like to have my name on a piece of paper so that he can see it continually as he can with the date. I have printed out familiar names to be kept on his notice board and will go over them each day.

Derek is complaining that his bottom is getting so sore and numb from all the sitting down he is doing so we went off for another walk down the ward and one more visit to the "loo" for the much needed, yet once again unsuccessful, sample which had Derek laughing more heartily than he had since before he had collapsed. He stated that these things could not be rushed.

3p.m. *Derek is sitting in his chair resting but still exercising his hand with the soft ball and listening to his music.*

Ten minutes later Derek suddenly drained once again of all colour so I put him to bed and he fell immediately into a deep sleep.

Derek has not passed urine since 11.30 this morning.

5p.m. *I had to awaken Derek to go to the toilet before his dinner (no success in passing sample.)*

5.45p.m. *Derek ate his dinner and asked if I would help get him ready for bed. He was able to wash his own hands but needed a little help with his face and body, he has improved tremendously with cleaning his teeth.*

Entered by Andrea Craig.

21.00hrs. *Derek was sleeping when I came into his room. He woke at 21.45p.m. and asked for the toilet. He opened his bowels a small amount.*

Derek sat out in his chair and talked about Andrea and George and how they are all going to have fish and chips. We talked about how bad the weather has been.

We put the radio on and Derek requested Radio One for the news, unfortunately there was only dance music on which he thought too loud and noisy so I turned it off and he seemed quite happy that I had done so.

Derek told me how physio is making him tired but knows that it is helping him become stronger.

Derek commented on how noisy and squeaky his bed was and agreed that it had a mind all of its own, which he thought was funny.

Entered by Gemma Grocott (Bank)

22.30p.m. *Derek seemed very tired so I asked if he would like to rest. He said yes and got into bed. He began to shiver and so I put on an extra blanket and he then settled.*

23.40p.m. *Derek got up and used the bottle and a urine sample was taken. Entered by Karen Kershaw.*

1.30a.m. *Derek got straight back into bed after using the toilet although he was unable to understand me when asking him to sit on the bed,* *he kept sitting in other places, however it was early in the morning. Derek settled shortly after and continued to sleep for a good period of time.*

Whilst awake his mood was very calm and gentle.
Entered by unknown.

4.15a.m. *Derek woke and used the bathroom for the fourth time, he took a drink and returned back to sleep.*
Entered by Gemma Grocott (Bank)

Saturday 7th July 2007

Derek woke again at 6a.m. we chatted about memories, Andrea and the past, which Derek seemed to enjoy.
Only once during our conversation did I have to remind Derek of previously
mentioned information.
Derek seems very clear in what he says and is in a lovely mood.
I found Derek exercising his arms and so gave him the soft balls to work with, although he does seem quite tired and may need a nap later on.
Entered by Karen Kershaw.

8.00a.m. *What a really lovely man Derek is. I was introduced to him this morning for the first time. He was so looking forward to seeing Andrea* *and going out with her for lunch. We talked about holidays, favourite foods, hobbies, including the tennis, and his children, Paul, Sarah and Max.*

I note that I look forward to meeting Derek again.

Entered by Becci Batey (H.C.A.)

10 a.m. *Derek had been showered and was looking forward to his little outing.*

Peter (staff nurse) explained that without Doctor Oates permission we may not be able to take Derek out. Derek's spirits have now dropped to an all time low.

I have explained to him that it is hospital protocol and that Peter is only carrying out his job and doing what is correct.

I explained to Peter that Mike (ward manager) already knew of our going and had given me some incontinence pants just to be on the safe side and to help Derek feel a little more secure.

I understand everyone's point of view entirely and will take full responsibility but I do firmly believe that this outing will do a lot more good for Derek than his not going.

I helped Derek dress in warm clothes and then played with the soft balls with him.

Peter had checked with Mike and we left the ward at 11.15a.m. Derek was a very happy man.

Entered by Andrea Craig.

2.30p.m. *We have just returned back with Derek from his friend George's home where we all had a lunch of fish and chips and peas, with curry sauce for Derek.*

Derek did fantastically well both getting to and into the car, he found it very easy and needed no assistance.

On the journey he was able to recognize where he was and knew the right directions we should be taking.

Derek was also able to recognize certain shops and road signs along the way and obviously enjoyed the journey very much.

There were a couple of steps leading into George's home which Derek was able to negotiate with ease, happily walking into the house, straight into the lounge and sat down again without help.

Derek ate a large lunch and had a drink. He seemed to visibly relax in his friend's home. He chatted easily and asked questions. We talked on lots of subjects and covered memories of people and places.

Derek did not have a sleep even though he was tired he said he was enjoying himself too much simply sitting around with his family once again.

I think Derek was ready to come back to hospital as he was so tired but naturally very sad also.

We talked a lot about places to go to in the future, especially us all going to Italy.

Again Derek had no problems either getting into the car or out again and was able to remember road names on the way back to 'Arrowe Park'.
Entered by Max. Payne.

2.30p.m. *Derek was very tired when he reached his room and only too willing to be undressed and put into bed after a visit to the toilet first. He was given his medication by a staff member then it was fast asleep as soon as his head touched the pillow.*

3p.m. *Sarah and Max have both left and Derek has just murmured from his bed that it has been his best day ever since his collapse.*

5p.m *Derek is still in a deep sleep and appears to be very relaxed.*

5.20p.m. *Derek awakened and asked to go to the toilet. He was able to wash his hands without help but struggled to dry them himself.*
On coming back into his room we spent a few minutes practicing finding the door handle and how to turn it to open the door and then closing it after he had walked through it. He finds this very confusing but is definitely becoming more used to it.
Derek was very good this evening at feeding himself with a spoon. Unfortunately Derek who is left-handed can no longer use this hand to hold the

spoon as it is too painful with the nerve endings (this is his damaged hand). But he is managing very well with his right hand if I first load the food onto the spoon he can then guide it to his mouth perfectly (this is a great improvement on last week).

Derek was feeling so happy with himself, said he felt as though he was nearly back to normal. The most relaxed I have known him for some time.

I helped to wash him and change him and he was able to clean his own teeth.

He then stated that he would like to go directly to bed as he felt pleasantly tired. He said that if I wanted to go he would be alright, he would watch a little tennis and have an early night. Derek we have all had such a beautiful day, goodnight sweetheart and God bless.

Entered by Andrea Craig.

21.00hrs. *Derek spent the hour after his wife left watching tennis.*

We then exercised Derek's hands using the soft balls and smoothing out his fingers. We spent the rest of the time talking at Derek's behest and because I thought he may be tired after his day out I wanted him to initiate all topics of conversation. These came thick and fast and all continuations of conversation pieces we had talked of at my last visit nearly three weeks ago such as decorating, my family and Mandy's hobbies etc.

I managed to introduce the subject of "Pelvic floor exercise" post catheter removal but Derek did not appear to have been advised to do any of these ----?

I suggest that these can be most beneficial.

Derek also mentioned that he would like a chess set and had forgotten to ask George for one.

Entered by Brandon Jones (H.C.A.)

I took over from Brandon and Derek and I talked about spiritual things, of how he felt whilst having his heart attack and the angels who were looking over him. He is very aware of being saved and being watched over. We talked about "Reiki healing" and he stated that he has a friend who does "Reiki". I suggested that he has some when he gets out as it is very relaxing, it would be good for him. Being a "Reiki Master" myself (in three different Reiki's) I would highly recommend it to anyone who has undergone something major happen to them.

This is the first time that Derek has met me but he told me he felt that I had been sent to him due to the above.

We had a very private conversation about what has happened to him and what has happened to myself in the past. He has needed to talk about it all so I let him.

22.20hrs. Derek is now tired and has gone off to sleep while using the soft balls for exercise. I lowered the bed and he dropped off with no problems. (pity really as there are fireworks going off in the distance and it's a great display, he would have loved it.)

Derek wakened for his pain killers etc. he took them all without problem. We had a small chat about the tennis, I told him that I had played back in Hawai. We laughed when I told him it was a long way to go for a game of tennis. It has now gone mid-night and he has dropped off back to sleep.

Derek used the bottle without any accidents.

5a.m. Derek woke and felt that he had had a good night's sleep. We went over the day's date, Derek managed that alright but found it harder with the names, Max being the only one he could read straight away.

Derek is able to recognize that he is at Arrowe Park hospital and likes the view from his window.

5.20a.m. Derek is in and out of sleep, he has passed urine and I now leave him to sleep again.

6.30a.m. Derek passed a large bowel motion and urine and has returned to sleep once more.

7.30a.m. Derek is still fast asleep.
Entered by S. Vanderbilt (Bank)

Sunday 8th July 2007

8a.m.

Derek was fast asleep when I arrived this morning. When he awoke I took him for a shower, he became a little confused as I took him to a different shower room. Thought it best to walk him to his familiar shower room that he is used to and Derek was much happier with this but he needed assistance with washing.

Derek was able to brush his teeth independently.

Upon returning to his room Derek listened to the T.V. whilst looking out of the window.

Derek managed to eat his breakfast of 2 Weetabix and 2 rounds of toast with help and guidance. We then talked about how he wanted to learn Italian and of how he would like to drive again and various other subjects.

We counted to one hundred and went over the alphabet, we went on to spelt out some words including the names of George, Sarah, Andrea, Max and Derek.

Derek has been given a suppository by student nurse and has not been effective as yet. Derek passed urine for the first time this morning at 11a.m. Upon returning from the toilet Derek spilt a glass of water onto the floor and got very upset over this. I reassured him that it *was not important but he had wanted to pick it up himself.*

Entered by Becki Batey (H.C.A.)

1p.m. *Derek was just finishing his lunch when I arrived and the first thing he said was how upset he felt at not being at home and how he wished he could be.*

He stated that he does not wish to do any games or exercises today because he feels too tired and would just like to sit quietly. Tears began falling down his face and I asked him if talking might help.

Derek began to tell me of how frightened he was incase he had not enough time left to him before he was well enough to come home. Next minute he asked for the toilet which was occupied so had to use the commode. Derek emptied his bowels and passed urine. He then said he would like to sleep.

1.30p.m. *Derek is in a deep sleep.*

2.30p.m. *Derek awakened very suddenly and said he would like to get up and was unable to understand why he was in bed. He is fed up and cannot say why. I asked if he would like to practice bouncing the large ball and he asked what was the point, he thought it was all so daft and a waste of time. I explained that he now found it easy throwing it to me but that he could not as yet* *bounce it, finally he agreed to have a go at this. After a short period of practice Derek managed to get the hang of bouncing the ball but soon became confused and disorientated with it so we moved on to the board and wooden pieces which Derek absolutely loathes. Again he claimed he could not understand why he was being asked to do such silly tasks and I went on to explain that it was part of his relearning to recognize, co-ordinate and focus once again, he then said he was willing to give it a shot but I could tell his focus was not good this afternoon so I brought it to a swift end.*

Derek said that he wished to watch the men's finals and enjoyed watching, with his eyes closed most of the time but definitely not asleep, he was listening.

Dinner was served right in the middle of the game and Derek said he would rather finish the match than eat. No problem I told him for just this once I will feed you as you continue to watch.

After dinner Derek became extremely emotional and believed that he had upset me by watching the tennis when he should have eaten his meal himself. This was not true but there was no convincing him of this.

Eventually he relaxed and went back to watching the game. He begged me not to go home this evening but I explained that I would have to eventually so that I could eat and get some sleep myself.

Entered by Andrea Craig.

Derek had a very settled night waking up twice to ask for the toilet.

6.50a.m. *Derek awoke and asked if I would open the curtains so he could see if the sun was shining, which it was.*

Derek and I had a good chat about Heswall, where he lives and I grew up, and we reminisced about the "old Heswellians". Derek even remembered "Robux", a lorry firm in Heswall which I can only vaguely remember, although I had lived right opposite!

Derek asked what I was going to do today and I explained that I was going for a scan as I am pregnant. He seemed genuinely pleased and congratulated me and then we went on to talk about our respective families, his son and which school he used to attend.

Derek asked me if I knew anything about "The Great War", and how appalling it was to see and live through such times, he even asked quite light-heartedly if the Iraq's were behaving themselves.

It has been fantastic having these conversations with Derek, to see him smiling and to hear his stories, as I looked after him during Derek's very first night on Ward 37. The difference is absolutely remarkable ------- keep fighting Derek, you're getting there!

Entered by Nicki Letts (H.C.A.)

Monday 9th July 2007

8.00a.m. *I sat with Derek for a short time this morning, he was in bed and asked to go to the toilet, we walked there and he was able to wash his hands when finished. Afterwards he sat in his chair and we chatted for a while.*

Entered by Laura McNab (H.C.A.)

8.30a.m. *I introduced myself to Derek as we had not met before. I helped Derek with his washing and dressing and then sat chatting for a while before breakfast was served. Derek managed to eat 2 Weetabix, 1 piece of toast, and bacon and scrambled egg with assistance and a little guidance. Derek said that the bacon was too fatty and that he did not wish to eat it.*

Following breakfast Derek brushed his teeth and gargled to freshen his mouth.

We looked out of the window and saw a beautiful rainbow, then down came the rain. We laughed at how I was going to get very wet if it continued.

Derek chatted about how much he had enjoyed watching Wimbledon and of how he had used to play tennis, he also told me of how he used to enjoy a good game of squash.

Derek carried out some exercises with the soft balls.

9.40a.m. *I asked Derek if he needed the toilet but he said that he was O.K. for now thank you.*

Derek and I discussed the topic of pets and then he chose his menu for tomorrow.

10.45a.m. *Physio's came and then we played Connect 4.*

Entered by Sue Ellis (Bank)

12.45p.m. *Derek looked and sounded very much brighter today but then he always does after he has had his physio. He told me that he had managed to walk up six steps this morning and had practiced walking up and down on the spot and that he had been on the exercise bike, my he was so pleased with himself and certainly uplifted.*

Derek had been talking football with a male nurse when I arrived and told me how good it was to have male company and be able to discuss football with a fellow supporter, even though Derek is an Evertonian and the nurse was a Liverpudlian. Derek enjoyed the football banter.

We exercised his hands with the soft balls and I read him his C.I.B.S. Journal, which was covering "Carbon emissions and Global warming". Derek was very understanding of it all and interjected with his own opinions on the said topics.

2p.m. *Derek asked to go to the toilet (passed urine) then said he felt tired. He went to sleep lying on his bed.*

4.45p.m. *Derek had a rested sleep and awakened asking to go to the toilet (passed urine) he then sat in his chair still very sleepy but happy.*

Derek was able to read out the date notice with a little help but at least he now knows where the notice board is each and every time which is an improvement. He was able to recognize several names but still needs a little prompting with each one.

5.15p.m *Sarah arrived from work and took over assisting Derek with his dinner.*

Entered by Andrea Craig.

5.45p.m. *Derek ate all of his dinner and then went for a walk down the ward with mum to top up his T.V. card. He seems to be in a good mood and wants to sit this evening to watch T.V. He has had a good sleep this afternoon and therefore is not ready to go back to bed just yet.*

He has been practicing a few Tai-Chi moves with mum, this was a hobby that he greatly enjoyed a few months ago and he seems to still get some pleasure from it.

Entered by Sarah.

18.00hrs. *I introduced myself to Derek who seemed quite settled watching the B.B.C. news on television. Derek enjoyed watching the sports review on "Look North" re: Alex Ferguson and*

Manchester United even though he told me he was a "True Blue" himself.

He also enjoyed the "Johnny Vegas interview" ------ he was amused by this.

I offered Derek tea but said he preferred water and he drank a glass full.

Derek was happily watching T.V. when I left.

Entered by Nora Alexander (Auxillary nurse)

20.10p.m. *Derek asked if he could hear some music so I put some on for him, he enjoyed listening to "Say you, say me" and sang along with it.*

20.25p.m. *Derek asked to go to the toilet (passed urine) after which he asked to go to bed.*

I helped Derek into bed where he fell fast asleep straight away.

Entered by Laura McNab (H.C.A.)

21.00hrs. *Derek was fast asleep when I arrived but woke for a urine bottle at 22.00hrs. He was relaxed and in a chatty mood talking about cooking, going back to sleep at 23.00hrs.*

Derek asked for a bottle on three further occasions requiring a change of bedding on one of these.

The movement and noise of the air-mattress would appear to be keeping Derek awake. He had a fitful sleep until 1a.m. when I decided to change the setting from (6) full massage down to (1) basic inflation. I wonder if Derek still needs an air-mattress? He is mobile, eating well etc. his "Waterlow" score will be much lower than on admission, it may be less disturbing for him on a foam mattress.

5.50a.m. *Derek woke and spent some time in the toilet.*

He stayed awake chatting about his time in Bootle, his development and my old home in Waterloo.

Entered by Brandon Jones (H.C.A.)

Tuesday 10ᵗʰ. July 2007

7.30a.m. *Derek was sitting in his chair looking out of the window when I arrived, we chatted for a while then I asked him his choice of wash or shower, Derek said he would prefer a shower. He was very willing in trying to wash himself. Derek is in very good spirits today. He has told me all about eating his fish and chips and how wonderful they tasted and how he had also been taken around the grounds of the park for a walk.*

We have been looking at his photographs. I said what a nice garden he had and he told me how they needed to now have a gardener for a while until he can get back to doing it himself once again when he is better.

9a.m. *Derek has just eaten all of his breakfast of Weetabix, toast, bacon and eggs.*

Derek managed to clean his teeth and use his mouth-wash without help.

9.40a.m. Derek said he would like to listen to some music and that he felt alittle tired. He fell asleep at 10.10a.m.

11.05a.m. Derek woke. The dietitian came to speak to him and said that they were going to stop the suppositories as he was now regular in his bowel habits.

We are now back looking at photographs and Derek seems very happy to see his family snaps.

We have also been working with the flash cards. Derek asked me what field I was specializing in and laughed thinking this was funny.

12.30p.m. Derek ate all of his lunch of Shepherd's pie, mash and veg. and was able to feed himself but I had to first put the food onto his fork.

After lunch I asked Derek to exercise with the soft balls, he said he would if he must but that his left hand is very painful and that he had a fall in the shower and got his arm caught which is still sore.

Entered by Mary Halligan (H.C.A.)

1p.m. Derek is in very good spirits today, he has eaten all of his lunch.

We walked up and down the ward several times as he said his bottom was numb from sitting for so long. He went to the toilet on the way back (Very small bowel movement and passed urine). Derek now automatically washes his hands after going to the toilet but still has trouble turning on the tap. He is still throwing paper towels on the floor because he cannot locate the bin but is now able to pick them up again himself and asks me where to put them, which is a great improvement on last week.

He is much improved with the opening and closing of doors and his walking is improving by the day.

Derek has expressed his desire to be able to wipe and clean himself so that he can be totally independent when going to the toilet but sadly I feel he is a long way from being able to do so.

We practiced marching on the spot (as recommended by Physio's) and he was much improved on last week.

I reminded him again of a very simple Tai-Chi movement using his hands only and he was very pleased that he was able to do this.

Afterwards I questioned Derek on the entire exercise set down by Rebecca Smith (speech therapist) and marked his score, again this was something else which was very much improved on last week and Derek completed the whole exercise before becoming tired, which I thought was brilliant.

Derek maintains that these exercises both annoy and tire him but that he does now realize and understand why he must do them.

He asked for the toilet and passed urine.

George came to visit and walked Derek up and down the ward and around the lift area several times which Derek so enjoyed.

Derek said that he had spent a very pleasant afternoon with him feeling as though he was a part of the human race once more.

After George had left Derek practiced using a pencil and paper with his left hand (Derek claimed it was very sore but I feel he must carry on as he is naturally left handed and vital that he begins using it)

Derek walked into the protruding rail on the end of the bed as I did myself a little later on. I feel this is very dangerous. I have placed a pillow over it for now and reported it.

6p.m. I took Derek to the toilet (passed urine) then afterwards washed him down before getting him ready for bed. He cleaned his teeth and rinsed his mouth which never fails to please him as this makes him feel a little more independent.

He has asked to go to bed as he feels tired but appears to be nicely relaxed and cheerful.

Can nursing staff please note that if T.V. goes off there is a new card to be found in Derek's locker.

Entered by Andrea Craig.

6.45p.m. *Derek was content watching T.V. I offered to make him more comfortable but he said he was quite happy as he was. He started to get sleepy, he rolled over onto his left side and went to sleep, I switched off the television.*

Derek had a short visit from his sister.

Entered by unknown.

21.00p.m. *Derek was asleep when I came in. He awoke at 21.40p.m. and asked to go to the toilet. Coming back from the bathroom Derek sat in his chair and we had a lovely chat.*

I told him how I had taken my children on a school trip to Chester Zoo, Derek asked about the penguins and said how he would like to visit the zoo himself when he is better.

He spoke about Max and Sarah and of how fantastic it would be to have grand children and how he loves kids but that he would like Max and Sarah to see the world before they settle down, Derek feels this is very important for them.

Derek worked with the soft balls in his left hand for ten minutes before saying he felt tired. He then tried to get back into bed but was confused over which way he should lie down and required guidance and assistance.

Derek had a drink of water before going to sleep at 22.40p.m.

Entered by Gemma Grocott (H.C.A.)

1.30a.m. *Derek woke and asked to use the bottle, after using it successfully he tipped the bottle over the bed by accident. I changed the bed and Derek's T-shirt and shorts and helped him back to bed. Derek very confused as to which way he should be lying and needed assistance.*

4.20a.m. *Derek woke up and asked to use the toilet (passed urine) he was confused on how to wash and dry his hands. Derek went back to bed by following my instructions quite easily and did very well.*

Entered by Paul Mannion (H.C.A.)

Wednesday 11th July 2oo7

8a.m. *Derek was sitting on the bed looking out of the window when I arrived. I asked him if he would prefer to sit in the chair which he did.*

8.30a.m. *I walked Derek down for a shower, he did well with my helping him to dry himself. He ate all of his breakfast after which he listened to the news.*

We went through all of the photographs with Derek being able to remember all of them.

Derek has brushed his own teeth without help and is now waiting for the Physio's to come for him. (He looks forward to this)

11.30a.m. *No physio's so we went for a walk across to the lift area and back.*

11.45a.m. *Occupational Therapy.*
Derek was a lot brighter than when I last saw him.

We played Connect 4, he could tell what colour each counter was and was able to pick them up. He had difficulty bringing them upto the board and placing them.

He was able to move away all the jig-saw pieces and put them back again in correct places with some assistance.

Entered by Emma Turnick (O.T.A.)

12.30p.m. *Derek ate and enjoyed a good lunch of Turkey roast followed by bread and butter pudding. He managed to place the fork to his mouth after I put food onto it for him.*

Entered by H. Howatson (H.C.A.)

1p.m. *Derek has been very chatty this afternoon and remembered that his sister had called in to visit him last night.*

Derek said he has missed the physio and his exercises and was feeling a little stiff from sitting about all day. We walked around the entire third floor area with Derek not wishing to go back to his room. He wanted to keep on the move so we did the round several times and then did some

Andrea Craig

marching on the spot when we finally did arrive back.

We stood and bounced the large ball between us. Derek can now recognize the word ball (he always used to call it a "bounce-bounce") and knows the difference between bouncing and throwing which he did not last week.

He was very happy playing this but quite suddenly his focus crashed and I knew that Derek was not seeing. I asked him if he was tired and he said yes, very. I put Derek to rest on his bed where he immediately fell into a deep sleep.

He had visited the toilet before hand to pass urine.

4.30p.m. *Derek woke up and sat in his chair and I read to him. Sarah arrived just in time to help feed him his dinner.*

6.45p.m. *Sarah walked Derek around third floor again for a little exercise.*
Entered by Andrea Craig.

18.30p.m. *Derek was sat in his chair watching the evening news when I came in, he was comfortable and laughing at the T.V.*

19.45p.m. *I took Derek for a walk to the lifts, down to the ground floor and out of the main entrance for a breath of fresh-air. Derek was very pleased to be out of his room and enjoyed talking about*

Andrea, he was very cheerful. Coming back he watched a further twenty minutes of T.V. then fell asleep in his chair so I helped him into bed at 20.20p.m.

Entered by Claire Kelly (student nurse)

Thursday 12th July 2007

7.30a.m. *there were no problems over night in my opinion. Derek seemed to sleep well. He got up to use the toilet a couple of times in the night to pass urine. He walked well with me.*

Derek seems to be very alert and responsive this morning, he has been asking me how long he has been in hospital for.

Entered by A. Whitehead (H.C.A)

I took over from Andy. Derek was very subdued, he claims that he is alright but tired, he is not very talkative at all (perhaps because I am a new face).

He ate all of his breakfast. I showed Derek how to scoop the food onto his spoon.

9a.m. *Derek has finished his breakfast and has requested the soft balls to do his hand exercises. I asked him if he preferred a wash or a shower, he refused either for now but has said he would like a shower a little later.*

We chatted about his daughter and his time spent in hospital. He told me I was too young to get married and that I should be enjoying myself.

10.00a.m. I took Derek down to the shower room where there were no problems. He has reported a rash but I could not see one, I have creamed the area which he indicated just incase.

I forgot to record that Derek had his bowels opened at 9.10a.m. there were no problems.

We continued our talk about families, marriage etc.

10.10a.m. I asked Derek if he would like to watch the news and he is now doing so.

11.15a.m. Derek has just returned from his physio. session. He is in good spirits but still very quiet. He seems concerned that they did not spend much time walking him instead concentrating on co-ordination, he explained that each session concentrated on different areas (I was a bit confused).

We then went on to speak about sport and swimming.

Derek ate most of his lunch and his yogurt with very little assistance. At 12.30p.m his wife arrived

Entered by M. Woodworth. (H.C.A.)

12.35p.m. *Derek was in the toilet with his nurse when I first arrived. He looked well and walked back into the room very perky and happy to see me.*

Derek sat and exercised with the soft balls, his left hand still very painful with nerve damage.

1.30p.m. *Derek and I had a game of draughts. He needed a lot of guidance but managed much better than I believed he would. Half way through his focus dropped again as it can (I believe tiredness is the main cause of this).*

2p.m. *Derek had two visitors (Marlene and Glyn). Glyn took Derek for a walk as far as the lifts and back. Derek was so pleased to see them both and we sat talking of Italy.*

3.15p.m. *Visitors have now left and Derek is lying down watching a news program.*

5.15p.m. *Derek has watched the news channel on and off for the last two hours he says he finds it all so informative and that he needs this kind of information.*

6p.m. *Derek ate heartily all of his dinner. I have helped to wash him down and dress him for bed. He cleaned his own teeth insisting that he rinsed his mouth also. I then flossed them for him and*

Derek stated that I would never make a dentist (what cheek!).

He is in a lovely relaxed and mellow mood this evening.

I applied a little prescribed ointment onto his rash, unless one knows where it is, it is difficult to see, it is right in the groin area of both sides just below the testicles. PLEASE NOTE THAT DEREK NEEDS ONE MORE APPLICATION LATER THIS EVENING.

Entered by Andrea Craig.

21.00hrs. *I introduced myself to Derek, he was just returning from the toilet when I arrived for my shift. Derek seemed to be tired and quickly settled down into bed. He has had quite a peaceful night only waking to use the bottle (which he managed successfully) and to walk to the bathroom once.*

6.15a.m. *Derek awoke and walked to the bathroom settling back into bed on his return. He seems to be in good spirits. We chatted about the weather and the model aeroplanes that he can sometimes see from his window. Derek soon fell back to sleep.*

Entered by Sarah Folley-Davey (H.C.A.)

Friday 13th July 2007

7.30a.m. *Derek was awake at the start of my shift so I left him in bed for a while as the O.T. is coming* in at 9.15a.m. to assess Derek washing and dressing himself to see how he is progressing.

Derek was up in his chair eating breakfast at 8.45a.m.

Entered by Claire Kelly (H.C.A.)

10 a.m. Occupational Therapy Assessment.

Derek was able to wash and comb his hair with prompts.

He had difficulty taking his dressing gown off/on.

He was unable to take off his T-shirt but was able to do better with prompts.

Practice ended at this point.

Derek is communicating well and telling me about watching T.V.

Plan is to continue with personal care practice.

Entered by Michelle Kozlowski (O.T.)

11.30a.m. Speech and Language therapy.

We had a really good session this morning. Derek did very well.

His orientation is much improved, conversational skills improved as has his recall and his memory.

Derek's reading skills are developing nicely and his vision is much better. I am really pleased with his progress.

Entered by Rebecca Smith (speech and language)

Derek has had a really busy morning and coped very well. He has eaten exceptionally well having more toast and egg and bacon after his O.T. session.

Derek helped me to write his menu for tomorrow by deciding for himself what he would like to eat. He is in really good spirits and looking forward very much to seeing Andrea.

Derek and I have enjoyed a number of conversations about sport and how he likes to play squash and tennis.

Derek's T.V. is not working again, Derek says, "not again" so I have phoned the operator who is sending someone out to look at it. Derek hopes it will be soon as he misses it.

Derek has had his bowels opened this morning normally and paid regular visits to the toilet to pass urine.

Entered by Claire Kelly (H.C.A.)

12.30p.m. Derek was sitting very cheerfully in his chair when I entered his room. The T.V. engineer arrived to look at the set and broke the news that Derek would be without a T.V. for a few days as the engineers did not work over the week-ends.

Derek said he felt tired so at 1.30p.m. he had a lie on the bed and fell into a deep sleep.

Sarah popped in mid-afternoon but Derek was very drowsy

3.15p.m. *Derek woke and got up when Doreen (a friend) came to visit. We walked with Doreen to see her into the lift at 4p.m. and on the walk back Derek voiced how disgusted he felt at not being able to tune into the news later on and how long the evening would be.*

Arriving back in his room I trimmed his hair and beard.

5.15p.m. *Derek managed to feed himself this evening (the best to date) using both a knife and fork but I did have to still feed him his soup. Derek explained how it took so much concentration in feeding himself but felt so pleased that he had at last been able to.*

Derek asked if I minded him going to bed early this evening.

I have helped wash and prepare him for bed and applied ointment to rash.

PLEASE NOTE ONE MORE APPLICATION IS NEEDED LATER THIS EVENING and could it also be noted that Derek has been telling me of how the lights at night are keeping him awake.

Entered by Andrea Craig.

8.30p.m. *Derek has spent a very settled evening since his wife went home. I spent time with him looking through his photographs, it is important for us to be reminded that our patients are human and live full lives outside of the hospital environment,* *this fact often gets lost in the routine that goes on.*

We shared nice conversations about his family, work and holidays. Derek can converse very well but gets a little muddled at times but does remember with a few prompts. He is also capable of asking questions of the other person about their lives and seems genuinely interested in their response, I found this very good, Derek converses very well indeed.

After a while he became very tired and I helped him into bed where he slept until the end of my shift at 9p.m.

I have noticed a marked improvement in Derek since I last nursed him and hope that this will continue.

Entered by Mandy (H.C.A.)

p.s. I have asked staff nurse about his family being able to bring in their own T.V. she replied that she would have a word with the ward manager and would let the family know the outcome. I know how fed up Derek must be without his telly to watch.

Derek was drifting in and out of sleep when I took over my shift with him and continued to do so until I was relieved.

Entered by (Kershaw. H.C.A.)

10.40p.m. *Derek woke wanting the toilet, he walked with me and was very smiley and happy,* *he came back and I offered him a drink but he only wanted water, he took his medications with this and was happy to go back to bed. I covered him up and he is now back asleep.*

Entered by (H.C.A. Wood)

Derek woke up to use the toilet and was in need of prompting throughout.

Apart from tossing and turning, Derek has slept well for the majority of the night.

Entered by (Kershaw H.C.A.)

Saturday 14th July 2007

8a.m. *Derek woke up in a very happy mood and was ready to have his shower. He put on fresh underpants, jogging bottoms and clean T-shirt. He has had his hair washed and enjoyed his breakfast of cornflakes, toast and bacon and egg.*

Mid morning Derek drank two full beakers of elderflower juice.

Derek has practiced his jig-saw and the different word lists. He practiced patterns using the Connect 4 counters. We did some silly exercises of "Simon says", followed by some walking and then we had a nice chat and told some funny jokes.

Derek is now having a rest before his lunch.

11.45a.m. *Derek ate his prescribed "Forticreme", followed by a strawberry fortified drink (all were taken without problem).*

For lunch Derek ate Turkey and ham hot-pot with sauté potatoes and peas followed by apple pie and ice-cream. He ate most of it.

We have been singing "Aga doo", "Hokey Cokey" and "Consider Yourself One of Us", Derek really enjoyed it. He claimed it was nice to keep light-hearted and do nice kind of things.

Entered by (H.C.A.)

12.45p.m. *I bought Derek a T.V. of his own and with the help of George who carried up to his room and the authorization of staff, we excitedly set about installing it for him only to discover that it would not work off the hospital system.*

Derek was so disappointed he said that he wants no more television and that in future he will listen to the radio.

George and I took Derek for a walk around the hospital and called in at the cafeteria, Derek said he was so pleased to be out of his room which was beginning to feel like his prison.

Returning to his room George attempted to show Derek how to put his jacket on and off. George failed to understand that Derek must be given very clear, simple and precise instruction otherwise he becomes very confused as his brain cannot digest and file the information received.

George sadly used too many words spoken too quickly and Derek became very agitated.

Once we were alone Derek asked if we might have another go at practicing with his jacket and this time he was able to take off one side over his shoulder but failed to be able to remove the other. I assured him that this was indeed a huge step forward, with which Derek replied with an "ummm".

5.15p.m. Derek managed his dinner very well once again. He is now able to use both knife and fork but says that his left hand is still as painful as ever but he wishes to work through this believing that it is important that he does so.

He actually worked it out for himself today that it is much easier if he turns the fork (or spoon) as he takes it to his mouth as it goes in without any trouble.

Derek was tired this evening and after I had washed and prepared him for bed I watched him brush his teeth and then rinse with the mouth wash, he was confused with the tiredness and instead of spitting it out Derek swallowed it giving himself a shock.

Derek was very willing in trying to undress himself this evening but I do worry about his Peg tube when he struggles with his pants. He has caught this several times and I feel it is only a question of time before we have an accident.

I have also noticed recently that when Derek is performing any task he is holding his breath as though he does not realize that he can do both at the same time.

We had a little talk about this and he says that the concentration necessary to carry out anything at all takes everything he has and he does not even stop to think whether he is breathing or not but that he will try to mindful of it in future.

I could sometimes cry at his willingness to do all that is asked of him, I can only hope that I do not expect too much of him. (I feel it is so much like being a parent all over again, how far should one push and how far does one step back in doing the right thing.)

He has asked to go to bed as he wishes to lie down.

Derek has tried so hard today, I could feel his determination. Well done my darling have a good night's sleep.

Entered by Andrea Craig.

6p.m. *Derek's wife left and I took over from her. Derek was already in bed and went straight to sleep, (wish I could do that). I sat and read the paper then at 7p.m I was relieved by another H.C.A. for an hour. I returned at 8p.m. to find Derek continuing to sleep well, although he tosses and turns a lot he soon settles down again.*

8.40p.m. Derek woke and asked to go to the toilet for a pee. I suggested that he sat on the toilet instead of standing to it as he is wobbly on his feet. Derek finds basic commands difficult to understand, you have to repeat command and also show him what he must do before I could get him to do it on his own.

I then stood outside of the door to give him his privacy checking on him at all times to finally ask him if he had finished. Unfortunately Derek had not been positioned on the toilet correctly and had wet the floor and his undergarments.

I helped to change Derek and put him back to bed where he fell back to sleep.

Entered by Mandy (H.C.A.)

9p.m. I took over duty and as soon as Derek woke up I read out aloud to him from the "Liverpool Daily Post" newspaper which we both enjoyed.

He has complained about the light at night keeping him awake and I explained that it was very necessary for the corridor lights to be kept on at all times because the staff needed to be able to see where they were going and that patients also needed the light s to see their way to the toilets.

Derek said he understood but that he was still going to complain about it in the morning. I made the room as dark as I could for him.

Andrea Craig

6.30a.m in the end Derek had a good night's sleep. He did wake to go to the toilet four times during the night.

He asked for the soft balls this morning and sat doing exercises with his right hand. Derek was a bit confused when I asked him to swap over to his left hand but he eventually got it right after a lot of explaining and prompting.

Derek has enjoyed a glass of elderflower juice but he has missed having a T.V. to watch and catch up on the news.

Entered by (H.C.A.)

Sunday 15th July 2007

8a.m. Derek and I have spent a pleasant morning together and we have chatted about lots of different things, we have talked about Scotland and how beautiful it is there. We have both visited Scotland and agree that it is a lovely place to go (albeit a little cold and wet.)

We have also chatted about Anglesey and how Derek has enjoyed sailing around there with his friend in his yatch. We agreed that it is also very lovely there but again it could be a little wet and cold.

Derek has talked a lot about his wife Andrea this morning and when I asked him how long they had been married he told me over twenty years and that they knew each other inside out!

He claimed he was so lucky in having such a supportive family.

Derek was able to dress himself this morning with a little help from me but he did struggle with arm co-ordination. He was able to lift the appropriate foot into each slipper very well.

I offered Derek a trim of his beard but he quickly told me that Andrea did that -----

So I will leave that to Andrea!

We are just sitting waiting for breakfast and Derek has said that he is hungry and that he prefers to drink water as he does not like tea or coffee, although he does enjoy the odd "Cappacino" now and then.

After breakfast which Derek ate all of we looked through photographs together, I like the look of Venice and Derek assured me that it is indeed very beautiful but can be very expensive.

We have been playing games. We thought of animals for each letter of the alphabet. Derek insisted on being very strict with the rules and would not allow me to have "Unicorn" for the letter "U", nor did he allow me "White shark" for "W".

We had great fun playing this game, although Derek was much better at it than I was. The best name Derek came up with was "Duck-billed Platipuss" I was very impressed!

Derek went to the toilet and had a slight accident (but he did open his bowels and it has been reported on chart) so we changed his pajama's and washed him down and he now feels more comfortable.

(Wet clothes and slippers are in a plastic bag waiting to go home).

We worked through some language tasks and Derek did very well. He is visibly tired now and is going to rest on his bed until lunch time.

P.S. Derek had a walk down to the ground floor earlier this morning (in lifts of course).

12.05p.m. *Derek is still sleeping, his bed is dry and he remains comfortable and happily settled.*

12.30p.m. *We had another minor accident but had to assist Derek to wash and change himself just in time for lunch.*

Andrea is now here assisting Derek with his Sunday lunch.

It has been an absolute pleasure working with Derek today and I wish him and his family all the luck in the world. xx

Entered by E mma Jenkins (H.C.A.)

12.45p.m. *I took over from Emma and was pleasantly surprised to see Derek sitting on his own feeding himself. (Emma was busily putting Derek's dirty washing in a bag).*

Derek struggles to put food onto his fork but is doing so much better than he was a few days ago when he could do nothing at all.

I brought in a radio which Derek is thrilled with but still frustrated because he is unable to change the stations for himself.

I found tablets still lying on the floor where they had lain from the day before, I felt very strongly about this and considered I must do something about it. I summoned Staff and requested that the room be thoroughly cleaned out and the tablets disposed of. I asked why Derek was allowed to administer his own medication and why had it not been noticed that he had dropped some of them, and left to lie under his chair and his bed. I was informed that Derek had not dropped them and it would have been the nurse on duty who had dropped them and then replaced them so that Derek in actual fact had not gone without his correct medication.

I accepted this explanation but as I pointed out to Staff, why had the cleaners not picked them up when they cleaned and swept Derek's room but it was obvious by the dust in the room and the fluff which had been allowed to build up on the floor that the room had not been cleaned. This I told her, I found totally unacceptable. I had been stopped from mopping out Derek's room which I had been doing on a daily basis as it did not meet with hospital protocol, "Where is hospital protocol now?" I asked.

While Derek was having his afternoon nap a domestic knocked on the door stating that she was far from happy having to come back and *clean this room as she had just been going home. She had already been informed about the tablets which had been on the floor since the day before and almost accused me of planting them there myself.*

I told her not to even dream of going there with that accusation and would she mind simply getting on with her task as quickly as possible. She seemed to have total disregard for a patient who was desperately trying to sleep. Two minutes later and realizing that she may have been a little hasty in her accusations she continued by sympathizing with Derek's "unfortunate dilemma" and "the dangers of dropped tablets and the harm they might cause visiting children", throughout the rest of the cleaning process.

I could only agree with her and expressed my sincere wishes in hoping that she was not held back too late in getting home. "All's well that ends well", as they say!

Derek thought the whole affair was hugely hilarious and said it had been worth missing his sleep for and who would have thought that only six months previously, five dropped tablets would have been the high-light of our day.

I would like to note that I had considered my mopping out Derek's room every day to have been a help to the domestic staff and a great therapy to myself as Derek took his afternoon nap. I also had the satisfaction of knowing that it was done and not forgotten as so often happened. Too bad that protocol had put a stop to it but I do still wipe everywhere down each and every time I come in.

I consider hygiene a priority in hospitals, not something which happens if there is time. (This is not a slur on the team of domestic's themselves but their management most certainly needs to be more vigilant).

2.30p.m. *I gave Derek four words to memorise, (apple, ball, comb and bell) and then repeat them back to me. First attempt he could not remember any of them, second attempt leaving a few minutes before I asked him to repeat them, he did so successfully.*

I had Derek doing simple exercises, (lifting right knee, lifting left knee, lifting his arms above his head, placing them by his side again and then clapping hands).

Derek is beginning to recognize that he has two sides to his body which he has not been able to do before. He can now recognize his head, his arms and his legs and both his body and facial features.

3.15p.m. *Derek is now resting on his bed he is tired but cheerful.*

4.30p.m. *Sarah, Max and myself took Derek down to the basement cafeteria for a walk and a drink which Derek so enjoyed, on arriving back at* *his room Derek became more and more subdued and then quite emotional.*

After Sarah and Max had left I asked him if he would like to explain to me what it was that seemed to be worrying him.

Apparently it would seem that he was left alone on the toilet last night and after shouting for help for some considerable time he claims he got himself into trouble. (He had a fall). Derek was extremely agitated whilst relating this incident and it certainly causes me more than a little concern.

Derek is on twenty-four hour watch and needs guidance in all that he does still, especially with his toiletry. It is important that his privacy is respected but must be given without him being left completely on his own.

Derek cannot as yet clean himself after using the toilet, his lack of co-ordination prevents this (as does the nerve soreness in his left hand)

I would like to bring to everyone's attention that work with Derek in this area has only just begun but will take time.

LEFT ON HIS OWN HE WILL BECOME UPSET AND UNABLE TO FUNCTION CORRECTLY.

This is not a complaint ------- only that the nurse on duty with Derek will understand more fully.

After getting this off his chest and my promising him that no-one will get into trouble, Derek had a rest until dinner was served. He managed very well in feeding himself, this is improving a little more each day but still always with assistance.

After dinner Derek was once again low in spirit and expressing a very strong desire to come home, (this is growing stronger now each day).

He did not want me to get him ready for bed this evening, said his nurse would help him later on.

Entered by Andrea Craig.

As per discussion with Andrea:

Derek was left alone in the toilet (refer to notes above) and it has been agreed with ward manager that at present Derek does indeed require twenty-four hour supervision, thus under no circumstances should he be left unsupervised whilst he requires special nursing care.

Entered by Rachel Lilley (Nurse in charge).

9p.m. *Derek got ready for bed after we had chatted about his day. He said he felt quite tired. Then he told me he is worried about going to the toilet. Andrea has taken his slippers home to wash and will bring others tomorrow.*

Will staff please remind him of this when he asks for his slippers.

Entered by Linda Kearns (H.C.A.)

21.00hrs. *Derek was asleep on my arrival.*

21.25hrs. *Derek awoke and I escorted him to the toilet (passed urine) and helped him back into* *bed. We had a short chat, his medication was given and he fell asleep once again.*

Derek had several visits to the toilet during the night (passing urine).

He slept well in between times and when he awoke he was able to read the date from the date board and several of the names. He then exercised his hands using the soft balls.

Entered by Joan Lomax (H.C.A.)

CHAPTER TEN

Medically Derek was improving, so much so that the night feeds which were administered through his PEG tube had now been stopped and thankfully he continued to gain weight which indicated that the removal of this tube was now possible. The PEG nurse felt it should be left in place for a further four weeks after his night feeds had stopped to make sure that Derek was nutritionally stable and that he could take all of his medication orally. His night feeds had been reduced to half on the 28th June and stopped all together on the 3rd July and so far he was doing well, except that I felt the tube was a great nuisance, for each time Derek went to the toilet and tried to pull down his trousers he would catch on it, I was a little concerned about this but his nurses thought it was not a problem.

Doctor Oates had requested from Doctor Silas, Derek's cardiologist, a further review and an assessment of angiogram if appropriate. I personally believed that this would clear up so much of what still remained unclear to Derek and myself.

Derek's MRSA infection seemed to be under control but each day I waited to hear confirmation that he was free of it and prayed that nothing more serious would strike and set him back on his road to recovery.

In spite of the tremendous progress being made, Derek seemed to be more and more emotionally down. His longing for home was quite natural and I believe this had deepened after his visit to see George. That first Saturday's visit had been a huge success. I had been more than a little concerned as to how we were going to manage getting Derek into the car but I need not have worried for he had needed no instruction whatsoever in getting into Max's car. Max brought the car around to the hospital side entrance where Sarah and I were waiting with Derek in his wheelchair, no sooner had Max parked up, when Derek was out of the chair, having no problem stepping off the curb (which I thought he might easily have slipped on) and in a flash had the door open and himself seated, as if to say, "what's keeping everyone!"

Leaving Sarah open mouthed with an empty wheelchair, I ran round to see if he was alright and to make sure he had not injured himself, to find that he had already closed the car door as normal as I or anyone else would have done. Had I really spent the last several days teaching him how to open and shut the door to his hospital room until I had almost despaired that he would ever be able to do so, we were all truly stunned. Having returned the wheelchair, Sarah slid into the back seat beside myself and we were away with Derek's words, "Away James and don't spare the horses", causing us all to laugh.

Derek was able to recognize the road we travelled and pointed out various landmarks and shops as we came to them and there was no disguising the excitement he was feeling, my only moment of anxiety came as we approached our own house. We had to pass this just two or three minutes before we reached George's home and I had no idea how Derek would react. We live in a house elevated high from the road with a flight of steps leading up through a long garden to the front door. Perhaps he would not be able to take it in, I thought or rather I hoped in one way that he would not, but as we turned the bend in the road in the run up to it Derek turned his head to the left and I felt his mood change dramatically. I sat forward and placed my arms around his shoulders to support and comfort him as he murmured, "One day I shall climb those steps no matter what anyone else says".

Derek's mood had dropped but two minutes later as we were parked in George's driveway with George standing at the front door waiting to greet us, his excitement soon returned. He was out of the car just as quickly as he had got himself into it and after shaking hands with George he deftly climbed the two steps into the porch, up another rather high step into the hall and then it was straight through into the lounge and into "his chair", which was the one he usually sat himself in whenever we visited.

Derek was doing much better than any of us had ever dared consider possible, the only help he had needed throughout the entire visit was in feeding and visiting the toilet. Yes the whole day had indeed been a great success, although Derek was actually relieved to get back to his room where he could have a lie down, he kept reliving the conversations that had taken place, of how much he had enjoyed the simple normality of the visit and of how being able to read a few road names had given him fresh hope.

It was two days later that Derek very tearfully told me just how much he longed to be able to go home. He whispered how very sad he had felt when we had driven passed the house on our way to visit George and how he had looked up and felt at the time that his heart was going to break, he also told me of how fearful he was that another heart attack might take him before he was ever able to return home. I could only listen and remind him as gently as I could of how patient we must continue to be and that although it must feel to him as though it would never be possible I believed it would be so.

On returning home that evening I wrote my second letter to Derek in the hope that it might once again give him the courage to continue his climb back. As in my first letter I addressed Derek with the nickname I always call him.

My darling Blue,

It has been strange over the past few months, what with the shock of you so very nearly being taken from me and how poorly you have been during the time since. You see, as well as feeling sad at times, I have also felt a sense of happiness I have never known before.

Each and every day I have witnessed the wonderful team of specialists, doctors and nurses around you, not forgetting all those lovely girls serving you with tea and coffee but most of all I have noted the effort that you have applied in aiding your own recovery and how during every moment you remained cheerful and uncomplaining, this my darling, has swelled my heart beyond belief.

I know that we have shared something very special these past two months, even more special than anything that has gone before for I feel our love has taken on a new and much deeper expression and in the process so much has fallen away allowing us to grow closer in God's Love. All is possible within His Love, my darling, and therefore we must hold onto that.

I long to have you home where you truly belong, surrounded by all that is familiar to you but I ask you to remember that no matter what the circumstance, we are as one always and as that saying so rightly states "home is where the heart is". My darling, darling Blue, I am at home with you in spite of circumstances that strive to keep us apart or the space that separates us physically, for you are held in the true home of my heart constantly. We must be patient and take things slowly, there is no rush for all will be taken care of in its correct time.

When you feel embarrassed and undignified, my darling, try to remember that you are actually showing a truly greater dignity than you could imagine. The nurses love your humility and gentle manner (has the lion truly learned how to walk with the lamb?) They have stated that you are a true gentleman and a joy to care for, so you see my darling boy, nothing, absolutely nothing is as bad as you imagine.

This phase will soon be over but we must both learn not to be afraid or embarrassed by it. I for one feel an overwhelming love when I am helping you and caring for you, especially with your toilet visits. No greater or more personal task can one person carry out for another, so therefore please know that I carry these out for you in love.

These accidents and happenings take you down and I know that your spirit drops, so my dear, lovely, wonderful boy, you must bounce right back up and allow your love to over-ride this phase of your recovery. It will pass and until it does remember you and I will cope. We will cope with everything together and with the help from all the wonderful people nursing you, your friends and family who are supporting you and the Love of God and that great strength of Spirit to uphold us, we will come through this, you will see.

My love is with you, around you and upholding you always. Know that I am in your heart and a part of you always, forever and beyond my darling. Remember that our homes are only the outer expression of what we hold within our hearts, rest in the love which you hold within your own heart and you will find yourself walking into the physical fabric of your home before you know it.

Yours always Andrea xxx

P.S. " In love there is no right nor wrong and all things that you so believe in shall be possible", a little thought that came to me as I folded up this letter and so I write it lest I forget. Good-night and God bless my darling.

I read my letter to Derek the following afternoon as he lay resting on his bed. He asked that he might keep it under his pillow for a while but later asked that I take it home to keep it safe for him. I suggested that I kept it with the first letter which he would ask me to read to him every so often, in my handbag, and then I could read them both to him if he so wished.

Derek had short term memory problems but he never forgot the letters I wrote to him and I include them in these records only because Derek maintains that they helped him tremendously during the times when he almost gave up.

Although this was a period of the most wonderful medical recovery and Derek was far exceeding every prognosis that had been made it must be remembered that he was still at high risk neurologically, also from further heart attacks, not to mention the MRSA which he was still fighting and from the numerous other infections invading our hospital wards these days.

We must also remember that everything Derek was doing, all those every day things the rest of us take for granted. He had to relearn them all one by one. It took so much effort for him to walk around his room, slowly discovering and re-learning what each item was. His locker was a total mystery to him. The word locker had been lost from his memory and his perception could not take in the locker as a whole. He was unable to focus on the objects placed upon the top of it and at times I believed he could not see them but then came the day when he picked up the little card which Harry had sent him from the hospital chapel and Derek asked me if I had read it as it was such a lovely card. I cannot describe how I felt when he had been able to single that one item out from all the others and recognize it, almost akin to witnessing a baby taking its first steps and you wanting to shout it out to the whole world.

These were the little opening windows which I held onto. Sometimes we would wait for days without any openings at all, then perhaps like the day that he picked up the card, we would have a small window open, or perhaps we would have several windows being flung wide open all at once. These were the days when it seemed Derek was taking three steps forwards then two steps back and the doctors had to keep reassuring me that although he was indeed following this pattern I should not lose heart because in fact he was actually taking one step forward on a continual basis. I could see that this was true but it was just beginning to dawn upon me that his recovery was going to be extremely slow indeed.

In the meantime daily entries in his diary were growing in content and Derek himself would often remind me that I had not written in them on that particular day and had I not better get on with it, but would always suggest that perhaps I should write them up after we had first taken a walk or carried out some other task he was eager to be getting on with. How could I argue with him, for I delighted in his eagerness to keep on going.

No longer allowed to mop out his room, I looked forward to sitting beside him as he had his afternoon rest and making my own entry into the diary. It was even more enjoyable and interesting to read the many other entries now being entered by the nursing staff and therapists who gave of their valuable time in doing so. As I have written previously, I feel quite certain this is not the type of diary that Dr. Pinder originally referred to when he suggested that we kept one.

However they are becoming more and more detailed in Derek's daily progress and outline each day's events in an order which became both simple and useful for myself and staff to look back on.

The following entries show how Derek was beginning to feel the boredom of being in isolation, the disappointment of no physiotherapy sessions, they had stopped suddenly at a time when he felt he had needed them most and the frustration he felt at not being able to go home permanently.

Monday 16th July 2007

Derek has enjoyed his breakfast this morning but did not wish to eat his bacon and egg. I assisted him with his shower, we filled in his menu for tomorrow with him declining on the bacon and egg once again.

All charts noted and recorded.

Entered by unknown.

12.40p.m *Derek was being taken for a walk up the ward when I arrived because his bottom was numb.*

He is so disappointed that he has had no physio again, he has asked me to check this out as to why.

When he came back from his walk and because he was so upset at getting no exercise I made up a program of some simple exercises i.e. stretching arms over his head and out to the sides (he does have difficulty copying my movements, I had to physically place his hands and arms where I wanted them to be but eventually he managed).

We practiced marching on the spot, lifting alternate knees up and walking briskly around the room concentrating on his posture. (He enjoyed this).

Afterwards we continued identifying and locating various items around the room and asking Derek to bring one or two simple items back to me. Derek thought this very silly but did agree that it was helping him to recognize his room and its contents more and this pleased him. He states that he feels much happier now that he can see things and know where he can find things such as his water and handkerchiefs.

1.15p.m *Derek asked to use the toilet and passed urine and had bowel opening.*

2.15p.m *Derek has worked hard and after playing bouncing with the large ball (no patient in next room to disturb) he is now so much improved in the control of this he has really amazed me, he is having a rest on his bed.*

3.30p.m *I read to Derek for half an hour and then he fell asleep and slept until Sarah came in just before dinner.*

5.15p.m *Sarah fed Derek his dinner with Derek attempting most of it himself.*

Entered by Andrea Craig.

6.20p.m *I took over from Derek's wife and Derek was sitting peacefully listening to his radio, he said that he would really like to be watching t.v. but couldn't as his was broken. I suggested that we could go to the day room to watch it there and Derek readily agreed.*

We watched t.v. until 8.30p.m watching various programs. Derek thought this was great as he had not been able to watch for a while.

Derek drank half a cup of water as he watched t.v.

8.30p.m *Derek said he would like to go back to his room. Derek got into bed and requested his radio be turned on and continued listening to it.*

Entered by Amy Staswik (student nurse)

9.00p.m *As I arrived Derek was settled in bed, I introduced myself to him (he did not recognize me although I had nursed him on two previous occasions but it was at a time when it would have been impossible for him to remember).*

I told Derek that I would be sitting with him tonight and he gave me a great big grin and said, "Hello love".

Derek has been mostly settled throughout the night, waking up a couple of times to go to the toilet.

Derek has not expressed any anxieties or concerns during the night.

It really is a pleasure to sit with Derek, as he is such a lovely, mild-mannered gentleman. I hope he continues to make wonderful improvement.

Entered by Mel Deakin (H.C.A.)

Tuesday 17th July 2007

7.30a.m *Derek was awake when I arrived. We had a chat about how he was feeling and he told me he was o.k.*

He went to the toilet and passed urine, he then showered and washed his hair with assistance. We watched breakfast t.v. afterwards Derek ate his breakfast of two Weetabix and two rounds of toast with jam.

Derek did some colour recognition exercises and built towers using the blocks.

We went for a walk (Derek said his bottom got very sore with all the sitting). He enjoyed having a good look around.

I rang the t.v. people to remind them about Derek's t.v. not working. Earlier he listened to his radio.

11.35 a.m   *Derek is sitting in the day room watching t.v.*

Entered by Liz Van'Derlean.

12.40 p.m   *I found Derek sitting in the day room with his nurse watching t.v. he had eaten lunch, his spirits were high and he told me how pleased he was to have been taken for a walk in the fresh-air earlier in the morning. We walked back to his room and Derek said he felt he would like a little rest.*

Once lying down Derek told me how disappointed he felt because no physiotherapists had been to see him. (Last visit was July 12th).

Claire (staff nurse) rang the physio's and they arrived mid-afternoon. I was invited to join them in the gym. We walked down one flight of stairs then took the remaining floors by lift to the ground floor.

Derek's focus was not as good as it had been yesterday when we played with the ball in his room, nevertheless there was some progress after a short period of time.

Derek walked back up the stairs surprising us as he took them all exceptionally well with no problems whatsoever. Derek really does come alive after his physio sessions, they lift his spirits and give him that encouragement he desperately needs.

After he was rested we had a game of Connect 4 and I saw the difference in his ability to pick up counters and place them correctly, he even enjoyed the game (which he usually loathes).

I have been advised to encourage Derek to use his left hand more so as to stimulate the damaged nerve.

Derek has visited the toilet several times, (passed urine and opened bowels).

Derek is still extremely frustrated and agitated at not being able to clean himself independently as yet, I have tried to tell him he is improving each day.

4.45 p.m Sarah arrived and manicured his nails and encouraged him with his dinner, she is very good with him and he looks forward to hearing her footsteps as she draws closer to his room. It amazes me that he can always tell it is her and I notice how his face lights up.

Entered by Andrea Craig.

18.00p.m I took Derek down to the day room where he watched what was going on in the rest of the country on the television.

19.15p.m Derek wanted to go back to his room

He is having a lay on his bed and is listening to his radio. Later told me he was feeling rather exhausted so I put him into bed and asked him if he would like any painkillers, he refused them.

Entered by Victoria Roberts (H.C.A.)

21.00hrs. *Derek is resting in his bed listening to his radio and dozing.*

I accompanied him to the toilet (passed urine) and helped him back into bed.

Entered by Joan Lomax (H.C.A.)

22.00hrs. *Derek had been asleep for an hour, he awoke at 23.00hrs. I made Derek a drink and he took his medication.*

I made Derek comfortable and he went straight back to sleep.

Entered by Beryl Cornmell (H.C.A.)

1.00a.m *Derek was in the toilet when I came on duty to relieve Beryl and was in need of a change of underwear due to a small accident. (I suspect that Derek is perhaps simply missing the bowl whilst on the toilet).*

However Derek settled down immediately afterward the incident.

s5.00a.m *Derek is sleeping but restless. He has visited the toilet once (P.U.)*

Entered by Karen Kershaw (H.C.A.)

Wednesday 18ᵗʰ July 2007

I took over at 7.30a.m Derek needed to pass urine once but went straight back to bed, he stated that he had spent a pleasant night but has no desire to get up just yet, he is now asleep.

Derek has been showered and eaten a good breakfast. (He is still having problems in the shower and needs prompting with all actions, he is never quite sure of where to place his legs and tried this morning to climb onto the shower stool, he seemed quite confused throughout).

Derek is very quiet this morning and says that he would rather sit quietly and not speak or do anything. He is sitting looking out of his window.

Derek's t.v. has finally been repaired, he has a card that will run out at 22.00hrs.

Derek has enjoyed his lunch and only required assistance with cutting up his chicken.

He has remained very quiet throughout the entire morning and has done no exercises at all.

Entered by Mike Woodworth (H.C.A.)

12.45p.m *Derek was watching his t.v when I arrived. I explained that Derek must not be allowed to sit in front of a television all day either in the day room or his own room. (Small amounts of viewing are one thing but too much could be detrimental to him) Derek should have quiet and gentle exercise during the day and if he wishes to watch t.v then he should be encouraged whilst he is sitting to pat his left hand and arm as often as he can to improve the nerve damage, he could also use the soft balls by squeezing them one in each hand. It is important that Derek be encouraged to use his left hand and arm as often as possible.*

Derek can be encouraged to undo bottle tops or pick up small objects such as dominoes or the coloured counters with his left hand, any small objects will suffice.

Bouncing the ball (large or small) to each other or better still by himself, he rather likes to do this. Depending on his focus and attention awareness Derek can be encouraged to throw the ball backwards and forwards but please be careful not to confuse him.

Please forgive what might appear to be my over fussiness and thank-you for noting the above.

1.00p.m Derek used the toilet to open his bowels and pee. (Please make sure that Derek sits well back on toilet seat to prevent wet accidents).

We practiced bouncing the large ball and then throwing it across the room with me taking up different positions in the room to improve Derek's focus and co-ordination.

We then went for a walk down to the ground floor, (via the lifts), out of the main entrance, around to the side entrance and then sat in the sunshine for a pleasant half hour.

Derek was happy to be in the fresh-air but was more than content to come back to his room and have a game of the dreaded Connect 4. He is now learning the concept of the game and is much improved in playing it, he managed to pick up two counters and play them before he had had enough, then he helped me to place all the pieces back into the box.

We played Dominoes, not the game but rather picking up the pieces from their flat side and placing them onto their sides. Derek thought I was daft and wanted to know why I wanted him to do this. I explained that I knew I was daft but I believed it was a little exercise that might help him to use his left hand and arm more and also might help to develop his concentration. He claimed it was far too simple and childlike and became very agitated when he discovered that he could not do this task. Eventually we had success. (He was quite pleased but grudgingly so).

4.00p.m Derek now extremely tired so I read to him while he lay on his bed and rested.

4.30p.m Sarah and Max arrived.
Entered by Andrea Craig.

4.45p.m Derek seems very relaxed and happy today, he also seems to be conversing with us better than ever, this is very good news.

Sarah has worked with him reading the names on the large sheets and he read out two of them spontaneously on his own.

Although he is obviously very tired I am so impressed with Derek's continued improvement, both mentally and physically.

Derek has never lost his sense of humour and has really made me laugh to-day by being cheeky to his lovely wife!

It has been so good listening to him talking about getting up the steps leading to his home and he has a conviction now that he will make it---we are certainly over the foothills of the steep mountain he is climbing.

Entered by Max Payne.

6.45p.m *Derek has fed himself this evening with a little help (but only a small amount of help was needed).*

He is now lying on his bed watching the news and is remembering to pat his hand as instructed. He has worked so hard today and claims to have had a very good day, one of the best so far. Here's hoping for a good night's rest my darling, sweet dreams.

Entered by Andrea Craig.

7.00p.m *Derek has spent a very good evening and has been supervised at all times.*

Entered by Mandy (H.C.A.)

21.00hrs. *Derek enjoyed the chatting between myself and my colleagues and joined in with no problems, he was lying on top of his bed at the time.*

He later asked to use the toilet (passed urine) and then got into bed to settle down. He got up

several times in the night to go to the toilet (each time to pass urine), otherwise had a restful night.
   Entered by Joan Lomax (H.C.A.)

Thursday 19th July 2007

7.30a.m *Derek is very happy this morning, we have made plans for the rest of the morning after breakfast. We are going to enjoy a walk outside with a short film to follow, then some exercise to finish.*
   He has eaten all of his breakfast and enjoyed it. (He has passed urine this morning but had no bowel movement).
   Derek did not watch the film as planned as we spent more time off the ward than we thought we would, we used free time exercising his left arm.
   Entered by Jackie Newcombe (H.C.A.)

12 noon. *Derek was just finishing his lunch when I first arrived. I am told he ate most of it unaided. He was in a lovely mood and told me all about his morning and that he had been taken to see a tree which had been planted by Jackie's relative.*
   Derek seemed fit, active and ready for anything so I walked with him down to the ground floor using the lifts. We walked down the corridor to the side entrance and enjoyed half an hour sitting on the bench outside in the glorious sunshine.
   Derek talked about how happy he feels today and how hopeful he feels with regards to the

future. He is especially pleased that he is having his angiogram to-morrow and that this is going to sort him out one way or the other.

(I tried to explain to him that it would hopefully tell us what had caused his heart attack and what condition his arteries were in, not that it was a cure for anything, I believe Derek understood my explanation but still said he was thankful that it was at last being carried out).

He went on to say how much he hoped that if anything needed doing to sort him out that they would do it there and then whilst he was in theatre. I told him this would be extremely unlikely.

As we continued to enjoy the sunshine Derek stated how much he was looking forward to moving over to Dr. Pinder's clinic at 'neuro rehab'. He is quite convinced a short spell there is going to return his brain back to normal, or as near to normal as is possible laughed Derek.

As we sat talking Derek's reasoning and conversation astounded me. He seems to have found a new surge forward within himself.

Walking back around the perimeter of the hospital we entered through the front entrance, up in the lifts and had just arrived back to his room when the physio's arrived and whisked him away to practice purchasing an item in the shop downstairs.

2.00p.m *Derek returned from his physio having purchased a 'Mars Bar', a treat for us to share* *with a cup of tea he said. (Apparently Derek was able to choose the item but was totally confused with the money).*

I trimmed Derek's hair after enjoying a drink and our "Mars Bar". I was allowed to brush and mop out the room because I had cut his hair. A wipe down completed my enjoyable task.

I suggested that Derek have a rest while I wrote out the alphabet letters but yet again he surprised me by stating that he would rather exercise a little if I did not mind. I was thrilled as this was the first time that I had witnessed Derek take the initiative and direct himself.

He marched on the spot for a little while then proceeded to walk around the room picking up various items and telling me what each one was (each one correct).

Derek then began to demonstrate what he believed were some 'Tai-Chi' movements (not even close but nevertheless very impressive). Derek seems so happy and pleased with himself to-day.

3.30p.m We have practiced the alphabet (Derek was actually able to recognize some of them). He is now sleeping deeply, flat out on his bed, a wave of tiredness suddenly hit him, this surprised him but I was beginning to wonder how he had kept going for so long. He has worked so hard today and been very upbeat the whole time. As he was dropping off he murmured how much he wished I could go down to theatre with him tomorrow.

5.00p.m *Derek is still sleeping soundly but will have to awaken him for dinner.*

Derek requested the toilet before he ate his dinner (passed urine but has not had a bowel movement to-day).

6.15p.m *Derek has eaten all of his dinner with very little assistance. There is a tremendous improvement here.*

Entered by Andrea Craig.

21.00p.m *Derek was in a very good mood when I came on duty and remembered me from yesterday and also that I had a daughter and a small dog.*

We chatted for a while and then watched a bit of t.v. (we talked about the things we were watching)

22.30p.m *Derek had a drink and used the toilet (passed urine) and settled into bed with help.*

Derek has had a good night's sleep getting up three times to pass urine. He has eaten an early breakfast of toast and juice. I got a great big smile from him when he first woke up and he seems to be in a very happy mood. He remembered that he was going down to theatre for his angiogram this morning. Hope all is well for him.

Entered by Christine Mephan (H.C.A.)

Friday 20th July 2007

8.40a.m *I came on duty at 7.30a.m and introduced myself to Derek, found him very quiet for a while. As Derek has an angiogram today his groin area needed to be shaved after his shower, this has been carried out.*

While Derek was having his groin shaved he joked about "Sweeney Todd" the barber except that he thought I was much better.

Derek seems confused when showering, he finds it difficult to turn on the tap, has difficulty washing, nor can he dry or dress himself. He needed help in all aspects.

Afterwards he was asked to remain lying on his bed so he watched television.

Entered by Jennifer Abbey (Flexi-bank).

10.15a.m *Another good session.*

Derek was able to tell me today that he lives in Heswall for the first time and also that Arrowe Park hospital now has a new name!!

Derek continues to be more aware and if he gives an incorrect answer he tries very hard to self-correct, which reinforces the need to give him plenty of time to answer questions.

We carried out a quiz using objects in his room, Derek had to say what they were called and then tell me what each one was used for, he did very well.

Entered by Rebecca Smith (Speech and Language Therapist)

11.00a.m *After Derek's speech session we went for a walk downstairs and stood outside to take in some fresh-air after which we sat for ten minutes in ground floor café (the one serving clinic's) talking about Derek's like of tennis, walking, holidays and where we both lived. Derek was very bright but said he thought we should get back to his room because of his angiogram appointment.*
Entered by Jennifer Abbey (H.C.A.)

11.15a.m *Derek is now feeling a little pensive so I suggested we sit quietly and I would read to him. Derek went down to theatre at 3.15p.m I was allowed to accompany him with the ward staff nurse. I signed his consent form and waited with staff until the test was completed, Dr. Newall took us both and Derek into a room and explained the findings of the test.*

We were informed that the test resulted in good and bad news. The good news showed Derek's arteries to be in much better condition than expected, comparable in fact to many twenty five year old males. The bad news proved that he had what was medically known as 'two vessel disease'.

'Cardiologist' not quite sure of the way forward at present time due to Derek's circumstances

being unprecedented but he has stated that Derek is responding well to his present medication.

On returning to his room Derek stated that he felt pleased with the results. He is feeling pleasantly relaxed but very hungry.

5.15p.m *Derek was helped with his dinner by Sarah.*

CAN ALL STAFF NOTE THAT DEREK IS NOT TO HAVE A SHOWER OR BATH FOR TWO DAYS PROCEEDING HIS ANGIOGRAM HE MUST HAVE A WASH ONLY. THANK-YOU.

Entered by Andrea Craig.

Saturday 21ˢᵗ July 2007

1.00p.m *I arrived to find Derek sat in the day room watching t.v. having had an accident in the chair (passed urine and had not known he had done so) I was a little surprised that his sitter had not picked this up as I noticed it as soon as I walked in. I have never known this to have happened before and feel a little worried.*

1.35p.m *I walked Derek back to his room, cleaned him and changed his clothes then spent time doing exercises, we worked with the wooden jig-saw pieces (which Derek loathes still), practiced the alphabet and finally ended with a game of Connect 4 which Derek stated he felt like flinging.*

Derek was not good today, he seems very tired and emotional, his focus is poor but he certainly tried hard.

3.15p.m *We walked for fifteen minutes and then he lay down on his bed for a rest.*

6.30p.m *Derek stated that he has felt strangely woozy today. He ate all of his evening meal, he fed himself very well.*

Derek has been very concerned as to how he could have had the little accident earlier on in the day-room and not known of it. He now seems a lot more settled

Entered by Andrea Craig.

Sunday 22nd July 2007

12 noon *Derek was having a lie down when I arrived. He had been for a walk and carried out his ball exercises.*

Sadly he is very down again and wishes to come home and was asking what is holding everything up.

Derek ate his lunch with very little help today.

2.00p.m *Derek went to the toilet and had his bowels opened.*

2.30p.m *George arrived and took Derek downstairs in the lifts and brought him back to his*

room by walking up one flight of stairs and then taking the lift for the next two floors.

Derek stated that the rash and itching in his groin was worsening and would I take a look at it. George said on seeing it, that it looked very similar to the one he had which had been caused by the particular "Statins" he had had prescribed for himself. His doctor changed his medication and the rash cleared up immediately. I have asked Mike, Ward Manager, to take a look at it.

4.15p.m Derek is having a lie down before dinner, he looks drained and very tired.

6.00p.m Derek fed himself this evening with just a little help from myself. He is able to use the knife in his left hand more now.

He stated that he was cold and tired and asked to go to bed. I washed and changed him, he cleaned his own teeth with a little guidance, went to the toilet, passed urine, and was then eager to get into bed. Derek still very disorientated when getting into bed but is now managing better than he did. He cannot position himself correctly and gets into a muddle with the covers.

I am leaving him watching the news on t.v. after handing him his box of tissues because of a very runny nose, he believes he has the start of a cold coming on but this has occurred before without a cold developing and I am beginning to wonder what is the real reason for it.

CAN STAFF PLEASE NOTE THAT DEREK CAN RESUME HIS SHOWERS TOMORROW MORNING, THANK-YOU.

Entered by Andrea Craig.

Monday 23rd July 2007

7.30a.m *On taking over duty I was told that Derek had slept well and peacefully.*

I helped to shower and dress him before breakfast.

Derek told me about having his angiogram and how he believes that stress had a great deal to do with him having had his heart attack.

All medication has been taken and his "Forticreme" eaten, we then went for a twenty minute walk around the hospital grounds. We did some exercises on coming back, played dominoes, connect 4 and draughts.

Derek requested lunchtime news be switched on at 12.00

Entered by M.Woodworth (H.C.A.)

12.30p.m *Derek ate his lunch unaided but needed just a little help with his knife in his left hand. He seems very alert which is pleasing but sounds very chesty and his nose is running more so than yesterday.*

2.30p.m *Sarah and Max came in with a cake to celebrate Sarah's birthday which is today. We* *spent a pleasant one and a half hours then Derek and I walked them both back down to their car. We took the lift down to the first floor and then walked down one flight of stairs. Derek is now managing the stairs very well and is so pleased at every opportunity to climb them.*

Derek said he was desperate for fresh-air all of the time, says he lies in his room longing for it. He enjoyed walking around the car park and on the way back from saying our farewells to Sarah and Max we had a little excitement in my showing Derek the new car I had bought. He touched it and said he liked the colour very much and made me promise to always drive carefully.

We walked up one flight of stairs before taking the lift once again Derek proved he could manage them with no trouble, except that he needs to concentrate very hard on what he is doing.

Derek still very lively at 5.00p.m he has been the most aware and alert to-date.

5.10p.m *Derek asked for the toilet before dinner (passed urine and small bowel opening).*

I read to him until the arrival of dinner which he ate all of and fed himself unassisted. Afterwards Derek said he felt very tired, I washed and changed him and put him to bed, he said he would clean his teeth later after his medications

Entered by Andrea Craig.

6.30p.m *I took over from Derek's wife, he was lying in bed watching his television and after five minutes or so he asked if I would please change the channel for him.*

He had a good drink of water at 6.30p.m and then another drink of juice at 8.30p.m.

He asked to use the toilet, I took him and waited (passed urine) after returning to bed he said he would rather listen to the radio but after ten minutes I switched it off as Derek is fast asleep.

Entered by Barbara Tollerton (H.C.A.)

Tuesday 24th July 2007

We had a slight accident on our way to the shower room this morning, I feel maybe that Derek is unaware of his need to pass urine until it is right on top of him, it would have been fine only for both toilets being occupied and Derek was unable to hold it.

10.30 *Peg nurse came up and informed Derek that they would be removing his peg tube next week and explained to him how they would carry out the procedure.*

Afterwards Derek had twenty minutes exercise squeezing the soft balls and bouncing the large ball on the floor, he learned that when he loses control of the bouncing he can catch the ball and hold onto it.

I assisted Derek with eating his lunch, observing Derek eating I feel he would greatly benefit from the use of a plate guard and suggest that one be provided with his meals. Derek has stressed his concern at the lack of Physiotherapy, feels he has been forgotten and let down.

Entered by M. Woodworth (H.C.A.)

12.45p.m I could not help but notice how alert Derek was today when I took over. I have queried Derek's rash once again but as yet still no answers.

Sarah arrived at 1.30p.m and played a game of connect 4 with him and placing the wooden pieces on the board. Derek was using his left hand which was pleasing. We tested him with the alphabet letters. He proved very good at calling out the whole alphabet and quite good at recognizing those we held up to him.

The physio's arrived to say that they would take Derek tomorrow if we could walk him outside today.

Sarah and I took him into the park. We walked him down one flight of stairs then took the lift to the ground floor, out of the side entrance and took our time slowly walking into the park where we played ball like three children and enjoyed it thoroughly. Derek amazed us with his ability to keep up with both the throwing and catching of the ball and trying to run for it when he missed it. We then found a spot where Derek found he *could bounce the ball on his own and kept it going for some considerable time (compared to what he could do in his room that is).*

Derek is over the moon with what he has done this afternoon, says he has had so much fun and feels better for it.

We walked back to sit down on the wooden bench outside the hospital side entrance where Derek said he loved the feel of the sun on his face, it felt so good and he did not want the moment to end.

Walking up one flight of stairs we then took the lifts back up to the third floor and back to his room. Derek claimed he was not tired, just pleasantly relaxed.

3.30p.m *Derek sat quietly whilst I read to him and then asked if he might lie down for an hour before dinner.*

5.15p.m *Derek went to the toilet (passed urine, stated that he was a little constipated).*

6.00p.m *Derek ate his sandwiches, cheese and crackers himself without any assistance, he said he had ordered these, as sandwiches were easier for him to manage.*

After washing and changing Derek into his night clothes he said he felt pleasantly tired and had spent a really lovely day and that wanted me to know how much he had enjoyed all the activity and how important that was to him.

I leave him very happy this evening.
Entered by Andrea Craig.

Wednesday 25th July 2007

Derek slept until 9.00a.m, he ate all of his breakfast and appears happy. I showered him and noticed a bruise on his inner thigh I thought I should report this to staff.

Derek and I did some ball exercises as he was unable to leave his room incase the physio's came for him.

I have no idea what kind of night Derek has spent, however this morning he does seem very tired and slow.

Entered by M. Woodworth (H.C.A.)

12.30p.m *Derek was just finishing his lunch when I arrived. He seems very cheerful but tired.*

It is difficult knowing if Derek is really asleep or if he is pretending to be, (just a feeling I have that he does not want to communicate at the moment).

His bruise has been checked out and is not considered important, certainly not related to the plug that was inserted in his groin after his angiogram.

Mid afternoon Derek was taken to the gym off ward 36, I accompanied him and was pleased to see how much improved he is with the steps and the different colours.

Dr. Pinder paid a visit to make a further assessment and gave what I considered to be a very brutal delivery when he announced that it was now certain that Derek would never make a complete recovery. This news has left Derek reeling and quite devastated. I have spent some time trying to encourage and uplift him and have suggested we go for a breath of fresh-air.

4.30p.m *I walked with Derek down to the ground floor, taking the lift to first floor and the stairs for the final flight. We walked out of the main entrance, around to the side door and back along the corridor to the lift which we took to the second floor and walked up the stairs to the third floor and back to his room.*

Dr. Pinder still recommends that the door to Derek's room be kept closed to outside distraction, also that we continue walking outside and listening to the news and topical programs for the much needed information that Derek requires.

6.00p.m *In spite of the upsetting news that Derek received this afternoon he claims he is now feeling a little better.*

Derek ate well and said that he felt much more comfortable since he has had his bowels opened.

I am leaving Derek washed and ready for bed and more settled than he has been all day.
Entered by Andrea Craig.

21.00p.m *Derek was in bed listening to his radio via his ear-phones when I arrived on duty.*

21.30p.m *Derek asked to go to the toilet, the one adjacent to his room has an "out of order" sign on the door. Derek told me it was "Kaput" and that there was another one just around the corner. We managed to locate it and Derek peed.*
I walked him back to his room and asked what he would like to do next, he said he would like to get back into bed and listen to his radio as it might help him get to sleep. I offered him a drink which he declined.

21.50p.m *I closed the curtains and put Derek's eye mask on for him to keep out the light which he finds disturbing.*

23.20p.m *Derek woke and asked to use the toilet, he pee'd and went back to bed.*

1.20a.m *Derek went to toilet again (p.u.) then straight back to bed.*

5.00a.m *Derek has been waking throughout the night but asleep at the moment.*

6.05a.m Derek woke and asked to use the toilet yet again (p.u.) I tucked him back into bed. What a cold and miserable morning it appears to be from here in Derek's room. (This is an extremely cold room).

It is raining outside and the trees are blowing strongly in the wind.

So far I have not had much conversation with Derek other than the few words we shared on our trips to the toilet.

Derek has only had sips of water during the night, he declined all offers of refreshment.

7.10a.m Derek has taken to full glasses of blood orange juice which he really enjoyed.

7.25a.m Derek has had a good practice with the soft balls using his left hand.

Derek spoke of his and Andrea's holidays in Italy which he loves but says next time he would like to go to France.

Have a great day, Derek.

Entered by Barbara Obenholzer (H.C.A.)

26th July 2007

Derek was lying in bed when I took over. A new T.V. card is needed as it ran out at 8.15 this morning leaving Derek very annoyed and disappointed.

He took all of his medication with no problems, ate all of his breakfast and drank a glass of orange juice.

I helped to shower Derek and have applied prescribed cream to his rash.

He has carried out lots of exercises this morning, walking outside, stairs, ball bouncing and hand exercises with small balls. We also included some throwing to each other with the large ball.

Entered by M. Woodworth (H.C.A.)

12.45p.m *Derek was feeding himself lunch when I arrived today and was really struggling so I gave him some prompting bringing in the use of his left hand with the knife. (His brain has difficulty recognizing that he has a left hand).*

Derek seems very bright and happy and states that he enjoys Michael's company as he does a lot of activity that Derek feels he needs. (Thank-you Mike).

1.15p.m *Derek visited the toilet (passed urine and opened bowels).*

He claimed he felt much better and believes that all the fresh fruit that he is now eating is doing the trick nicely.

1.45p.m *Sarah arrived and peeled Derek an orange which he ate followed by a dish of strawberries and yogurt, which he thoroughly enjoyed.*

Sarah worked with him using the alphabet cards and the quiz sheets.

4.00p.m *We all took a walk down to the shop on the ground floor where Derek enjoyed a good look around (although he soon seems to get disorientated with the business in there).*

On returning to his room Derek had a lie down and fell asleep until dinner was served. He ate well with a little assistance.

Entered by Andrea Craig.

6.30p.m *Derek fast asleep when I came on and had not awakened by the time I was relieved at 9.00p.m.*

Entered by Linda (H.C.A.)

21.00p.m *Derek was asleep with his radio head-phones on when I came on duty this evening. He was not in bed but lying on the top with his dressing gown on. I will help into bed and settle him after his medication, I am loathe to disturb him at the moment as he looks so peaceful.*

22.15p.m *Derek has just been to p.u. he claims he was not asleep but just resting his eyes. I helped him into bed and put his eye mask on so the light does not disturb him.*

Each time I come in to sit with Derek I see such a huge improvement, he is doing so well, especially when I think back to when I first met him when he was first in bay one a few months ago (I can't remember the exact date). He should be so very proud of himself.

Derek has been up a few times during the night to visit the toilet (P.U.) each time, otherwise he has had a good night.

Entered by Angie McCormick (H.C.A.)

27th July 2007

Derek was awake but in bed when I came on, he got up for breakfast which he ate well with no assistance whatsoever. I helped him shower and applied cream to his rash.

I took Derek for a little exercise, we walked down the stairs and around the park. This was quite a long walk which took approx. thirty minutes. Derek did well and thoroughly enjoyed it.

Entered by M. Woodworth (H.C.A.)

11.10a.m *Speech and Language Therapy.*
Derek is continuing to improve.

He remembered my name and my job straight off without any prompts.

We did a word finding test, we read and discussed newspaper article about alternative therapies, Derek was teaching me how to pronounce some of the homeopathic remedies.

Entered by Rebecca Smith (Speech and Language Therapist).

11.30a.m *Derek's sister came and took Derek for a little walk, I also finally managed to obtain a plate guard for Derek. Please place on plate for every meal with the guard positioned on the plate closest to him. Please remove and wash after every use BUT DO NOT REMOVE FROM ROOM, THANK-YOU.*

Derek ate well and with the guard he needed no assistance at all.

Derek has had a very busy morning and has worked hard. I noticed Derek's

T-shirt was covered in cut hair which I have tried to remove.

Entered by M. Woodworth (H.C.A.)

12.45p.m *Derek was very happy and upbeat when I took over. He was able to remember a lot of things which had occurred during the morning but not all.*

He enjoyed a freshly juiced glass of pineapple and ate a fresh orange.

Derek then found his toothbrush in his soap-bag himself but needed a little help with locating his toothpaste. He struggled with putting toothpaste onto the brush but managed to clean his teeth unaided. He finally rinsed with mouthwash and started laughing whilst doing so. When asked why he was laughing he came back with the time when he had swallowed the mouthwash instead of spitting it out and how horrid it had tasted.

I told him that if was not careful he would be swallowing it again or choking on it if he carried on talking before he spat it out.

Derek then asked me if I would mind him having a rest as he felt a little tired. It was now my turn to laugh as reading and hearing of all that he had carried out this morning I felt he should feel exhausted more than just a little tired.

1.45p.m *Derek now fast asleep having laid on his bed for twenty minutes before exercising his hands with the soft balls.*

3.15p.m *Derek awoke and asked for the toilet (P.U. and opened bowels).*

We practiced Derek following my movements for a few minutes and went on to him locating various objects in the room, he did exceptionally well in spite of still being very tired. I suggested he had another lie down.

4.00p.m *Derek has been lying on his bed for half an hour in a deeply thoughtful mood. He began to ask questions about home and talk about how much he is missing it and the life he had lived before his collapse.*

I have once again tried to explain that we must be patient and work through this chapter in our life as philosophically as we can. The tears fell as he explained that he felt deeply emotional rather than low or depressed and that there was a huge difference between these feelings.

4.50p.m Derek said he needed to get up, we played draughts until 5,30p.m.
Derek played very well (best to-date).

5.45p.m Derek drank his soup and ate his sandwiches and fruit unaided with no problems. After dinner he washed and cleaned his teeth with the minimum of instruction.
(I was disappointed today as Derek's aftershave has disappeared from his soap-bag).
Entered by Andrea Craig.

18.30p.m I was asked to move from ward 38 to sit with Derek. I have sat with Derek on two previous occasions, once when he was first admitted to bay one and secondly in room 23 where he is still.
The improvement in Derek is massive and it is really so good to see him progressing so quickly.
On this occasion he has been singing along to a tune on the radio. He looks so rested whilst all cuddled up in his fluffy dressing gown, bought for him by his daughter. What a tremendous improvement.

19.40p.m Derek asked to go to the toilet (P.U.) He went again at 20.35p.m and I prompted him to *wash his hands on both occasions which he was able to do himself.*

Returning to lie on his bed he asked for the soft balls and exercised his hands for approx. fifteen minutes whilst listening to his radio. I asked him if he would like to get into bed but he replied that he would in half an hour or so when the night staff came on.

Entered by Angie Benton.

21.00hrs. *Derek was lying on his bed listening to his radio when I came on this evening, he looked very relaxed.*

22.00hrs. *He asked to use the toilet (P.U.) then took his dressing gown off and got into bed. I assisted with his eye mask and he settled very quickly.*

Derek got up several times in the night to use the toilet but generally he had a good night.

Entered by Joan Lomax (H.C.A.)

28ᵗʰ July 2007

7.30a.m *I came on duty to find Derek sleeping.*

Derek ate his breakfast and then had a shower, afterwards he asked to use the toilet (P.U.) he was encouraged to wash his hands which he was able to do. Derek is in a very pleasant mood, we enjoyed a good talk.

Derek was able to clean his teeth, he recalled his swallowing the mouthwash and remembered that he had to spit it out.

We went for a walk around the hospital, both "Annabell's" and "Bowman's" cafes were closed so we called in at the shop where Derek chose a drink for himself. Derek climbed all of the stairs back up to his room on the third floor. He asked to use the toilet (P.U. and opened bowels).

Derek has been using the small and large balls doing exercises which he says he has to do and that they are helping him.

Derek has eaten and enjoyed his lunch.

Entered by Maureen Clark. (H.C.A.)

12,30p.m *Derek was cheerful, rested and said that he felt good today. George had come along with me this afternoon and we took Derek out for the afternoon back to George's bungalow. After we had enjoyed afternoon tea Derek had a lie down and fell into a relaxed sleep for an hour. He woke up and knew immediately where he was and said that he felt so happy. We had no problem returning to the hospital and he stated that he felt the visit had done him so much good.*

4.15p.m *Derek asked for the toilet on arriving back to his room (P.U. and opened bowels). Also visited the toilet whilst out to pass urine.*

Derek is now relaxing whilst waiting for dinner.

5.30p.m *Derek fed himself soup followed by sandwiches and gateaux, he managed very well with only a little help with the soup.*

CAN I ASK THAT WHOEVER TAKES DEREK FOR HIS SHOWER THAT THEY CHECK HE HAS PUT ALL TOPS BACK ON SHAMPOO AND SHOWER GEL ETC. AS THERE WAS A MIS-HAP THIS MORNING WHICH MADE FOR A VERY MESSY SOAP-BAG. THANK-YOU.

Entered by Andrea Craig.

6.30p.m *Derek was asleep when I took over from his wife, he woke up at 6.50p.m and asked if he could walk to the toilet as he needed to pass water. I escorted him to the toilet and he went immediately back to bed on returning to the room, he is now in bed listening to his radio via the head-phones.*

7.15p.m *Derek asked if he could go to the toilet again (P.U.) He is once again listening to the radio and exercising his hands with the little soft balls.*

He is singing along with the radio and seems to be in very good spirits.

NOTICE TO NIGHT-STAFF: please could you assist Derek with putting on his eye mask, as he needs complete darkness to enable him to sleep, thank-you.

Derek has been in a very good mood this evening. He has been singing "Somewhere Over the Rainbow" he is very relaxed and happy at the end of my shift. Good luck Derek !

Entered by Jan (H.C.A.)

21.00hrs. Jan had taken Derek to the toilet when I came on duty, I brought him back to his room and assisted him into bed and placed his headphones on as he wished to listen to his radio.

Derek soon fell asleep but woke up at 22.40p.m to go to the toilet (P.U.) I gave him his medication and he soon went off again.

Derek woke several times in the night to visit the toilet and also kept losing his eye mask whilst asleep.

7.30a.m Derek woke and asked for the toilet, he is now back in bed wide awake listening to his radio.

Entered by Angie (H.C.A.)

29ᵗʰ July 2007

7.30a.m Derek was listening to music on his radio when I arrived. Derek has eaten all of his breakfast and after visiting the toilet he washed his hands and dried them without any prompting or encouragement.

A little later I helped Derek take a shower, he made a good attempt at drying himself, but *found it very difficult in dressing. He did manage very well at cleaning his teeth and gargling with mouthwash.*

PLEASE NOTE DEREK NEEDS MORE TOOTHPASTE.

Derek is in a pleasant mood.

We went over the first four letters of the alphabet and Derek seems very familiar with the letter A.

Derek has been exercising using the small and large balls.

He has successfully recognized all of the flash cards that I showed him and enjoyed a walk around the hospital.

Derek has just finished and enjoyed his lunch.

Entered by Maureen Clark (H.C.A.)

12.45p.m *Derek was in such a lovely happy mood when I arrived and I told him he was in for a wonderful surprise this afternoon. I did tell him that Sarah and Max were coming in and that we were going to take him out. He said he was happy to be going to the park. I told him he must wait and see.*

2.00p.m *Sarah and Max have arrived and we are leaving the hospital for a couple of hours.*

4.15p.m. *We took Derek to visit his own home. He was that elated he practically flew up the steps* *which I had been so worried about. A handrail had been installed up the steps in anticipation of his homecoming but he claimed that it hurt his hand too much for him to hold onto it (with the nerve damaged left hand) he was alright coming back down the steps as he held on with his right hand.*

Derek walked from room to room, stopping now and again to touch something or other, I asked him if he remembered these items or were they unfamiliar to him, he replied, "How could I forget any of these things, they make up my home, this is me and where I belong and I was beginning to believe that I would never see them or my home ever again".

After Derek had completed the tour of the house he sank back into his chair, just as he had done in George's home, only this time the smile on his face said it all, this was his chair in his very own home.

Derek did mention whilst sitting enjoying a cup of tea that it suddenly felt as though he had never been away.

A few tears were shed before we came back but he says that it has been such a happy day and the most wonderful surprise he has ever had.

Derek visited the toilet on returning back to his room and said that he felt so tired he just wanted to rest. He is now fast asleep and I will wake in time for dinner.

(Derek had his bowels opened earlier this afternoon).

21.00hrs. *On arrival I found Derek to be fast asleep on his bed. After fifteen minutes he woke up and I introduced myself to him and he claimed that he remembered me from the other night which I thought was very good.*

I assisted him to the toilet (P.U.) He asked to listen to his radio whilst lying in bed.

22.15p.m *Derek settled down with his eye mask on but at 22.45p.m asked to go to the toilet (P.U.) He went two more times before finally settling into a good sleep from 12.30a.m until 5.50a.m. when Derek got up and walked to the toilet. He walked well but needed guidance.*

Entered by Angie Benton (H.C.A.)

30th July 2007

8.00a.m *Derek was awake on my arrival. He commented on how well he had slept throughout the night. He talked about how nice it looked outside and asked me what I had done over the week-end.*

He did not want a hot drink, just water with his breakfast when it comes.

Derek is still in bed just dozing on and off.

I had a nice long chat with Derek about various things.

He went to the toilet (P.U.)

He enjoyed his breakfast, saying he was hungry, finished off with toast and water.

We have had a game of dominoes and gone over colours.

10.15a.m *Derek has just had a shower and washed his hair. He helped to wash his face and interacted throughout. He managed to dry his upper body with some prompting and encouragement. We are just listening to the radio and having a little rest.*

Derek is sat in his chair in a happy mood. We have been outside for some fresh-air, we sat on a bench for about twenty minutes and chatted and watched the people going by

On coming back in Derek stated that he would like to walk back up all the flights of stairs to the third floor so we have and at 11.25a.m we are back in Derek's room where once again Derek is relaxing listening to his radio.

Derek has eaten his lunch, he did very well feeding himself, just needed a little help at times.

Entered by Stephen Gisborne (H.C.A.)

12.30p.m *Derek had eaten his lunch and appears very quiet, he says he feels very thoughtful perhaps more deeply than ever before he thought.*

I trimmed his beard before he went down for his "field test" at 1.50p.m.

Whilst Derek was gone I made up some two and three letter words to practice with him and wrote out some more date sheets.

2.30p.m *Derek was brought back up from clinic, he asked to use the toilet (P.U. and opened bowels).*

Dr. Oates cheered Derek enormously by consenting to allow him home leave at week-ends. He claims that Dr. Oates is a very positive person and manages to strengthen him a little more each visit. (Well done Dr.Oates that takes a little more than medical knowledge or medication and you are helping to heal two people here not just one).

3.15p.m *Derek asked that he might lie down and soon fell into a deep sleep.*

5.30p.m *I had to wake Derek up to eat his dinner. He ate all completely unaided, well done Derek. I helped to wash and change Derek and am leaving him lying on his bed having to clean his teeth later on when night-staff come on duty. Derek says he might have a little something to eat for supper so no point in cleaning them now.*

Entered by Andrea Craig.

Derek has had a quiet night, he has slept well getting up the toilet four times (P.U. each time and opened bowels twice).

Entered by Cathy Robinson

31ˢᵗ July 2007

7.30a.m *Derek and I have spent a most enjoyable morning together chatting about holidays, travel and hopes for the future. Derek appears to be in very good spirits and was telling me about the "love of his life" Andrea his wife.*

Derek was awake when I arrived but still in bed. He informed that he was having a lie in.

9.00a.m *Breakfast eaten well (3 weetabix and toast/marmalade) a hot drink was refused—water given instead. Derek managed very well with his breakfast and needed minimum assistance.*

11.30a.m *Derek had a shower including hair washed, again minimum assistance given, mainly prompting.*

We visited a young lady on the main ward who has spent six weeks in Clatterbridge Rehab-Derek got some really positive feedback from her and is now extremely keen to get there. I think this has lifted his spirits no end.

We are planning a walk later on. A really enjoyable morning has been spent.

12.10p.m *Derek seems a little tired now so is having a little quiet time listening to his radio, I think I have talked him all out !*

Observations stable and all recorded as per chart.

12.30p.m Derek ate all his lunch and fed himself. I have phoned PALS to see if we can request talking books for Derek as he has expressed some feelings of boredom and frustration at not being able to read or concentrate.

12.45p.m PALS are going to bring up talking books and machine to play them on.
Entered by Taara Das (H.C.A.)

12.45p.m Derek was enjoying his conversation with Taara when I arrived and said he was keen to continue with some work or perhaps go for a walk but Taara told me that she thought Derek was very tired.

1.10p.m Derek asked if we might have a walk in the sunshine whilst it looked so lovely outside. I walked him down the stairs, (all flights to the ground floor) along the corridor and out of the side entrance where we sat on a bench and enjoyed glorious sunshine for forty-five minutes.
Derek said he would like to exercise and keep moving so we walked around the perimeter of the building and back through the main entrance. We walked all of the stairs back up to the third floor (I had to stop for a rest half way up but Derek said I was not fit like him and that he could keep going further if needs be) and back to his room.

2.25p.m *Derek is now asleep on his bed looking very relaxed. I have noticed over the last few days that Derek's colour has returned to normal once more.*

While we were out walking Derek told me that he thought yesterday was his best day so far. (Dr. Oates helped to restore Derek's confidence and his will to carry on, along with her permission in allowing him home Saturdays and Sundays. He has certainly picked himself up again).

2.45p.m *Lyn. came up with a talking book for Derek which he should enjoy if it can hold his attention, sadly Derek's attention span is very short.*

3.00p.m *Derek has said he wishes to finish his sleep out and has settled down once more.*

3.10p.m *The dietician came in to check that all was well before Derek has his PEG tube removed.*

After this visit Derek decided to give up on his sleep and said we might as well do some work, so we practiced going over the alphabet and a few simple words but Derek found this extremely difficult (too tired I feel).

We did some stretching exercises and marching on the spot, Derek enjoyed these tasks much more.

5.30p.m *Derek fed himself this evening, he ate soup followed by sandwiches and cheese and crackers.*

Sarah and Max visited.

I am leaving Derek this evening very tired but happy.

Entered by Andrea Craig.

21.00hrs. *As I arrived on duty this evening Derek was lying on the bed looking very relaxed and at ease. As I came into the room Derek greeted me pleasantly with, "Hello Dear".*

I immediately, and sincerely, commented to Derek on how each time I see him he always looks a lot better than on the last occasion I spent with him.

Although we did not sit and chat, Derek did seem pleased that I had noticed his improvement and flashed me a nice big, friendly smile.

As Derek's previous sitter was leaving I asked her how he had been doing as it was about four weeks since I had last seen him. She told me that he was good but a little tired and felt he needed to settle down for the night with which Derek readily agreed. I asked if he would like a drink which he refused as he felt too tired.

I assisted Derek into bed and helped him to move up as I did not want him squashing his toes on the bottom of the bed. Derek laughed at this and despite being very tired seems very relaxed and in a happy mood.

I am very impressed with Derek considering how he had been on my previous shift with him when he had not been able to position himself in the bed and had had no co-ordination or sense of direction at all.

Once settled Derek requested his eye mask. I settled his pillows and he sank back into them comfortably. I explained that I would be with him all night and that if he should need anything he should not hesitate to ask.

21.30hrs. *Derek is sleeping lightly on his left side.*

21.55p.m *Derek woke asking to use the toilet. After making sure that he was sat correctly on the toilet I stepped outside leaving the door open just a little. He washed his hands, needing assistance, and then returned to his bed thanking me for respecting his privacy. Just a little thing which obviously meant so much to Derek, he went on to say that it is the little things which give him the determination to get things back to the way they once were and how he would never take anything for granted ever again.*

Derek asked me for the time and pointing to the clock I told him it was ten o'clock, noticing how Derek was looking straight at the clock I realized how much he was improving because previously he had not been able to focus upon it.

Once again I asked if Derek would like a drink before he went to sleep but he politely declined saying he really was too tired.

I helped Derek back into bed asking him if he had had a good day. He replied positively by saying very much so but adding that perhaps he might have overdone things today ,as he felt overwhelmingly tired.

Just as Derek had settled back down in came his medication and asking if he would like a hot drink to have with them he said no, just water.

Ten minutes later as he was settling down he chuckled saying that good old water was his favourite tipple and added what a shame that people took it so much for granted and did not appreciate it for its goodness Within minutes Derek was fast asleep.

23.25p.m Derek woke politely asking to go to the toilet (P.U.) on getting back into bed Derek apologized for being so sleepy and said he was hopeful of us having a good chat in the morning. **3.50a.m**

Derek woke from a very restful sleep, needing to go to the toilet, once again Derek's privacy was maintained, although he was observed at all times.

I left the bathroom door ajar slightly allowing me to observe for his safety at the same time as *giving him his privacy and dignity he so rightly deserves.*

During all visits to the toilet Derek has managed to pull up his shorts requiring assistance only with the straightening of them for comfort. Each time Derek walked over to the wash-hand basin and automatically washed his hands without assistance or prompting. Derek was able to recognize that the paper towels had to be taken over to the bin but was unable to place them inside. I realised how difficult this was for him as there is no foot pedal to the bin (it has broken off).

Unable to open the bin Derek placed the towels on the top of it.

Under the circumstances could this not be looked into at all? (Maybe I'm just being a wimp!!!).

6.30a.m *Derek woke to pass urine walking to and back from the bathroom with ease, I thought this was marvelous considering he had only just opened his eyes.*

He went straight back to bed and fell into a light sleep before I had even straightened his sheets for him. (I am so jealous that he is able to sleep!)

Although we did not get the chance to have a chat and "put the world to rights" I was so pleased Derek had such a peaceful and restful sleep. Not only does this reflect a relaxed and happy patient but it is the perfect time of self-healing which is helping Derek along his remarkable recovery process.

Keep going Derek, your hard work really is show

Entered by Nikki Letts (H.C.A.)

1st August 2007

7.30a.m *Derek was asleep on my arrival and continued to sleep for over an hour.*

9.00a.m *A good breakfast was eaten and water given to follow.*

Derek is in very good spirits today and is very positive about the future. I weighed Derek (75.8kg) and recorded per chart.

I assisted him with washing his hair and showering, mainly by prompting. Derek told me how much he is struggling with dressing himself.

Jill the PEG nurse came at 10.30a.m to inform us that Derek's Peg feed will be removed on Friday 3rd as it was unable to go ahead today due to Derek having eaten breakfast. Derek to have nil by mouth from midnight Thursday 2nd also

Andrea needs to consent before treatment.

10.45a.m *We are leaving the room to go for a walk around hospital grounds.*

11.30a.m *We had a wonderful walk and sat on the bench outside putting the world to rights!*

Derek had retained a lot of the information I had given him yesterday which I think is excellent. He remembered that I love my holidays and travelling around the world experiencing different cultures. Derek tells me there are places he would love to go with Andrea – so we made a mental list: it is getting longer as the day goes on.

We took the stairs for our walk, there and back – Derek's co-ordination was excellent – I was most impressed, I think I was definitely the least fit climbing the stairs out of the two of us!

12.30p.m *Derek ate most of his lunch, desert and his cheese and biscuits to follow. He drank both a full glass of orange juice and a glass of water afterwards.*

Derek enjoyed his meal apart that was for the hard roast potatoes.

Entered by Taara Das (H.C.A.)

12.45p.m *Derek looks very relaxed but is a little disappointed as he had believed his Peg tube was due to come out this morning*

1.00p.m *Derek asked to use the toilet (P.U.)*

1.30p.m *We walked downstairs (via the lifts) out through the main entrance and around to side entrance where we sat on the bench chatting for fifteen minutes before walking back around to the main entrance. We paid a visit to the shop where*

I experienced my first fright. Derek had selected a flapjack to have with a cup of tea and walked to the till with me to pay for it, he had not got sufficient money and as I went into my purse to make up the difference he disappeared.

I fled the shop apologizing for my hasty retreat to discover Derek was nowhere to be seen, I was panic stricken not knowing which way he would have taken. Rationalizing that if he had taken the indoor corridor route he would be safe, I ran in the opposite direction towards the main entrance feeling extremely anxious knowing how busy an area this was at all times. I could not believe how quickly he had managed to disappear and was afraid of how confused he would be when discovering that he was alone. The thought that he might just keep walking, perhaps right out into the road made me shudder. My mind was in a whirl with the many possibilities, when suddenly I spotted him outside of the main entrance heading back in the same direction from which we had just walked.

He seemed to be totally oblivious to what was going on around him or that he had done anything untoward and when I tried to explain that he should never have walked out of the shop without me he simply laughed saying he did not know what all the fuss was about and that he had known that I was settling up and that he was just heading back to his room, believing that was, that we had come out of the side entrance and therefore that was the way he should head back.

The confusion set in when I turned him around and took him back through the main entrance, as Derek had forgotten that we could return via either main or side entrance, on reflection I should have perhaps allowed Derek to continue walking back his own chosen way.

2.15p.m *Safely back in his room. Derek headed straight to the toilet (0pened bowels). He is feeling very tired and is now resting on his bed listening to his "talking novel".*

3.20p.m *Derek wished to get up and get on so we did some stretching exercises and moving objects around the room. It is so good to see Derek is now able to recognize most things in his room and is beginning to manage moving his table to wherever he wants it.*

Having moved the table into position he then took the game of connect 4 from the window sill and placed it on the table in front of me. I was amazed, firstly because Derek was able to carry out these actions with purpose and ease and secondly because I know how much Derek loathes this game and yet here he was, without any suggestion or prompting from myself, only too willing to play.

This is something I have never witnessed before and feel quite staggered by Derek's progress.

After our game (Derek still struggles with this and gets himself agitated and upset) we continued with placing the wooden pieces in position on the board. Derek proved a lot more aware with this than previously

We went on to work with the flash cards and words. We must keep these going as I notice a remarkable improvement.

5.15p.m Derek managed to feed himself with just a little assistance with his soup and then his fresh fruit and ice-cream.

I feel today has been a good day in spite of my fright.

Entered by Andrea Craig.

5.45p.m Derek went to spend a penny and opened his bowels again.

6.50p.m Another visit to the toilet (P.U.) he is now back on his bed listening to some music.

Derek has lay on his bed listening to his radio visiting the toilet and P.U. each time at 7.15, 7.45 and 8.45p.m. He dozed on and off throughout.

Entered by Sue Griffiths.

9.00p.m Derek was lying on top of his bed with the blanket over him when I arrived. He had his *eye mask in place and appeared settled. He was awake so introduced myself and asked if he was warm enough.*

10p.m *Derek requested the toilet (P.U.) He returned to bed and got under the covers. Derek has not slept well and was unsettled tossing and turning until 3.0a.m. He got up to visit the toilet three times in total.(P.U.)*

7.0a.m *Derek has been asleep for a short while but is now awake, he asked to visit the toilet and is back in bed resting but not asleep.*
Entered by Stephanie Gisborne (H.C.A.)

2nd.August 2007

7.30a.m *Derek was dozing when I first arrived and he awoke at 8.30a.m in a lovely mood. I have been so impressed with the amount of information that Derek has remembered from yesterday (especially as he has only just woken up).*
We had a conversation yesterday about Florence Nightingale and Derek was able to recall every aspect of the conversation perfectly this morning.
Derek has eaten a good full breakfast and opened his bowels, observations stable and recorded as per chart.

Full shower was taken with minimal assistance. Derek managed to brush his teeth and gargled without prompting.

We went for a short walk in the hospital grounds and Derek made me walk up three flights of stairs, once again he was laughing at my fitness level (or lack of it). He put me to shame!

We have returned to his room as Derek is due to be seen by Physio/OT's at 11.00a.m. Derek is now listening to his radio.

Physio's have taken Derek off the ward.

On his return Derek informed me that he had been to the shop and bought a banana and some crisps, he was able to recognize a pound coin but struggled with other smaller denominations. He seems a bit tired now but happy within himself.

12.30p.m *Derek has eaten a good lunch of chicken and mushroom pie with sauté potatoes, mixed vegetables and broccoli. Derek ate all of his sticky toffee pudding and custard. He refused a hot drink and chose grapefruit and a glass of water instead.*

Derek requested that his radio be put on and is now quietly resting listening to it.

Entered by Taara Das (H.C.A.)

I found Derek to be alert and very relaxed today. I would state the most I have seen him since his first being admitted, long may it last.

It was mutually agreed that before we do anything more, Derek should have a rest and is therefore now relaxing contentedly on his bed.

1.30p.m Sarah arrived and Derek is still resting.

2.15p.m Sarah and I took Derek out into the park and practiced bouncing and throwing the large ball for a good forty minutes, Derek was so keen and eager and one could see his competitive streak coming to the fore as he ran to catch the ball (tried to, but nevertheless, his attempts were brilliant).

I noticed Derek tire, this came on very quickly and therefore we strolled very slowly back to his room where he was eager to have a lie down stating that he could not remember when he had enjoyed himself so much. (Bless him).

4.00p.m Derek awake and wanting to get on so we went over the flash cards and played a couple of games. Derek is maintaining his alertness in all that he does, once again a tremendous improvement I feel.

5.15p.m Derek ate all of his dinner and I encouraged him this evening to start using his left hand to feed himself, (Derek is naturally left handed but has so far been unable to use this hand very well) he says that he finds this extremely difficult and that it actually hurts both his hand and his *head when he tries. I thought he managed very well and will encourage him to persevere.*

Derek did manage successfully to feed himself in spite of the difficulty he claimed to be having.

5.45p.m *I helped to washed and changed Derek ready for bed. He cleaned his teeth and gargled without any assistance.*

Entered by Andrea Craig.

6.00p.m *Derek seems to have tired himself out today but says that he has had lots of fun. He has been lying on top of his bed resting and relaxing listening to the radio at the same time singing along with it. Derek is now dozing on and off.*

Entered by Sue Griffiths.

9.00p.m – 7.45a.m *Derek has spent a restful night and slept peacefully, awakening four times to visit the toilet (P.U. on each visit).*

Entered by Laura O'Sullivan (H.C.A.)

3ʳᵈ August 2007

12.50p.m *Poor staffing levels on the ward meant that no-one has been available to sit with Derek throughout the morning. Regular checks have been made and no problems encountered. He has played with the small balls this morning before he showered with the assistance of Lisa Barnes (H.C.A.)*

Andrea Craig

Derek has had his PEG tube removed this morning and required sedation for the procedure. I am now sitting with Derek to observe him after this procedure and at the moment he is sleeping.

Entered by Paul Jones (staff nurse).

12.50p.m Derek was sleeping when I arrived but awakened at 1.10p.m, he was very dozy but said that he felt happy that the PEG tube had gone at last. The last tube to disappear, he said he felt liberated but extremely uncomfortable with the hard bed. This is the first time I have heard Derek complain about anything but he is really very cheerful.

1.40p.m Derek sat up in bed relishing his beef sandwiches, cheese and crackers, he ate with no problems.

2.15p.m Derek asked to go to the toilet (P.U. and opened bowels). The most pleasing thing to-date is that Derek stated quite out of the blue that he would like to wipe himself afterwards. He struggled but with a little prompting managed very well. This has worried me for some time as to how he would ever relearn, if ever he could, to carry out this personal function for himself. Well done, my darling, you really are getting there.

On returning to his room Derek remembered a "Mars-bar" and "flapjack" that he had in his goodie-box and ate them both with relish. He is *now once again resting on his bed but stated that he has no wish to get back into it.*

4.15p.m *I walked Derek down the ward to the lift area and back.*

We spent a quiet afternoon with Derek nodding off now and then but he is looking forward to going home tomorrow after breakfast and says he feels quite excited.

He ate sandwiches again this evening and fed himself with left hand without prompting.

Entered by Andrea Craig.

18.00hrs. *Derek is alright after having had a little walk seeing off his wife Andrea.*

Derek is going home tomorrow and is to get up early so that he is showered and ready as Andrea is calling for him approx. 9.30a.m. Andrea has left Derek's clothes all ready for him in his wardrobe together with his underwear and socks.

Derek has had his PEG tube out today so cannot bend at all, please note.

Derek is resting and relaxed.

Entered by Victoria Roberts (H.C.A.)

21.00p.m *Derek was asleep on my arrival. He awoke at 10.30p.m and asked to use the toilet (P.U.) and then fell straight back to sleep on his return.*

Derek woke a number of times throughout the night and was continually disturbed by the patient in the room next door who was very noisy shouting out loudly all night.

I feel Derek will be very tired today because of this.

Entered by Claire Kelly (H.C.A.)

Saturday 4th August 2007

Derek was awake lying on top of his bed when I arrived this morning. He remembered me from the other night and asked how I was as I hadn't felt very well when we last met.

He is very excited about Andrea picking him up at 9.30a.m to-day to take him home for the week-end. He was talking about the lovely meals she would be cooking for him and about his friend, George, coming to visit. He told all about how he and Andrea first met and of how much he was looking forward to a good night's rest in his own bed.

8.30a.m Derek has had his shower and washed his hair with some assistance. He is now sitting in his chair awaiting his breakfast. Andrea has just arrived.

Entered by Stephanie Gisborne (H.C.A.)

Although it has not been entered into the diary I must mention here, that on arriving to pick Derek up on Saturday 4th August I had to tell him that, although he was being allowed home for the

Saturday and Sunday, he would in fact have to be taken back to hospital each evening. Clearly disappointed with this news he nevertheless remained upbeat. I went on to explain the reason for picking him up so early was so that we could spend as much of the day at home as possible and that we would do the same tomorrow.

Derek was in high spirits leaving the ward. We took the lifts down to the ground floor and slowly made our way to the car-park. Once arriving at the correct aisle in which I had parked he had no trouble in pointing out our car. I was amazed that he had been able to remember it. I had changed the vehicle whilst Derek had been in hospital and he had only seen it in passing on two previous occasions as we had walked him through the car-park on our way into the park. I knew he had been very fond of the colour as he had selected it himself just prior to his collapse and thought perhaps this might have jogged his memory but I was also at the point of realizing that I had no way of knowing just what Derek could or could not remember. I had been told that his short term memory was impaired and yet here was an example when this appeared not to be the case, at other times Derek had little or no memory at all, long or short term. I often felt quite confused by it all.

If I had ever had any doubts as to how Derek would ever manage the many steps to our front door I need never have worried, he almost ran up them as soon as he got out of the car. He entered into the hallway almost in reverence unable to believe that he was at last home. We walked from room to room with him touching pieces of furniture as he passed as if checking that they were real. I asked if he would like to rest and he replied only when he had been upstairs and completed the tour.

It was a beautiful warm and sunny day so we simply sat outside and relaxed with Derek stating that all he wanted to do was simply enjoy being home. He actually got a little sun-burned. I had applied sun-cream to his face and arms but he fell asleep and spent a little too long outside. He was not at all bothered about it, in truth he was thrilled with the fact that he was going back to hospital looking a lot healthier than when he had left. I on the other hand was rather worried to what the staff might have to say about my taking their patient back suffering with sunburn.

I cannot describe how good it felt for me to have Derek home at last and to watch him sink back into all that was familiar to him and know that he was able to recognize and relate to it in terms of his home and where he truly belonged. In complete contrast to how I felt at having him home on that first occasion came the feeling I experienced in having to take him back once more to his hospital room. I can only imagine how Derek must have felt.

It was also brought home to me that Saturday just how difficult the rest of the climb back was going to be for him, for although Derek had wandered with ease around his home when going in no particular direction, it became a completely different matter when needing to find his way directly to a room such as the dining room or perhaps the toilet, he then became disorientated and confused. He needed help in sitting down on a dining room chair when it then became impossible to position him correctly to the table and I found it easier to move the table to him. At home he no longer had the use of a plate guard and found it extremely difficult keeping the food on his plate, a trivial thing but one that caused great upset to Derek. This of course could be remedied by asking the hospital if I may borrow a plate guard when Derek next came home at week-ends.

Using the toilets at home also proved difficult. Not being the same type (as in model) as the hospital toilets, Derek claimed they felt different to sit on and seemed almost afraid to use them. I found this a little strange as he had used the toilet when visiting George without any trouble whatsoever. I questioned was it perhaps over excitement at being in his own home? Was he afraid of accident? I had no idea. Very often the answers were never to be found and it simply needed time to resolve the dilemma.

The kitchen proved to be the most confusing and upsetting room of all to Derek. It is, like many other homes, the most used room in our house and the one in which Derek spent most of his time as he enjoyed cooking and pottering about in it. I saw his face light up when he first walked in but could not fail to notice how quickly that light was extinguished and replaced with a look of confused dread. Trying but failing in his attempt to open the many cupboard doors or even locate or pull open the drawers, he felt lost and bewildered. I asked him to watch as I opened and closed each one stating that tomorrow I would help him to understand what was kept in each cupboard.

"No... no...no, I don't need to know," he shouted. I knew then it was too much and he was unable to take it in. I helped to sit him down at the kitchen table while I made a cup of tea. The doors were open onto the patio and I found my mind going back to the last time Derek had sat at that table one warm sunny morning three months ago only all had been well on that occasion, or so we had believed, little had we realized that we were just a few short hours away from the disaster which had cut straight across our lives.

Everything ever since that fateful day carried mixed blessings and emotions with all that had taken place, the joy and elation felt with each new phase of progress. My heart swelled with pride as Derek mastered each relearned task and warmed, especially that Saturday morning, with thankfulness because he had survived and been allowed to return back to his home. These were the blessings experienced along with the heartache of having to watch the hard struggle and deep frustration as Derek came to terms with how little he could do for himself. In hospital he had progressed so well and climbed so high and yet here at home he seemed more vunerable than ever.

At the end of the first day at home I knew Derek had enjoyed himself beyond measure and in spite of the confusion and slight agitation he had at times been subject to I felt it had been a tremendous success and looked forward to the next day. I went to my bed that evening with the full realization that I had as much to learn as Derek and that we were truly walking a pathway in recovery together.

21.00hrs. Derek was settled in his bed when I arrived for my shift and apart from several trips to the bathroom he remained settled throughout the night. Sadly the man next door starting shouting very loudly causing Derek to wake up early but he did manage to drop back off again.

a.m. After a shower we sat and talked about politics and foreign affairs with Derek contributing greatly to the shared conversation.

Derek spoke about how much he is looking forward to going to Clatterbridge Rehab. as this will be the final step to him going home.

I was really pleased with the improvement I see in Derek since we first met, especially as he was able to remind me of conversations we had held weeks ago.

Entered by Karen Kershaw (H.C.A.)

Sunday 5th August 2007

7.30a.m *Derek is fine this morning, he is very chatty and talking to me about his son and daughter and the family holidays in Cornwall.*

Derek had been showered and dressed when I arrived and has now eaten all of his breakfast.

Entered by unknown.

Again it has not been recorded in the diary but Derek was taken home for the day. Once again I picked him up early and took him home where we enjoyed a relaxing couple of hours before going off for a walk with a packed lunch. We enjoyed picking blackberries, which we thoroughly enjoyed eating later with a little ice-cream. The weather was glorious and all seemed so hopeful and Derek so happy. I felt wonderful although we both felt rather subdued as we made our way back to the hospital. Still next week was his birthday and I knew that all being well Dr. Oates had said that Derek could spend a long week-end at home as a birthday surprise.

21.00p.m *Derek was awake but all ready for bed when I arrived. His eye mask was in place and he was lying on top of the bed.*

Derek was up to use the toilet three times in the night. He spent a very disturbed and restless night due to the patient next door shouting for most of the night.

6.30a.m *Derek is still lying here wide awake but states that he feels fine.*

Entered by Stephanie Gisborne (H.C.A.)

Monday 6th August 2007

7.30a.m *Derek is in bed dozing on and off. He got up for his breakfast. Derek looks very well with his suntan and told me how much he enjoyed his day at home yesterday and Saturday, but yesterday was the best.*

Derek showered with minimal assistance. I applied cream to his rash area.

Gill took Derek for a walk around hospital grounds.

He is now happily relaxed dozing in his chair listening to his radio.

Entered by unknown.

12.45p.m *Derek was practicing bouncing the large ball when I came in and he was doing very well continuously bouncing it with one hand.*

Derek has been familiarizing himself with the newspaper and picking out various letters which he can recognize. Derek seems very much more alert today and eager to learn and practice.

We covered the alphabet, flash cards and the name sheets which Derek is beginning to recognize more easily now.

The date sheet is becoming much more familiar to him but he can still get confused with it.

We took a break and went for a walk, down the stairs to ground floor where we visited the shop and purchased a "Bounty Bar", Derek chose this himself but did not have the confidence to go to the till to pay for it.

We then walked around the outside of the hospital to the side entrance and sat in the sunshine for half an hour. We returned to his room after walking up the three flights of stairs, Derek manages these floors with no problem whatsoever (I on the other-hand have to stop to regain my breath after two flights).

Back in the room we had a drink and continued with a questionnaire, which proved the best to date.

Derek has been at his best today but is now showing signs of tiredness. He has for the first time used his left hand (automatically) putting pen to paper but got very frustrated because he can no longer write or use his left hand without pain.

Derek tried so hard to keep going. I could so easily have cried for him.

4.15p.m *Derek is now having a much deserved rest on his bed.*

I believe that his weekend at home has done him the world of good. At first he was deeply emotional causing me to believe that perhaps it was too soon but he soon settled and was quite excited in the fact that he was able to recognize everything as it had always been. He was amazed that nothing had changed in all the time that he had been away and stated how concerned he had been that nothing would be the same. He said that it felt as though he had been away for years rather than months.

Derek showed a much improved ability in his verbal expression but being at home showed his vunerability more so than when in his little room within the hospital. The main cause of concern being that Derek believes he is more able to do things than he actually can at this present time and this could so easily have knocked his confidence but I believe his excitement over came this.

The weekend was a huge success with us both enjoying it immensely. We look forward, hopefully to being able to celebrate his birthday at home next weekend without my having to take him back for the evening.

5.30p.m *I had to awaken Derek for his soup and sandwiches which he ate himself unaided. He is now washed and ready for bed of his own choosing. He brushed his teeth and rinsed his mouth with no assistance.*

Entered by Andrea Craig.

18.00p.m *I took over from Derek's wife who had already helped prepare him for bed. He is lying on top of his bed listening to his radio.*

Derek has been to the toilet twice (P.U.) but is not ready for bed. He is sitting in his chair listening to his radio.

CAN NIGHT-STAFF PLEASE PUT EXTRA BLANKET ON TONIGHT AS DEREK WAS VERY COLD LAST NIGHT.

Entered by Carole Wright (H.C.A.)

21.00hrs. *Derek was lying on his bed listening to his radio. I unfortunately had to leave him and go onto the ward due to shortage of staff so Derek said he would get into bed. I returned to find Derek asleep and stayed with him for the remainder of the night. He awoke for the toilet three times during that period.*

Entered by Joan Lomax (H.C.A.)

Tuesday 7ᵗʰ August 2007.

Derek was sitting in his chair when I came on duty this morning. He enjoyed his breakfast and has showered with minimal assistance. We went for a walk, looked around the shop on the ground floor and then continued our walk outside in the grounds. We walked down the stairs and back up again, all flights.

Derek is now resting and relaxed listening to his radio.

Entered by unknown.

12.45p.m *Derek was going to walk to meet me today but unfortunately I arrived before he had left the third floor, so we walked back to his room to sort out his laundry and clean clothes and then we continued with his walk.*

We walked down the stairs and sat on the bench outside but soon discovered that the wind was too cold.

Having walked back to his room up the three flights of stairs Derek is now leafing through the newspaper relating anything that he recognizes. (He is happier doing this than he was yesterday).

He was able to recognize various letters (no words as yet) several pictures and was able to identify the sports pages and crossword. He claimed that it held too many adverts and too much rubbish.

We then went over the alphabet, flash cards and practiced holding the pen in his left hand.

The biggest improvement was in Derek's ability and focus in bouncing the large ball. He manages a far greater control of the ball now than he once did and is capable of moving around the room keeping the ball bouncing at the same time.

Derek becomes very confused when asked to come forward or move back but is much more able to assess side movements than he was a week ago.

We had a rest and a drink.

3.30p.m *Derek is practicing drawing holding his pencil in his left hand. (Derek believes he is drawing but actually he is only holding his pencil, but Rembrandt must have started somewhere!)*

Derek seems quite aware of topical events and states that he enjoys listening to the news because it feeds him information he is eager for.

4.00p.m *I had to request that the room be cleaned today as it was extremely dusty and collected fluff on the floor.*

Room was given a thorough good clean whilst Derek was resting. (I do miss my therapy!)

I noticed that whilst Derek was lying on his bed his right hand turned very blue, I must query that.

5.45p.m *Derek is very agitated incase he should be left alone again this evening.*

He states that last night he could not find his way to the toilet nor locate the alarm buzzer to summon assistance and got himself into a state.

DEREK MUST NOT BE LEFT ALONE.

I leave Derek having eaten his meal and ready for bed but not wishing to get in to it just yet.

Entered by Andrea Craig.

21.00hrs. *Derek very peacefully resting on his bed listening to his radio, he went to the toilet once (P.U.)*

Entered by Carole Wright (H.C.A.)

21.30p.m *Derek was asleep when I arrived, he awoke to use the toilet (P.U.) went back to bed and requested eye-mask and is now sleeping peacefully.*

Derek has refused to get under the covers and states that he would prefer to stay out of bed with his dressing gown over him.

12.00hrs. *Derek has been up to use the toilet and is once more asleep on top of his bed.*

7.00a.m *Derek woke up in a good mood this morning and was very chatty. Although he did sleep well he woke up several times to (P.U.) and asked the time.*

Derek is now sitting in his chair waiting for his breakfast.

Derek had an accident last night when he went to the toilet, he did not pull his pants down far enough and wet them a little, this upset him so much.

Entered by Elaine Ibberson (H.C.A.)

Wednesday 8ᵗʰ August 2007.

Derek was sitting in his chair listening to his radio when I came in this morning. We went to the bathroom where Derek had a shower with minimal assistance. Derek asked if we could go for a walk so we walked down the stairs and sat outside for a while enjoying the fresh-air but we could not stay long as Derek needed to get back for his breakfast.

A full breakfast followed by a glass of water was taken and enjoyed.

We played dominoes but Derek did not enjoy this.

10.30a.m *Derek visited the toilet (bowels opened).*

Entered by unknown.

12.35p.m *I arrived to find that Derek had been taken for a walk after his lunch.*

1.10p.m *Derek arrived back to his room in fine spirits. He told me that Dr. Newall or Dr.Pinder had been in to see him but was not quite sure who, and that whoever it had been, needed to see myself regarding something, but that he could no longer remember what it was about. (In fact it had been Dr. Newall who had called to see Derek just after I had left last evening re: the appointment with Dr. Palmer at 'Broadgreen Hospital'). I was so pleased that Derek had been able to remember so much of this incident.*

1.30p.m *Derek and I worked with monetary coins, I was pleasantly surprised to find that he had quite a good memory of them but he was confused at putting stated amounts together.*

I find that although Derek is very willing to learn, his attitude changes dramatically when not able to do the things he feels should be so easy for him to do.

1;45p.m *Derek tells me that he feels very nauseous once again as he did when he first woke up this morning. He says that it had worn off but has now returned and wonders if it might be because he did not sleep very well last night as he had felt strangely disturbed all night.*

He is now lying down and has fallen asleep.

3.15p.m *Derek woke and asked that he might exercise his left hand and arm which we did. We went on to practice his balance and bouncing the large ball.*

He is managing very well with his right hand now so we are concentrating more with his left, which he claims is extremely painful but says that he is able to tolerate it. He has done very well for his first attempt at this exercise.

We continued working with the alphabet and the flash cards and as soon as I noticed him tiring we stopped.

Derek asked if we could go for a walk and a breath of fresh-air before dinner.

5.15p.m *Derek is sitting in his chair exercising his hands with the soft balls whilst awaiting his dinner.*

I have found Derek to be very clear headed today and would note that his sickly feeling had disappeared after his sleep.

Derek fed himself with just a little help in changing over the dishes and placing each one before him.

I helped him to wash and get changed for bed but he is now totally independent in cleaning his teeth and is so happy at being able to do so but states that there is still so much more he wishes he could do for himself.

Entered by Andrea Craig.

9.00p.m *I came on duty to find Derek already in bed. He has slept soundly for most of the night, only waking to use the toilet (P.U.) after which he settled back to sleep.*

6.30a.m *Derek awoke and asked if he could sit out in his chair. I assisted him to put on his dressing gown and slippers and walked him to the toilet (P.U.and B.O.)*

We sat and chatted and Derek told me how he was looking forward to Andrea coming and how they sit outside on the bench watching the world go by.

Entered by J. Rylands (H.C.A.)

Thursday 9th August 2007

Derek was sitting in his chair chatting to Jean when I arrived. We went through to shower and washed his hair, came back and dressed and then we sat and did some crosswords while waiting for breakfast which Derek ate heartily and then we went for a walk around the hospital grounds sitting on the outside bench for twenty minutes or so.

11.00am. We returned to his room and Derek sat listening to his radio.

Derek has eaten 90% of his lunch and enjoyed it.

I would note that Derek has a very runny nose today but he states that he always has one lately!

Derek has taken lots of drinks, mainly water and one glass of grapefruit juice.

Entered by Helen Howatson (H.C.A.)

12.45p.m Derek was so bright and cheerful when I entered his room today but was over the moon when I told him that I was going to take him home this afternoon and that he was going to stay home until Monday morning. I explained that this was so that he could celebrate his birthday at home. He did not know whether to laugh or cry, instead he eagerly helped me to carry his bags to the car. It was too hot to sit outside so on returning to his room I managed to persuade him to have a lie

345

down so that he would not be too tired when we were finally able to go.

I have taken all of Derek's clothes to be cleaned and have permission to borrow his plate guard I will return it on Monday without fail.

Derek has stated that the best birthday present he could ever have would be waking up in his own bed.

Entered by Andrea Craig.

CHAPTER ELEVEN

We sat waiting for the pharmacist to make up Derek's prescription for the weekend leave and although Derek was lying down resting he was far too excited to sleep. The afternoon dragged on but thankfully Derek had an electric cooler unit in his room which was turned on full, otherwise it would have been unbearably hot.

When it seemed we were not going to be leaving in a hurry I tried to persuade Derek to practice some reading and writing but he was not interested in anything other than walking through the door which would take him back into a world he was so afraid of losing touch with.

I read to him, but every time a footstep was heard outside his eyes would dart to the door in anticipation, sadly I could only watch as he sank back in disappointment as they walked into the other patient's room next door or to collect something from the store cupboard situated opposite Derek's room.

Finally I decided to walk him around the third floor, knowing that we could easily be found when needed, but he would not be budged. No way was Derek going to be found missing when the pharmacist did arrive so we sat it out until five minutes past five when at long last the door opened and in walked the pharmacist accompanied by a nurse to check that his medication was correct and in order.

We left that evening with not only every conceivable aid that the staff felt we might need but with a bag full of birthday cards and a heart full of warm wishes from them, all hoping that we would spend a wonderful weekend along with the reassurance that they were only at the other end of the phone. I felt deeply touched, as did Derek, but with the thought of soon being on his way home overshadowing all else, he bid a hasty farewell to the staff and we were at last on our way.

The memory of that weekend will remain with me always, just as the memory of that previous weekend in April, when Derek was so nearly taken from us will always remain with me, but this time, thank God, he was returning, not just on a quick visit but also staying where he belonged for four whole nights and three full days. My excitement equalled his.

Just as he had done on his first visit, Derek walked around his home taking everything in as though he were seeing it for the very first time. He wandered slowly from room to room whilst I prepared the evening meal. A little later we sat where we always sat when dining alone, at the kitchen table and but for the plate guard around Derek's plate, it was a very normal setting, apart that was from the anxiety which could be detected on Derek's behalf. It took all of his concentration as he tried so hard to do everything as it should be done. He need not have concerned himself for he managed well.

At nine o'clock we were both extremely tired and I suggested that we should both go to bed as it had been a long day. It was only then that I realized I had not yet sorted out his medication. Opening the small case in which the tablets had been brought home I was suddenly taken aback with the huge amount of drugs which had been prescribed for him. Thankfully the hospital had printed out a morning, lunchtime and evening table which made it simple for me to follow, but nevertheless I could not prevent the tears from flowing as I sorted them into their groups and was hit with the sudden realization that Derek's life now depended upon this brightly coloured collection of pills laid out in front of me. I reminded myself that I was tired and must not allow him to see me upset and that all would be so much better in the morning. I gave Derek his evening tablets and after switching off the lamps and checking that all was secure for the night, we made our way to bed.

Halfway up the stairs Derek came to an abrupt halt. I asked him if he was alright but received no reply. He swayed slightly as though uncertain of which way he should be going. I knew his attention had gone,(or that he was having a mini focus crash as I called these such moments), so putting my hands to his back in order to steady him I called out the instruction for him to move his right foot onto the next stair. I pushed him gently trying to keep him moving forward but failed, Derek was going nowhere. Beginning to feel a little desperate I shouted out more instructions remembering that I must keep them clear and distinct.

"Keep going Derek... Place your left foot on the next stair... Lean forward. No", I shouted, "Not back...Forward... Just try to keep going... Hold onto the rail with your left hand". I quickly realized that my instructions were falling on deaf ears. Derek found it difficult to follow instruction at any time but when his focus dropped he found it impossible. There was just enough room for me to squeeze passed him on the stairs but I was afraid to move from behind him in case he should fall backwards. I began to feel his full weight leaning back on me and wondered how long I could support him this way.

I felt helpless and vowed in that moment that I must always carry a phone with me in future. I realized that at any moment we could both so easily go toppling down the stairs and despaired of what I should do next when I suddenly remembered that if I could clap my hands in front of him as I had once been told to do when he had these crashes then he might snap out of it.

I was not in a position to face him and knew that if I took my hands away from his back then he might indeed fall, so wedging my body as firmly as I could to support his back this then enabled me to very briefly remove my hands and I managed to give two very quick, short, sharp claps to his right ear.

"Why are you pushing me?" demanded Derek as though nothing out of the ordinary had taken place, "I'm going as quickly as I can".

Thanking God was all I could think of as we proceeded to climb the rest of the stairs. We managed with no further problems and Derek knew nothing of what had just taken place.

I had imagined Derek would be better sleeping in our own bed beside me, this way I would be aware of his needs and ready to assist him in and out of bed.

My one major concern had been the location of the toilet with its doorway adjacent to the top of the stairs and what might happen if Derek should ever get out of bed without my knowing and mistakenly miss the doorway to the toilet and topple down the stairs. Bearing this in mind and after helping Derek get ready for bed, (which took longer than in his hospital room) I had the brain wave of positioning a chest of drawers across the landing thus blocking off the passageway to the stairs. This gave me the security I needed from the threat of accident but it took a lot out of me lugging it from the bedroom and down the landing to where it would now live for the foreseeable future. At least from its new position I had only to push it across the top of the stairs each evening and then each morning move it back against the wall leaving a clear passageway both up and down the stairs.

As I showered that night I found myself unable to control the many mixed emotions that were taking over. Normally a person who copes well, I found myself wondering if I was going to be able to cope with what I was only just beginning to realize would be expected of me. Again I told myself that it had been a long day and that I must never start feeling sorry for myself. It was late and time for some much needed sleep.

Derek was already fast asleep as I slipped into bed beside him and I prayed that we would both have a good night's rest. Sadly that was not to be as soon afterwards he woke confused and wanting the toilet. I helped him to the toilet where he seemed unsure of what he was doing. A slight accident occurred, which embarrassed and un- nerved Derek although I tried to assure him that it was only because he had missed the toilet and caught his shorts by mistake and that we would soon have them changed with no harm done. I managed to get him back into bed but he kept repeating that he had thought this type of thing would all be over just as soon as he got back to his own home. No amount of reassurance would calm him and thereafter he spent a great deal of the night repeatedly asking for the toilet and for me to check and ensure he was sitting correctly before he would use it.

During the early hours of the morning, those deepest hours of darkness just before dawn with Derek sleeping soundly at last, I felt alone and scared. No amount of scolding or telling myself how fortunate I was compared to the many others who were going through so much worse than I did anything to change how frightened I felt. My fear was based on doubt. Doubt as to whether I would be strong enough or wise enough to look after this wonderful man, but dear God I was certainly going to try, with my whole being I was going to try.

The following morning was Derek's birthday, Friday 10th August, a glorious sunny morning which quickly swept away the fears, doubts and traumas of the night before. A morning we had at times doubted we would ever see again. We enjoyed a leisurely breakfast and opened his birthday cards sitting outside in the sunshine, after which we went for a short stroll. This was the first walk Derek had taken outside of the hospital grounds and I came to realize how difficult it was going to be for him crossing roads. It would seem that he had no perception of traffic or its speed and he suddenly came to another abrupt halt in the middle of the road, frightening the life out of me and a driver who had somehow managed to brake just in time. Once again, Derek had no idea of the near miss and wondered what all the fuss was about.

I am still to this day not medically or mentally sure of what happens during these lapses but I call them Derek's focus crashes. His focus, awareness and attention span suddenly drop, as it still does to this day but thankfully not as often and no way are these lapses as severe as they used to be but unfortunately we never know when they are about to occur.

We met two of our neighbours during our short walk who both expressed how well Derek was looking, this pleased him tremendously and he said afterwards that he must have appeared normal to them, at the time I really did not take in the full meaning behind his words but came to understand later just how afraid Derek really is of appearing stupid or retarded in some way when meeting anyone. Thankfully we met these people separately so Derek only had to deal with one person at a time.

Sarah and Max were holidaying in France and I had already informed family and friends that it was to be a quiet few days leave so we received no visitors except for his sister later that afternoon. On seeing how tired Derek was, Elaine kept her visit brief, but it must be said how much he enjoyed seeing her and the sense of humour she brought with her, she really cheered him up.

While Derek slept I prepared the evening meal and set the dining room table as we were not going to eat in the kitchen on his birthday. Earlier that week I had asked Derek what he would choose to eat as a special treat and his reply was a good, tender steak with all the trimmings and chips of course, he added sheepishly. Poor Derek, in all the years we had been married he had never been served chips or red meat and had never once complained. In hospital he had previously drooled over fish, chips and mushy peas and now steak with all the trimmings but tonight was his birthday and he was in for a surprise, for that was exactly what he was going to have.

We sat that evening by candlelight, the table decorated with fresh flowers, listening to his favourite music as we ate our dinner. Afterwards he asked me to dance with him and then added how sorry he was that he had, sadly, forgotten how. I stood up and taking his hand I quietly told him that it would all come back. At first we simply stood and held each other as we swayed to the music, then slowly, ever so slowly Derek began moving his feet until we were actually moving around the room.

Derek and I had always loved to dance. We felt we moved so well together and being the romantic man that he is it was always a joy to dance with him. That evening of his birthday was extra special, perhaps because we thought we might never be able to dance again, perhaps because every single moment we now spent together was a bonus granted by the Grace of God, perhaps with everything else stripped away we were experiencing nothing more than the true, deep love which binds two people together, the merging of one heart with another, who knows, all

I know for certain is that I had never felt love as I felt it that night.

Our moment began to slip and emotion began to overwhelm Derek as Chris Du'burgh sang his way through 'Lady in Red' and it finally shattered when he began singing 'Missing You'. The words of this beautiful song proved too much for Derek to bear and he broke down and sobbed as I had never heard him sob before. I held him and cried with him, some would say this was a moment too precious for me to be sharing but I do so because I believe that crying can be healing and proved to be just so for Derek and I that night. We felt as though we had cried away most of the pain and the shock of what had befallen us last April.

"Some birthday, Blue", I murmured as I finally wiped away his tears.

"I have just spent the best birthday a man could ever have", he replied as he dabbed away at mine, "I really don't know what I have ever done to be so lucky".

"What a daft pair we make, don't you think", I said trying to be light.

"We always were", he added laughing, "or me at least". Suddenly turning very serious he asked, "Andrea, do you think others will look at me and believe that I am daft?"

"They who know you will already know that you are".

"No seriously", with his tone much more subdued he continued, "I would hate to think that people will look at me and take me for an idiot, will they, do you think?"

"No Derek, they will not", I replied, noting that he had mentioned something similar earlier that same day after our walk. I knew he felt deeply disturbed as to how he might appear to other people and felt unsure as to how I should deal with it but not wishing to spoil the evening by dwelling on the subject I suggested we both settled down for a hot drink before retiring to bed.

What was left of the evening we spent sipping our drinks and chatting over the pleasant times we had shared on previous birthdays. Derek stated that this was the best birthday he had ever spent or could ever have wished for and he felt so extremely happy. What more could I ask for? In that moment my own happiness was complete.

Unlike the night before we had no trouble in climbing the stairs, Derek took them with ease but whilst getting undressed I noted that Derek became a little agitated and asked if everything was alright?

"Of course it is", he replied a touch too sharply and then immediately asked, "Where am I sleeping tonight?"

"Where you always sleep" I replied.

"Do you think I should?"

"Why ever not"? I asked in return. Without another word he continued to get ready for bed. He accepted my help and guidance throughout and ignoring my attempts at discovering what had prompted his questions he rather reluctantly allowed me to help him into bed. Rather strange after such a lovely day, I thought. Once again Derek was fast asleep before I slipped into bed. He was sleeping soundly but again it was not to last, for less than one hour later he needed to go to the toilet. Frequently throughout the night we made our visits to the toilet, sometimes no sooner had he got back into bed and he was asking to go again, this was something far from normal. I began to wonder if he might have a bladder infection but something seemed to be telling me that it was more likely to be anxiety. The following morning we were both exhausted but with no pressure upon us to be anywhere or to be doing anything we relaxed outside in the garden for most of the day.

On our third night, Derek suggested he should sleep in a separate bedroom where he might feel more relaxed and at the same time not disturb me. I argued this point stating that it would be easier if he was with me, but after seeing how agitated he was becoming I finally agreed to give it a try. I closed all other doors leaving his, mine and the toilet door ajar. I left a light on in the toilet and knew that he was safe from stumbling down the stairs. Derek had no problem finding his way to and using the toilet on his own but what I had not realized was that he had forgotten how to use toilet paper on the roll. In hospital the toilet paper came in separate pieces which pulled out of a holder and he had successfully learned how to use this method, with perhaps one or two pieces falling to the floor, so imagine my surprise when I awoke to discover the toilet floor and the landing strewn with toilet paper. The whole roll had completely unraveled reminding me of the 'Andrex' advertisement where the little puppy dog manages to run off leaving a trail of paper behind him. I could not help but laugh and thankfully Derek saw the funny side also.

I did not sleep, I was too afraid to drop off even for a minute, in case I should miss him needing my help, but I did allow him to find his own way to the toilet and gave him the privacy which he had recently become accustomed to in hospital.

Getting back to his room and into bed was another matter. Derek found this very confusing and needed guiding in the correct direction and assistance with getting back into bed. In his confusion he could not tell the top of the bed from the bottom and was certainly not able to cover himself over, even though there was only a duvet to deal with. In sheer desperation for some sleep I had to insist that he come back into my bed and after explaining that I could perhaps relax more easily if he were right next to me he agreed, but very reluctantly. The new arrangement made not the slightest difference, Derek still made his visits to the toilet just as frequently and I found it impossible to drop off for even five minutes.

Sunday was our last full day at home and we were much too tired to do very much except enjoy a little more of the sunshine we were experiencing at that time and try to catch up with as much needed sleep as possible. Fortunately Derek slept well for most of the day and I was able to catch up in the afternoon.

As the day wore on, Derek became more and more subdued and refused to say what was bothering him and I found myself wondering how on earth I was going to cope if I was to have another sleepless night. Later during the evening Derek finally blurted out how he found it impossible sleeping in the same bed together, that he had become so used to sleeping alone and how upset he felt at disturbing me every time he had to go to the toilet and he had thought that coming home would mean that he would regain his personal independence.

I needed to think. We both desperately needed sleep and neither sleeping with me nor sleeping in a separate bed had enabled us to get any sleep at all. In hospital Derek received twenty four hour care, with frequent shift changes. At home he had me watching him around the clock for twenty four hours every day with no break at all. I could not help but wonder how this arrangement could possibly work.

Believing as I did that most of this problem was caused by anxiety I wondered how I could best ease this situation when I remembered the incontinence pants that the hospital had provided me with should I need them.

I wondered how Derek would react to using them but considered it was worth a try. I suggested that if he wore them instead of his night-shorts he may feel more secure. I went on to explain that I believed he was naturally overly anxious and concerned because of the few accidents which had occurred since the removal of his catheter tube and that the wearing of this protection would give him freedom from the worry and fretting about it all.

I explained that he must still use the toilet whenever he felt the need but that he must try to go to sleep knowing that he would not have an accident whilst wearing these protective pants. Derek said he was willing to give anything a try and that night we put it to the test. The result, Derek slept well, waking only four times. Did I sleep? I am afraid to say not at all and Derek did worry about this but I was able to tell him that I felt so good about how well our little plan had worked I did not feel tired at all.

In spite of the difficulties encountered and the exhaustion experienced we both thoroughly enjoyed our first weekend spent at home, until Monday morning arrived and we had to return to hospital. Derek spoke very few words that morning and I could feel that he had distanced himself, a little later he told me how he had had to cut off from everything or he could never have brought himself to go back. We arrived back in his room where he stated how tired he was and that he wished to lie down. He murmured that he now knew how Sarah must have felt each time she took herself back to university after being home for the weekend.

As Derek lay upon his bed I sat reflecting on the days we had spent at home and although I appreciated how far Derek had come in his recovery I fully realized just how much further he had to go. (This was to become a familiar pattern along a very long road.) I felt exhausted and despondent. I had never felt so inadequate at being able to help someone in my entire life. I wanted to scream but had no-one to scream at.

The following entries record how increasingly difficult Derek found it each time he had to return to hospital and how subdued and reluctant he would be to carry out his exercises. Usually by midweek he came out of his low mood and would be as willing as ever to crack on with whatever was put before him. Thursday's were obviously the best days because he would know that the following morning meant home once more.

Monday 13th August 2007.

12.30p.m *Derek has enjoyed his weekend at home and I believe it has done him so much good, but I would like to state that I have come to realize that in spite of how far Derek has progressed he still has so much further to go. He has conquered the domain of his little room in Arrowe Park very well but seemed so lost and fragile in his own home.*

Derek is so totally dependent on myself and others for all his needs, although it must be noted that he is trying so hard and is doing so well.

He is lying down awaiting lunch. He has been quiet on his return.

2.10p.m Derek ate all of his lunch and was willing to practice his writing until now.
He has asked to lie down again.

3.40p.m Dr. Oates made her round and stated that she thought four day leave was a little too long and that Derek could continue his weekend leave provided we cut it back, perhaps taking him home on the Friday afternoon and returning Sunday evening.

It was also stated that Arrowe Park could do no more for Derek except looking after his well being and at the same time appreciating that Derek is still fully dependent on someone else.

I fully understand all that Dr. Oates has stated and agree entirely, medically they can do no more for him but I cannot help the way I feel at this present moment and would like to express how strongly I feel that Derek was so badly let down before April 28th which was when he suffered his cardiac arrest, by having to wait so many weeks for his angiogram appointment and I cannot help but feel that he is being badly let down once again. Not by Arrowe Park, (I cannot thank this hospital enough for all that they have done for Derek) but having to wait so long for the expertise training he badly needs right now. (I probably just feel like lashing out at someone.)

Derek has worked so hard and deserves the chance and opportunity of training and rehabilitation that I sadly cannot give him. (How I wish that I could!)

I do understand the dilemma of bed shortages at the Neuro-Rehab Unit but how long should anyone have to wait for their chance. I am led to believe that the first months in recovery are vital for these people suffering brain injury.

This is all probably down to my sheer frustration and fatigue showing through and having to now explain to Derek and help him to understand why it seems that nothing is being done for him.

This is as down as either of us has felt so far.
Entered by Andrea Craig.

Derek was asleep when I came on duty.

He has had a good night's sleep, getting up three times (P.U.) and going straight back to sleep again.
Entered by Sue Griffiths (H.C.A.)

Tuesday 14ᵗʰ August 2007

I met Derek for the first time this morning and we had a lovely chat about the weather.

8.15a.m *Derek got up and sat in his chair. I gave him the soft balls to exercise with while waiting for breakfast.*

He ate all of his breakfast, taking a cold drink instead of a hot one.

9.35a.m I took Derek for his shower and he did very well with washing and drying with just a little help needed. He managed to brush his teeth.

We played games and used the flash cards also.

Derek has been telling me how he is waiting for a bed in Rehab and that he is ready to move on so that he can get home.

He told me that he has been home for the weekend and how hard he found it to come back.

Derek took drink of water 200mls.

Entered by Sarah Wycherley (H.C.A.)

10.45a.m Occupational Therapy.

Derek told me all about his weekend at home for his birthday.

We practiced with the flash cards and object recognition.

His communication skills have greatly improved since last visit.

Entered by Michelle Kozlowski (OT)

10.50a.m Derek and I went for a walk, both up and down the stairs around each floor. I also took him to see the chapel and he said he would like to go to a service. I showed him the hairdressers and picked up a pricelist, he said he would show it to Andrea. We came back and had a cup of tea *and a cake which he enjoyed. We played games before lunch.*

We had such a good morning and Derek is such a lovely man who wants to get himself better and get himself home. I hope he does because I know this will make him very happy as he is beginning to feel very low and fed up now.

We played with the blocks. Derek was able to build a tower of eight blocks in total and was also able to tell me the colour of each block. This is a very good game for eye skills and balancing skills.

11.55a.m *Derek waiting for his lunch and said he did not need the toilet.*

12.35p.m *Derek ate all of his lunch and fed himself independently. He is visiting the toilet before his wife arrives.*
Entered by Sarah Wycherley (H.C.A.)

12.45p.m *Derek was much more emotionally stable than he had been yesterday. He has been very chatty and able to recall so much.*

We practiced putting on his socks and slippers. This proved to be impossible and caused a lot of distress to Derek. I must check this out with OT's.

We turned the pages of a newspaper which proved quite successful with Derek attempting to describe each pages layout to me and pointing out any letter or word that he was able to recognize. He is improving in this exercise.

We moved on to the flash cards with Derek able to recognize seven words.

Moving on to the wooden piece board I found Derek's attention span had dropped and he was struggling. I called a halt to the exercise but Derek said he wished to continue for a little while longer and he improved a little. After a few minutes we stopped.

3.00p.m *I asked if Derek might like to lie down and he said definitely not, so we continued with throwing and catching the small balls. This is the first time with the small balls, we have always used the large ball for this exercise, so much easier for Derek to see and focus upon, but he has done exceptionally well and stated that he enjoyed it so much more than with the large ball as it has kept him on his toes.*

We then did some simple exercises e.g. stretching and then following my instruction as I call them out such as: lift left leg, put hands on head and so on.

He is much more improved with this but still experiences difficulty in differentiating between left and right.

I have noticed a tremor to his left hand which he also claims to have noticed but stated that it is no longer as painful as it used to be.

4.30p.m *Derek broke out in a cold sweat so I insisted he lay down and rest. He did not wish to but I insisted.*

I gave him a manicure and pedicure before dinner.

Dinner was late this evening which meant that Derek had a good rest. He ate all of his dinner independently.

I helped Derek wash and get into his night clothes but not into bed.

Entered by Andrea Craig.

6.15p.m *Derek was very chatty this evening and held conversation well, occasionally mixing up the odd word.*

19.30p.m *Derek went to the toilet without any problems except that he tried to take off his shorts instead of just taking them down. I observed him for a few minutes before asking him if he needed my help, which he did!*

Derek finished in the toilet and walked back to his chair where I assisted him into his dressing gown.

Derek is sitting exercising his hands with the soft balls whilst waiting to listen to the football on the radio.

Derek appears to be a little tired.

20.30p.m *I asked Derek if he would like to get into bed but he said he was o.k. for the time being.*

Entered by Angela Baker (H.C.A.)

21.00p.m *Derek was listening to his radio when I arrived (It was the Everton match). He asked me if I wanted the light on because it was getting dark.*

Derek is happy because Everton won the match.

He retired to bed at 22.00p.m. He was able to take off his dressing gown and slippers himself but managed to get into bed upside down, we had a good laugh over this.

He asked for his blackout eye shield, settled down and soon fell asleep.

Derek requested the toilet three times during the night but was a bit confused pulling up his shorts.

6.00a.m *Derek woke and asked to sit in his chair.*

Derek was able to remember the football results from last night's match which I thought was very good.

Entered by Christine Mepham (H.C.A.)

Wednesday 15th August 2007.

On arrival I found Derek listening to his radio and patiently waiting for his breakfast which was a little late this morning. He enjoyed all of it and stated that he would prefer Marmite on his toast but was happy to settle for Marmalade!

Derek tried very hard to wash himself in the shower but finds juggling the showerhead and the shampoo bottle very difficult. Skills which he still cannot grasp but time will help Derek to improve on this.

He did manage to pull up his left sock and put on his left slipper but he could not manage the right sock and slipper, he found this difficult and could not understand why!

Afterwards I asked Derek if he would rather work with the cards or go for a walk and he chose to go for a walk. We walked all the way downstairs to the basement and stood for a while by the push-bikes and motor-bikes by the Personnel Department. Derek told me that he once owned a motor-bike.

We then went to have a look at the new lift and discussed them in some detail. We continued walking up the stairs and he said he would enjoy going down in the new lift, which we did.

We walked around to the main entrance and enjoyed a coffee in the WRVS tearoom, where also a flapjack went down a treat. After our drink we made our way back up the stairs and onto the ward and finally back into Derek's room.

11.00a.m *Derek is now sitting having a snooze in his chair. He has been exercising his hands with* *the soft balls while listening to his listening tape (Dick Francis' Wild Horses).*

Derek seems rested although he does have a constantly running nose as though he may have the start of a cold?

The Listening Tape people came in to change the tape for Derek.

A doctor paid a call to see Derek and asked how he was doing and Derek mentioned tingling in his fingers.

Entered by Angie Benton (H.C.A.)

12.45p.m *Derek was very much brighter today when I arrived and tells me that Angie has worked well with him this morning which has made him so happy.*

Derek has been reading through the newspaper and greatly surprised me by recognizing several pictures of well known people and reading out several words but was a little confused with the word "ostrich", but he did finally get it.

1.30p.m *We began exercising with the flash cards but Derek was obviously tired*
and needed to rest.

He is now lying down listening to the afternoon play on his radio.

Derek does not seem to be drinking his fluids as once did and simply states that he does not wish to. (I feel this might be because if he drinks more he thinks he will go to the toilet more!)

3.00p.m Derek awakened wanting to go to the toilet, he took himself (P.U.and O.B.) He was able to clean himself, pulled up his trousers but forgot that he was wearing underpants, which got rather tangled and he became quite confused but this was soon sorted and then he automatically washed his hands and dried them but forgot to flush the toilet. He apologized saying that there was still so much for him to learn but that he felt he was getting there.(Indeed you are Derek)

He found his own way back into his room and then we went to post a letter in the postbox on the ground floor. As it was sunny we walked outside and sat and enjoyed the fresh-air.

3.45p.m We are now back in the room waiting for the speech therapist.

3.50p.m Speech and Language Therapist.

I came to see Derek and talked to him and Andrea about his progress, they both seem pleased with progress being made but are looking forward to further work at rehab.

We looked at orientation, Derek needed clues to use his board. He was helped by Andrea and therapist.

Andrea talked about her being able to input in helping Derek with dressing and washing, I will ask nursing staff re. occupational therapy input.

We will see Derek again next week.

Entered by Rachael McCann (S.L. Therapist).

4.30p.m *Derek and I did some stretching and balancing exercises with Derek using both hands and arms.*

Derek is now able to recognize his body parts very well and enjoys any exercise asked of him.

5.20p.m *Derek fed himself with the aid of the plate guard and I noticed he is now able to use both hands to eat his meal. This is excellent.*

Derek has said that he would like to start going down to the day-room to watch a little television if this is possible, feels he is going mad confined to his room.

Please note that Derek is in clinic early tomorrow morning so I have left clothes out ready for him.

Entered by Andrea Craig.

21.00p.m *Derek enjoyed watching television in the day-room and is not yet ready to go back to his room. I made him a Horlicks drink.*

Entered by C. Wright (H.C.A.)

Derek was watching T.V. in day-room when I took over and he stayed until 22.00p.m. He needed assistance with undressing when back in his room and was settled down by 23.30p.m.

Derek got up to use the toilet a few times in the night and was able to do almost everything for himself.

6.00a.m *Derek got up and requested to sit in his chair, he needed help in putting on his slippers and dressing gown.*

Entered by Christine Mepham (H.C.A.)

Thursday 16th August 2007.

8.30a.m *Hello there, accompanied by a porter, we took Derek down to the eye clinic for his appointment, where I stayed with him throughout. Derek knew where he was and why he was there and told me how he had become compliant with waiting around in hospital and gets less "cheesed off" these days!*

Derek had difficulty in differentiating between which chair was his, in clinic this morning, on his return from seeing the doctor and he nearly sat on the lap of a little lady who, bless her, had a good sense of humour.

10.30a.m *Finally we arrived back on the ward at which stage Derek was feeling very hungry, as unfortunately we had to attend clinic before breakfast was served. He wolfed down cereal and toast as we discussed our mutal passion for "Marmite".*

Derek was given eye-drops in clinic which have enlarged his pupils and can make his vision slightly blurry, so we are now enjoying listening to the radio.

His ear phones fell loose around his head so I left Derek to try to sort them out for himself whereby he had one placed behind his right ear and the other on his forehead ----- I soon put him in the right direction!

We enjoyed funny little chats this morning and Derek was quite amused with what your average twenty three year old female keeps herself entertained with.

I told him that there was a new Simpsons film out which I had seen last week and he laughed heartily at the question of me asking if he had ever watched the Simpsons, at which stage he added that perhaps he had seen the odd one or two episodes in the past.

Derek has been singing along enthusiastically to every song he recognizes on Radio 2, so far I have heard a rendition of an Elvis Presley song sang quietly to me and a song called "Boxer" by Simon and Garfunkel I think!

Derek went to the toilet at 10.45a.m after which he pulled up his own trousers but forgot that he was wearing underpants which were still around his knees. He knew something was not quite right though and was amused when I told him what he had done ---- soon put right.

12.00 noon Derek and I have just returned from a pleasant walk around the hospital, tackling as many flights of stairs as I could manage! I kept asking, "Are we nearly done yet", but no he carried *on and on, Derek appears to be much fitter than I am.*

He is resting in his chair now and trying to remove the lining from his trouser pocket which I believe he thinks is his hankie!

Derek asked for his soft exercise balls which he told me were to strengthen his legs, I politely told him that I thought he meant his arms and he said yes that was exactly what he meant.

Derek is a polite and charming man who is certainly aware of all that has happened to him yet remains humbled by the fact that people care for him and believes that through rehabilitation he will continue to strive towards a happy life once more.

Entered by Jo McGrath (H.C.A.)

12.45p.m *Derek was sitting having just finished his lunch when I arrived today, he is not quite as lively as usual. He told me what a delight Jo has been and how thoughtful a person she is, thank-you Jo.*

When his nurse had left I went to give Derek a hug and he broke down, stating that he could not say why he was feeling the way that he was and that he did not even know how he was feeling. He went on to say that it might be because he was worrying about his heart or the fact that he could no longer do anything for himself anymore. He simply did not know anything anymore except that he felt deeply upset and weary with everything and of how tired, very, very tired he felt and that all he wanted to do was close his eyes and sleep.

1.15p.m *Derek is now lying on his bed in a deep sleep.*

2.15p.m *Derek awakened to go to the toilet (P.U.and O.B.) He stated that he wished to go back to sleep and did not want to talk to anyone.*

4.30p.m *Derek got up to go to the toilet (P.U.) and said that he wished to remain up. "Just as well", I replied, "as dinner will be served shortly".*

Derek fed himself and ate all of his dinner. He is not talking and has said that he simply wishes to listen to his radio.

Before I left Derek said that he would like to go down to watch some television later on in the day room.

I helped Derek to wash and change so that he is ready for bed, he tells me that he will clean his teeth later.

Entered by Andrea Craig.

7.00p.m *Derek was listening to his radio, I offered him a drink which he refused. He asked if he might go to the toilet (P.U.)*

We are going down to the day room to watch a little t.v.

Entered by unknown.

21.00p.m *Derek was watching T.V in day room when I took over, we stayed until 10.30p.m chatting to the other fellows off the ward who had been watching T.V. with also. Derek so enjoyed the other male company and the banter etc.*

Derek slept most of the night, he went to the toilet five times but went back to sleep each time.

He is managing quite well but needs reminding to flush the loo!

Entered by night staff.

Friday 17th August 2007.

8.00a.m *Derek had just been given his breakfast when I arrived on duty, which he really enjoyed. After he had finished I asked him if he would like a shower to which he answered yes.*

Derek found it difficult to hold the shower head so I helped him by holding the shower head whilst he washed himself. I also gave him assistance to get dried and dressed.

Derek was able to brush his teeth and said that he always used an electric toothbrush, I had to explain to him that it must be at home as he only had an ordinary one in his toiletry bag.

Not long after this the domestic came in to clean Derek's room so we went for a walk around the hospital grounds, which Derek said he enjoyed. We sat in the reception area for a while watching all the comings and goings.

Derek told me how much he was looking forward to going to Wirral Neuro. And how much he thought it was going to help him.

Back in Derek's room where he is listening to his radio and exercising his hands with the soft balls.

I asked Derek if he would like to play any of his board games which he declined saying that he was so fed up with them all!

Derek is now having a snooze while waiting for lunch.

Derek ate and enjoyed his lunch but struggled putting the food onto his fork. His plate guard has been taken from his room which caused a problem as this was helping to assist Derek a lot in feeding himself.

Derek's wife has just arrived and boy has Derek's face lit up! I am going off duty now after what has been a lovely morning.

Entered by J. Rylands (H.C.A.)

12.30p.m Derek is so much better today, I felt quite concerned about him when I left last night. He is much more upbeat and a lot brighter and is looking forward very much to going home later.

He tells me that he is now so bored with all the old exercises and games in his room so this morning I have devised my own "questionnaires" so as to try and encourage broader conversation with Derek.

Derek was weighed and has once again gained weight. Staff pleased with him.

2.00p.m *Physio's arrived with the wonderful information of how the girls had been over to the Neuro. Clinic and come back armed with physio more fitting to Derek's condition. Ten out of ten to Arrowe Park for bringing this about, we shall now continue our efforts with renewed spirits.*

All we need now is a little more input from Occupational Therapy regarding help with Derek learning how to dress himself or even showing me how best to help him. (Especially with his socks, which is proving the most difficult of tasks for me to tackle, although I must say that he made a wonderful attempt at doing so the other day. Derek had sat so pleased with himself and asked me what I thought of the job he was so obviously proud of, when I turned to look for myself I could not help but laugh for he had only spent the last five or ten minutes fitting a sock and slipper onto his right hand.

It had been known for some time that Derek did indeed have a problem recognizing his body parts and that he was having particular problems differentiating his hands and arms from his feet and legs and this incident brought it home so clearly just how difficult it was for him.

I told him how well he had done except for the fact that he should have put them on his foot which was to be found at the end of his leg which was at the bottom of his body. I gently asked him if he could have another try.

Derek was eager to do so, saying that he now understood, I could not believe it when he immediately proceeded to put the sock on his head. His explanation being that he thought the top of his body was in actual fact the bottom and that his head was in fact his foot and that I needed to make myself more easily understood in future.

There are times when I laugh and a great many times when I cry but that was a time when we both laughed so much we cried.

At last we have now received instruction as to what is really needed to work his left hand. I feel pleased with this information and Derek feels uplifted because he believes that at last something is now being done.

After one of our most emotional weeks and especially yesterday when Derek said how low and worried he had been feeling, I feel this is a good end to the week.

3.00p.m *Derek went to the toilet, he took himself there and I left him to see to himself. He returned with his trousers only half pulled up but was as pleased as punch because he had remembered to pull up his underpants, adding, "You can't have it all and who knows, perhaps next week I'll get them both right".*

Hopefully next week will see a great improvement, I feel we will.

Derek is now having a lie down as he seems a little tired after his physio but I cannot stress enough how much he enjoys his physio and the difference I notice in him each and every time he has it.

The eye clinic have asked if I will make an appointment with Derek's optician as soon as possible for a normal sight test.

4.00p.m We are leaving the ward as Derek is going home for the weekend. We will return Monday morning.

Entered by Andrea Craig.

Monday 20th August 2007.

11.30a.m Derek spent a very good week-end at home but was very reluctant to come back this morning. I talked it into a positive situation explaining that he still needed to train his focus and attention along with further development of his co-ordination whilst awaiting Rehab. He said he fully understood and realized how patient he must be and has seemed more positive since returning.

12.00 noon. Derek has sat browsing through the newspaper indicating any words that he is able to recognize.

Derek fed himself his lunch but was unable to cut up his meat.

2.15p.m *Derek has worked really hard on the alphabet, flash cards and the drawing of shapes, drawing circles came quite easily to him but he found squares more confusing, nevertheless he has greatly improved all round.*

Derek asked me if I can teach him how to tell the time as he can now recognize the clock which is on the wall in his room. This has pleased me so much for until now Derek has been unable to focus on it and therefore has not been able to see it.

I have drawn out a clock face and cut out fingers to work with but have suggested that he must continue to look at the clock on the wall and continually ask whoever is with him to help him read the time at that moment.

Derek has been in a very positive mood today and has worked so hard. He is understandably very tired now and I notice that his right hand has turned blue again.

Derek is resting on his bed and has fallen into a deep sleep.

3.15p.m *Derek had no sooner fallen asleep when Dr. Oates and her team arrived. Derek woke up and after the doctors had left Derek went to the toilet (P.U.) and went straight back to sleep once more.*

4.45p.m D erek awoke and went to the toilet (P.U.) he sat in his chair on returning, waiting for his dinner.

5.50p.m Derek fed himself and managed very well. I helped to wash and change him ready for bed.

As there is no nurse to sit with him until the later night shift I have agreed for Derek to sit in the day room to watch the television. Derek seems delighted with this arrangement.

Entered By Andrea Craig.

Derek went to the toilet once in the night and needed no assistance except at getting back into bed.

4.50a.m Derek requested the toilet again (P.U.) and went straight back to bed and slept well throughout the rest of the night.

Entered by Paul Mannion (H.C.A.)

Tuesday 21st August 2007.

Derek was awake on my arrival, he was very cheery and settled, he fed himself and needed minimal assistance with showering. Derek and I have been chatting all morning. He has been reflecting on a lot of past experiences e.g. holidays and family events.

Derek managed his lunch with no problems. His wife arrived at 12.45p.m and Derek is now very bright and cheery.

Entered by Sarah Crawford (H.C.A.)

12.45 p.m *Derek was very chatty and alert when I arrived and told me how much he had enjoyed chatting to Sarah his nurse.*

2.00p.m *Derek complained of feeling stiff so we went for a walk.*

Derek has voiced a very definite opinion that he would prefer being taught by someone other than myself in future, someone more trained to his situation.

I have told him that I respect what he has said and that I will stand back from now on. (I do not of course mean that but I want Derek to know that I do respect what he is saying).

I believe that Derek is anxious and worried about tomorrows appointment at Broadgreen hospital with Dr. Palmer.

Derek has been complaining about the pain he is getting down the left hand side of his neck and how it is getting worse instead of better, also his left shoulder is still very painful.

3.00p.m *We have returned from our walk and Derek is sitting reading (or browsing through) the newspaper. Once again he was able to recognize several words and photographs and placing them* *together he was able to relate a little from two incidents which had taken place. He was pleased with this.*

Derek has gone from cheerful and chatty to being quiet and agitated as the afternoon wore on. He is unsettled somehow. (However I do feel it is regarding tomorrow).

6.15 p.m *Derek enjoyed his dinner and is washed and ready for bed later on, says he will clean his teeth just before he gets into bed.*

Entered by Andrea Craig.

21.00 p.m *Derek very chatty and told me about how well Andrea cooks.*

He has had a good night's sleep. He got up to the toilet five times and went straight back to bed with only a little assistance.

Entered by Unknown.

Wednesday 22nd August 2007.

11.45a.m *Derek apologized for his behaviour yesterday and for being so awkward, and was eager to inform me that he would continue with his exercises and that he was willing to push on and learn more, even if it meant working with me. I did try to point out to him that regrettably he really did not have much choice and that I, apart from* *his therapist once a week, was the only teacher he had right now.*

I further explained that I felt sure it was due to his anxiety regarding his appointment this afternoon with Dr, Palmer, Derek nodded his agreement to this.

12.30p.m *Derek has eaten and enjoyed a hearty lunch, he was able to feed himself but needed help in cutting up his meat, he simply cannot direct or control both his knife and fork at the same time.*

6.00p.m *It has been a long afternoon but Derek returns very pleased with his appointment and felt that Dr. Palmer had gone to great lengths to explain to him in layman terms just what was going on with his heart and arteries. (His medical diagnosis was Two-vessel coronary artery disease, out-of-hospital cardiac arrest secondary to myocardial infarction with subsequent neurological deficit.) As Derek was responding well on medication at the present time it was agreed that he should undergo his rehab.at Neuro. before anything further be considered.*

Derek feels the news was very positive and is now looking forward to rehab. as soon as possible.

Derek was very hungry and relished his soup and sandwiches for tea.

I have helped to wash and change Derek ready for bed but he wishes to go to the day room to watch the England match with the other men at 8.00p.m.

I will walk him down to the day room and leave him after notifying staff.
Entered by Andrea Craig.

Thursday 23rd August 2007.

12.45p.m *Derek is very quiet today but seems happy. He is browsing through the newspaper.*
We attempted various exercises but Derek's attention and concentration seems very poor, he did say that he is able to recognize this fact and said he had not been able to focus very well this morning.
Deciding to leave everything we went for a walk in the sunshine which I believed might be more beneficial to him.

3.30p.m *Back in Derek's room and he now seems much more alert than he did before our walk. He said that he gets so stiff and aches from sitting for such long periods of time and that he had enjoyed his walk tremendously.*
Derek has been singing to himself since we returned and tells me that he feels more positive and happy today with his progress, but wishes that he was able to dress and undress himself.
I wish that I could help him more in this direction but feel so inadequate in being unable to

do so. I only wish that someone could teach me the retraining skills needed so that I in turn could help Derek.

I feel that I am lost and floundering in that same deep, dark ocean that Derek is struggling to keep afloat in.

6.00p.m *Derek has enjoyed his evening meal and says that he enjoys Thursdays more than any other day because he knows that he is going home the next day.*

I have washed and changed him ready for bed and will walk him down to the day room where he now looks forward to going each evening.

I will leave him after first notifying staff that I am going home.

Entered by Andrea Craig.

Friday 24th August 2007.

Joint session (Speech and Occupational Therapy.)

Orientation --- Derek continues to improve. He was able to give home address for the first time.

Word tasks (thinking of words with similar meanings.)

We held a newspaper discussion on smoking ban.

We had a very good session today and are very pleased with Derek's progress.

Have a nice weekend Derek.

Entered by Rebecca Smith & Michelle Kozlowski.

8.00a.m – 1.30p.m. *Derek managed to shower himself quite well this morning and attempted different dressing tasks.*

We worked on the word cards which he did very well with.

Derek had his Therapy session at 11.00a.m (see above) then we went for a brisk walk outside where Derek began to jog a little, he seemed to be really enjoying himself, however I could not say that I was, as it meant me jogging to keep up with him! Ha.

Derek has seemed very positive and focused on returning to full health today and I also sense that he is excited about his weekend leave.

Derek managed his lunch with ease.

Entered by unknown.

Monday 27th August 2007.

11.45a.m *Derek was not emotional on his return this morning as he has been in the past, in fact he seems to be in a very positive mood.*

He browsed through the newspaper as I put his clothes away and he ate his lunch without any help whatsoever, but still needs his plate guard.

Derek is managing very much better with the using of his knife and fork but still finds it difficult because of the tremor in his left hand, at least he is able to co-ordinate them both together more.

1.00p.m   This afternoon, Derek has practiced drawing various shapes, e.g. squares, circles, triangles and oblongs, he is able to differentiate but now gets confused with triangles which are relatively new to him.

1.30p.m   Derek is asleep on his bed which gives me the opportunity to write up his week-end leave, which he enjoyed so much, I must add that we both thoroughly enjoyed it.

I noticed that Derek is now able to cope so much better with so many tasks, little tasks, but nevertheless each small task tells of improvement. I noticed that Derek can now take himself to the dining table and seat himself, pulling up his own chair and that he is waiting for everyone to be seated before he begins, instead of ploughing ahead regardless, this is the Derek I am familiar with and feel so pleased to see each small return to his former self, no matter how small this might be, each breakthrough is important.

I do realize of course that it took everything Derek was capable of, to focus on eating, let alone having to consider the etiquette of table manners, but to now witness the reappearance, so to speak, of something which had been such a normal part of his everyday life, was wonderful and filled me with renewed hope.

I found Derek unbelievably improved with his toilet and was able to witness the tremendous relief within him at now being independent once again in this way.

Although I must stress that he still has great difficulty in dressing himself correctly after each toilet visit.

Derek believes that everything is in order and fails to comprehend that his clothes are in such disarray. He takes guidance with great humility and is so eager to get it right. I am impressed with his progress so far, the improvement has been tremendous.

Night times are also improving but the frequent toilet visits must be disturbing his sleep and is a great concern to me. Getting back into bed is now a lot easier but Derek can still get into a huge muddle and becomes easily disorientated.

Sadly I get very little sleep, if any, and have to try and catch up the following afternoon when Derek has his rest period.

Derek can pass various items to me in the kitchen. He finds it difficult to fill the kettle as he feels severe nerve pain in his left hand, but he does try and is doing quite well.

Sunday I witnessed Derek's focus crash, when this happens, Derek cannot function and it is almost as though a light has been switched off within him.

I immediately put him to lie down and he slept and slept the rest of the day and evening through.

This morning, being the following day, saw Derek very much brighter and his alertness restored, hence the new positive mood, possibly.

2.45p.m Derek awakened in not such a bright mood unfortunately, stating that he does not wish to write, read, draw or play any silly games. I reminded him that he was renaging on his promise to continue working hard.

He stated that he considered me unable to teach him further and that he would sooner wait until he got to Neuro Rehab, where they will be specially trained to teach him. He has decided that he does not wish to discuss the matter any further and is definitely not speaking.

I shall leave him to settle down.

4.00p.m Sarah has arrived and Derek is still remaining quiet.

4.30p.m Dr. Oates arrived and once again brought an air of optimism and a sense of positiveness with her, to which Derek responded and very quickly became his old cheerful self.

Afterwards he enjoyed a head massage and said that he felt much more relaxed but a little tired and would like to lie down and rest before dinner, and then perhaps later he could be taken for a walk when his dinner had "gone down".

5.15p.m *For the first time, Derek has eaten his meal using both his knife and fork*

but without the aid of a plate guard. He has done brilliantly!

He has come round and is in a much brighter mood. I took him for a short walk for a little fresh air before helping him to wash and change ready for bed. Sarah and I will walk him down to the day room, where he says he would like to watch the football later on.

Entered by Andrea Craig.

21.00p.m *Derek was in the day room watching football (Liverpool playing). He was cheerful and chatting about his weekend at home.*

As soon as the match was finished he said that he was ready for bed so we came back to his room.

Derek got confused when trying to undress but we soon realized that he was already changed for bed. He managed to get into bed with a little help and I helped him with his eye mask.

Derek has slept well throughout the night, only getting up four times to P.U. which shows a marked improvement from when I was last here with him. He is also now able to flush the toilet after each use and wash and dry his hands without the need for prompting.

I have noticed a huge difference in Derek this time.

Entered by unknown.

There is no recorded entry for Tuesday 28th August but whilst Derek slept in the afternoon I sat and wrote him one of my letters. A letter I hoped would encourage him and help him to know that he was not alone, not for one moment.

To my wonderful, darling boy,

I want to thank-you from the very bottom of my heart and the very depth of my soul for being the unique, beautiful being that you are. These past weeks have been so difficult for you, probably the most difficult you have ever lived through in your entire life and yet your smile has continued to radiate through your pain and anguish not wanting others to see how afraid you truly were.

In spite of the emotional roller coaster that we have both been riding I for one feel that we share a far greater closeness now than ever before. It is as though all barriers have completely disappeared and the trust you once found so difficult to place is now so readily given and I feel so blessed to have it.

I will never abuse that trust, my darling, not ever, and my love shall be with you throughout all time and beyond.

Whatever trials and traumas we find ourselves up against in this life, they are as nothing within the light and power of love. You have recently expressed how worried you are at no longer being able to care and protect me, but I ask that whenever you doubt your physical strength being capable of keeping me secure then please know that I rest completely, absolutely and securely in your love for me and the knowing that God's Love holds us both fast unto himself.

We are both secure within Him and I also believe that it is so often through trials such as we find ourselves facing at this time that we are brought, as I stated a little earlier, even closer together than ever we were before.

Some people have said how horrendous a time this must be and yes it certainly has not been easy or pleasant in any way and yet I feel it has been a very precious time, a time lived out in love, truth, commitment and the being at one with our own innermost beings.

I love you so completely and yet feel so inadequate in being able to help you more but I do know beyond doubt that we are both being healed in and during this special time in God's presence. We must through this difficult period hold true to our own inner light and trust that God's much brighter light will light up the way ahead for us and pray that His Holy Spirit will work His miracles so that all are touched and none left out.

We must be strong and brave and develop our patience and remember that all is taken care of in its rightful time. I pray for guidance when I feel weak and I ask that both God and yourself forgive me when I fail you both as I so often do.

If the weekends we now spend together are a glimpse of the times we shall spend together eternally, then my heart almost bursts with the very thought of it. I feel so fortunate and so very happy. Would, or indeed could anyone believe that I feel so happy during what is your greatest struggle.

Please know my darling Blue that I shall be by your side to hopefully uphold you, to share with you as well as to infuriate you and madden you but always to love.

I am with you always my darling,

Andrea xxx.

Wednesday 29ᵗʰ August 2007.

7.30a.m Derek was sitting in his chair when I arrived, we greeted each other and he came across as being very cheerful. We chatted about different countries and places we had visited and what food in other countries that we enjoyed.

Derek went to the toilet twice between my arrival and 8.30a.m, he was able to flush the toilet and washed and dried his hands without being told.

He remarked how late breakfast was this morning and when it did at last arrive

he noticed immediately that he had not been given a fork. Derek ate all of his breakfast without help.

10.00a.m *Dr. Pinder came to see Derek, he had a chat and asked several questions.*

10.20a.m *After Dr. Pinder's visit Derek and I sat chatting for a while.*

11.15a.m *Derek had a shower with minimal assistance required, he part dried himself and dressed with a little help, I put his socks on and he was able to put on his slippers. He is very happy and cheerful.*

Derek is now drawing shapes and he is doing really well.

12.15p.m *Dinner has arrived, I have put the plate guard on and Derek is using his knife to cut through his boiled potatoes, he is really enjoying his lunch and no assistance seems to be needed. Derek has a very good and healthy appetite.*

I have really enjoyed my shift with Derek and have seen a huge improvement from three months ago when I first met him.

Entered by C. Fitzpatrick (H.C.A.)

12.45p.m *Derek is a very different person today, very bright, keen and alert. He states that he has spent a very good morning and has explained Dr, Pinders visit.*

He says that he now feels very hopeful as a result of this visit and says how he longs to hear of news that a bed is ready for him at rehab.

As he has not been for a walk, I took him down the stairs, out of the side entrance and around the perimeter of the car park and back through the main entrance, up the stairs and back to his room. (Around the car park is my idea of introducing Derek to traffic and attempting to re-teach him road sense in a more controlled environment). The traffic did not seem to confuse him but he definitely has no concept of the dangers or the fact that cars might not have the time to stop just because he suddenly decides to walk into the road.

When I suggested that he had a rest he readily agreed stating that he thought he needed one before he started his exercises.

Lying on his bed Derek told me of how he had been practicing drawing shapes during the morning and how he himself had decided to do so without being asked by someone else and went on to explain that this was the new directive and assertive Derek and how he had thought it was time for him to be so. I told him I was delighted to hear this and that he must keep it going.

2.15p.m *Derek is now fast asleep. I would note that I have witnessed his left hand and arm is still being used and that he is still able to use them in conjunction with his right hand and arm. I feel that the exercises we have been doing each day are really beginning to pay off, I sincerely hope so and that thois progress is permanent. We will* *continue with them when he wakes up, he loves his exercises, there again exercise was always such a part of Derek's life.*

Derek has been telling me how difficult he finds it to write, he claims that it actually hurts his brain dealing with it. He added that he finds everything back to front or upside down and I have become more than a little concerned that perhaps I may be confusing him even further.

4.00p.m *Derek awoke and I decided that a little sit in the fresh air, enjoying the sunshine would do him more good than exercising anymore today.*

We sat outside on a bench and he is very upbeat and happy. One of the doctors stopped for a little chat and said how well he thought Derek was coming on, this pleased him even further.

Sadly I must leave a little earlier this evening so must hand over to his sitter before dinner, but I will wait until it arrives.

Entered by Andrea Craig.

5.55p.m *I took over from Derek's wife. Derek enjoyed his meal which he ate without assistance.*

Entered by (H.C.A.)

21.00p.m *Derek was in the day room watching television when I arrived on duty. Unfortunately there wasn't anything of interest on so at 10p.m* *we returned to his room where Derek listened to his radio until he took his evening medication.*

Derek was restless in bed throughout the night and got up to go to the toilet four times.

Derek got up at 6.45a.m to go to the toilet and afterwards sat in his chair and listened to his radio and had a cup of tea.

Entered by Joan Lomax (H.C.A.)

Thursday 30th August 2007.

8.00a.m *Derek and I said hello, I introduced myself and then Derek continued to listen to the radio through his head phones. He has his eyes closed and does not seem to want to talk.*

8.25a.m *Derek started chatting, we talked about his wife and his son who lives in Germany. Derek seems very happy this morning.*

Entered by Sue Collinge (H.C.A.)

8.30am *I took over from Sue, Derek was listening to his radio. He ate breakfast at 9.00a.m.*

Derek went to the toilet and had an accident through not pulling his underpants down far enough. No problem, we showered and dressed with only a little help needed. However Derek feels that he cannot co-ordinate this morning.

11.20a.m Occupational Therapy. *We practiced bed transfers. Derek managed to get* *himself into and out of the bed and was able to talk through his actions while he was doing them.*

Derek was talking about his son, Paul, working in Germany.

He was orientated to time and able to say the day and month.

We practiced telling the time on the clock, but he did have difficulty seeing the little hand.

Entered by Michelle Kolowski (Occupational Therapist).

I took Derek for two walks around the hospital this morning but refrained from going outside due to bad weather.

Derek is eating his lunch with minimal assistance.

Entered by (H.C.A.)

12.30p.m *Derek was eating his lunch when I arrived, I was pleased to note that he was doing so without the aid of the plate guard.*

I am taking him to keep an eye appointment with his own optician at the request of the eye clinic.

3.30p.m *Derek's eye sight was declared normal to his last prescription, which was April just prior to his cardiac arrest.*

Derek had said it would be lovely if we could have tea and teacakes before going back so that is just what we had. He so enjoyed this treat which he thought he might never experience again. Amazing how such ordinary everyday happenings such, as popping into a coffee shop, take on a much more enjoyable and colourful meaning. The coffee shop was in our local village near to the opticians we had just visited and Derek voiced how normal this had helped to make him feel.

Derek is now having a lie down after a busy day but he is stating quite firmly that he is not in need of a rest. I know that he is and have been equally firm in insisting that he has one.

3.45p.m *Derek now in a deep sleep, (so much for him not needing one!)*

5.45p.m *Derek is now well and rested and has eaten all of his dinner, which he thoroughly enjoyed. It was eaten without assistance or plate guard.*

I helped to wash and change Derek ready for bed later.

Entered by Andrea Craig.

5.45p.m *Derek was listening to his radio, some music he said he liked.*

Later he listened to the news but he says that it is always such bad news.

We walked down to the day room at 7.00p.m to watch television and I left him there with the nurse on night duty.

Entered by Victoria Roberts (H.C.A.)

21.00p.m *Derek was in the day room when I came on tonight, watching t.v. He went to bed at 10.15p.m and had a good night's sleep. He only got up twice to go to the toilet, this is a tremendous improvement from when I first met Derek three and a half months ago. Well done Derek!*

Entered by Cathy Robinson (H.C.A.)

Friday 31st August 2007.

Speech Therapy Session.

I began a Language Assessment with Derek, he found it challenging but he worked very hard.

Entered by Rebecca Smith (Speech Therapist).

Derek was awake when I arrived this morning, he was very chatty and happy.

He was able to shower himself with a little assistance and help was required with dressing, he was very chatty throughout and said he had enjoyed his therapy session a little later.

Entered by unknown.

12.30p.m *Derek was bright and happy when I arrived and very excited at going home. He has related all that took place with Rebecca.*

We are ready and waiting for the handover of his medication.

Entered by Andrea Craig.

CHAPTER TWELVE

It has been four long and extremely emotional months since that almost fatal Saturday morning of April 28th. During that time, Derek has struggled and stumbled to find his way through the foothills of a mountain he once thought far too high to even contemplate its ascent, but now with the help of a wonderful medical team, the caring and encouragement from his first class nurses, but mainly I believe, through his own steely determination, he is successfully well into the climb.

Nevertheless there have been times when Derek's fears of failure were very nearly proved to be justified, times when indeed the climb became too arduous and he was no longer able to maintain his grip or keep his footing. It was the afternoon of Wednesday 25th July that he experienced one such time. He found himself, symbolically of course, careering in freefall down a rock face, too sheer to offer any hope of salvation.

We had been sitting in his room working on the alphabet and word cards when suddenly he began trying to explain to me how very desperately tired he was feeling in the unrelenting effort it was costing him each and every waking moment and that he felt he could no longer carry on.

I sat quietly listening to him and in my mind's eye I saw before me the image of Derek clinging by his finger tips to the side of a mountain with a look of sheer terror on his face as though he were about to lose his grip. I began to lean forward to beg him not to give up, to plead with him to keep on but something held me back and I found myself looking in horror as the image before me changed and I realized that I was looking at the steepest and sheerest of rock faces I had ever seen stretching up far above him. I was looking at a rock face as smooth as silk with not the slightest indent for him to place a foot or for him to grip hold of. I found myself lost for words, for this image was showing me that this mountain was indeed too steep and impossible for him to climb.

I could see no way, yet I knew there had to be one, there simply had to be, I could not allow this wonderful man who sat before to simply slide into a dark abyss. I struggled to find the words, knowing that as I spoke they would not be capable of lifting him up high enough to clear that sheer rock face I found impossible to remove from my vision. Derek kept apologizing for feeling so pessimistic, but try as he might, he could do nothing to ward off the feeling of exhaustion which seemed to be overpowering him. It was at this point he actually told me that he felt he was losing his grip and feared that he was about to lose the fight.

I sat trying to raise his spirits and somehow feed him the strength he so desperately needed, I described how he was not alone, that we were climbing this mountain together with the help of and support of the most wonderful team of people anyone could possibly have. I was beginning to feel the strain as my words began echoing lifelessly around the room, and I found myself wondering how much longer I could continue holding him up when I heard a knock upon the door and in walked Dr. Pinder.

His presence during those early days always unnerved Derek, who believed he was being tested, which of course was true, but in spite of his anxiousness, Derek felt that his whole life depended upon this man. He believed that this was the man who was going to help him climb the remainder of his mountain, right to the very summit. He desperately wanted to prove to this doctor just how ready and capable he was, but at the same time he realized full well his inability to do so. He used to tell me how totally inadequate he believed himself to be when being assessed and how wide open and very vunerable he always felt.

I found Dr. Pinder to be a man of few words, he wasted none and those he spoke carried full meaning. This was a doctor I respected on first meeting him, a man I later discovered had climbed his own mountain in life, which I believed enabled him to have that special empathy I felt him to have with his patients along with the dedicated medical knowledge and expertise with which he has helped so many. Whereby he unnerved Derek somewhat, he instilled me with a strength and confidence I might not otherwise have had at that time. I believed he was the only person who could guide us along the treacherous journey which lay ahead.

Dr. Pinder walked across the room to where Derek and I were seated and motioning us both to remain where we were, he sat down on the bed opposite Derek. He talked to Derek asking him what day of the week it was, could he remember any of the topical events being reported in the news etc. Occasionally he asked me to pass him a letter of the alphabet we had been working with or an object which had been lying on the table, that he might use with Derek, otherwise I simply sat back and observed.

I felt Derek was showing much greater improvement on his last assessment and was therefore so taken aback when Dr. Pinder abruptly completing his assessment, snapped his file closed and on swiftly rising from the bed announced that it was his medical duty to inform us both that it was now clear that Derek would never make a full and complete recovery. I vaguely heard him telling Derek how he could be helped to live within the limitations he would now find imposed upon him. I heard the words but they sounded as though they were coming from somewhere far, far away. I was much more concerned with the man I saw in front of me falling, falling as though in slow motion right before my eyes and I will never forget the look of abject desolation etched upon his face.

This man was my husband, a man who had been hanging on with all of his might until he had felt his fingers slipping from the solidness he had been clinging hold of. In that moment I realized how far up his mountain Derek had climbed for the distance he covered as he fell was great. He was not panicking at all or struggling to find a hold, nor was he concerned at the thought of what lay awaiting him, it was as though the life had gone from him and it was all too much. I could only sit by helplessly unable to do anything as I watched him drop, this man who had against all the odds and direst of prognosis, worked so hard to achieve so much, suddenly plummeting before my eyes towards, if not to his doom, then a very dark place.

I could not believe what I had just witnessed. How could this doctor, this man I so respected be the one who had caused Derek to finally lose his grip. Instead of encouragement and nurturing him at a time when he needed it most, this doctor might as well have stamped on those fingers which were clinging so desperately until the blood almost ran, for he was definitely the one who caused Derek to finally lose his hold.

From far away I heard the words, "How extremely lucky you have been, Derek", but these were just words, hollow notes bouncing around the room which had now turned quite cold.

I was aware of Dr. Pinder leaving the room but I was more concerned for the man, whose body now slumped forward in his chair holding his head between his hands rocking from side to side and sobbing like a baby. Quickly pushing the table aside I knelt before him and held him tight and all I could do was cry with him. All the effort and hard work of the last three months were suddenly as nothing. I was holding a man from drowning. I knew he was drowning for I had seen him plummet down the side of a mountain into a great, dark, crashing sea. How could this doctor have been so cruel and how could I have been so wrong in my judgement of him?

A little while later after Derek had calmed down I swilled my face and managed to persuade him to do the same and suggested we went for a walk. It felt better being out in the fresh-air and we sat taking in the last of the sunshine before it finally went down and was lost behind the hospital building. We talked calmly over the news we had just received and Derek asked if I would explain once again exactly what Dr. Pinder had meant. He listened intently and then very quietly told me that he would find it very difficult continuing with life the way it stood and that he no longer felt he had the energy to carry on.

I gently hushed him and told him that we both needed time to allow the news and its implications to sink in and that I felt sure it would not be as bad as we believed it was going to be at that moment. We returned to his room and I stayed with him longer than I normally did after dinner but he had no desire to talk to anyone that evening and said that he simply wished to go to bed early and go to sleep.

I made my way home and after completing the washing routine which was still in operation each and every evening because of the MRSA infection I found myself too tired and emotionally drained to eat my evening meal so I showered and climbed into bed where I immediately felt myself falling, falling totally unable to stop myself, I knew that I was not yet asleep and still I continued to fall until at last I hit something which at first felt to be as hard as concrete but then realized that I had in fact fallen into deep water. I knew instantly that I had crashed into the same dark sea that I had witnessed Derek plunge into earlier that day.

I looked around desperately trying to find Derek, who I knew would be floundering in the great surge and swell of water as it crashed against the rocks. I felt certain we were both about to drown, or be crushed to death against the side of this dark foreboding mountain as it rose up out of the sea, looming high above us. Then quite suddenly I felt the waters calming, the swell was settling and instead of the icy coldness which had almost claimed my last breath, I felt a warmth wrap itself around me, inviting me to surrender and rest. I lifted my eyes and looked up to where we had fallen from and thought how, in God's name, are we ever going to be able to climb back up there, for all I could see was a sheer vertical rock face which looked impossible to climb, even if we had had the energy, which we had not.

I was far from happy with Dr. Pinder, whom I considered had pushed my husband into a position from which there appeared to be no return and I could not help my last uncharitable thoughts as the protective warmth saving me from the cold, cold waters drew me into sleep. I remember hoping that if I were now resting in this newly felt warmth, then Derek would be also.

The next couple of days were spent encouraging Derek to see the benefit of continuing with his exercises and therapy program, and outwardly it worked for he soon appeared to be his usual happy and cheery self once more, but inwardly it was a completely different matter. Derek was a broken man and continued to be deeply disturbed regarding the recent news Dr. Pinder had delivered.

During the afternoon of July 30th Derek declared that he felt more thoughtful than he had ever felt before in his entire life but felt he could not share these feelings with anyone, not even myself, in fact he did not wish to talk at all so I left him to sit quietly until it was time for him to be taken down to the eye clinic to have a 'field test' carried out. Later when the porter had delivered Derek back to his room I asked him if he felt ready for a drink to which he replied with a whispered, "Yes". I poured out a glass of water and as I handed it to him I nearly dropped it as Derek fell forward with great heart rendering sobs. Quickly placing the glass down I knelt before him begging him to tell me what was bothering him. Between his sobs he at last managed to confide how lost and afraid he was feeling and how he felt as though he were drowning in a sea from which he could find no escape.

I made no attempt to dry away his tears for Derek had a lot to cry out of his system, instead I chose to share with him my experience on dropping off to sleep the previous night. I was still trying to console Derek when I heard a knock upon the door and in walked Dr. Oates and her entire team. Dr. Oates saw immediately that all was not well with her patient and moved quickly to our side of the room. I stood up and moved back allowing room for her to sit directly before Derek. Her medical team remained on the far side of the room observing and noting.

Derek was too emotional and unable to explain what it was that was troubling him and so looking to me, Dr. Oates asked quietly what was wrong. I began to relate what had transpired during Dr. Pinder's last visit. My explanation was brief as Dr. Pinder had himself used very few words in his delivery but at the same time I did feel the need to convey my heartfelt regret with the manner in which he had chosen to deliver them.

I also begged the team of young doctors to note the effect that delivering bad news could have on a man. I asked that each of them when finding themselves in a position of delivering such news should try to remember that whilst bad news needs to be delivered, it should not be done in a way to destroy or demoralize the patient. I ventured to add that 'learned knowledge' was nothing when compared to what had still to be learned from that vast ocean of the unknown.

Dr. Oates and her team afforded me the grace of listening to my every word that day and after I had finished speaking Dr. Oates leaned forward and very gently taking hold of Derek's hands spoke the words which managed to forge their way straight through to Derek's heart, affecting both Derek and myself deeply and I will remember them for the rest of my life.

It is not too strong to say that room 23 was emotionally charged that afternoon. A still silence filled the room except for Dr. Oates words. Her words carried an authority which transcended medical knowledge and helped to hold up a man from drowning in waters which were threatening to claim him.

Her words, although spoken quietly, were directed strongly as she begged Derek to look at her. Slowly Derek raised his head as the doctor took him back to the early days of his recovery when I had been told it would be unlikely for him to survive, "But you did", she stated, "I was also there right at the beginning when your wife was told that if you did survive then the outcome would not be good. That you would be severely brain damaged and perhaps live in a permanent vegetative state and once again you proved us wrong. Every prognosis that was made you managed to prove us wrong and now I'm asking that you do the same once more. I ask that you take what Dr. Pinder has given you and digest it with the respect it so rightly deserves and then, Derek I want you to move on and prove him wrong, just as you have done with the rest of us". The doctor holding Derek's complete attention continued, "I have just listened to your wife talk about a vast ocean of the unknown and I would tell you this, that right from the start I have watched you steer your own unique course through unchartered waters and we doctors in Arrowe Park Hospital are having to run extremely fast to keep up with you".

Throughout the whole time this wonderful doctor talked to her dispirited patient I never once took my eyes from my husband and what I looked upon that afternoon raised my spirits sky high as I witnessed Derek's spirit lifting up out of the dark cold water. I watched spellbound as he continued to rise way up and beyond the very rock face which only hours before had caused me to believe there could be no way of ever overcoming this sheerest and steepest of obstacles. But Derek had been lifted up and helped to rise above his latest setback and it showed in his facial expression, his eyes shone with life and renewed hope, he was back on his pathway climbing his mountain once more.

I left Derek that evening more excited than I had ever seen him. He had been told before Dr.

Oates had left his room that he could celebrate his birthday weekend at home which he claimed was the best medicine he could ever be given. Driving home I could not stop myself from laughing at how he had begged me to go earlier tomorrow as he was keen to crack on as soon as possible with his therapy program. Derek was feeling so much better and I was feeling a lot happier. So happy in fact I came to realize that I had done Dr. Pinder a great disservice with the harsh thoughts I had harboured and can only say that those thoughts were never directed from my heart, only from the tormented mind of a woman lashing out against the cruelties of life and how easily those fates come to almost breaking each and every one of us.

On waking the following morning I also realized that if Dr. Pinder had not knocked Derek from the position he was struggling to keep a hold of then Dr. Oates would never have been able to lift him above it. I began to think perhaps Dr. Pinder had not been cruel in his delivery and perhaps experience had proved to him that before a man can move on he must first be knocked down from the position he is stuck in. Sadly he had the unenviable task of doing that and I am so pleased he had the strength to do it. I believe that each doctor played an equal part in helping Derek clear that difficult and seemingly impossible part of his climb and I thank both of them from the bottom of my heart, each for the very special part they played.

With my newly acquired realization would I still ask a young doctor to take note of their deliverance of bad news? My answer is yes I would. I believe Derek could have been knocked down, so to speak, without being crashed into a dark sea of despair.

No matter what I found myself doing during the mornings at home my thoughts were never far away from Derek and the morning following Dr. Oates' visit proved to be very much the case. I felt lighter than I had felt in a long time and had awakened, not only happy with my renewed faith in Dr. Pinder, but also remembering the last part of the message I had received at our evening of meditation during the week prior to Derek's collapse. I had been told that I would have to be very brave and very strong but most of all I would have to be so very, very patient in the days ahead. A message I was obviously unable to share with Derek at that time but do so now in the truth that it was given. I was told that Derek was about to begin laying a pathway that others would follow, except of course that the choice of others to follow is theirs and theirs alone and I can only suggest that when like Derek, you find your own pathway too difficult, do not give up even when you feel you might be losing everything and you are losing your grip on your own upward struggle. Please do not fear that you may fall, for if you do there may be a need for you to do so before you can raise yourself that much higher.

The past four months entries into Derek's diaries have recorded the general daily happenings over that period but what they cannot truly register are the deep lows and the lofty heights of his recovery, the heartache, the despair or the many tears shed by Derek who was mourning a loss so great he could neither fathom nor understand it.

The many tears I shed with him and, when on my own, those I shed for him and selfishly those I shed for myself mourning the loss of a life we would never live or know again, for life as we had both lived it had been good and was now gone and sadly, all loss leaves one grieving. But if we would as individuals only take the time to look deeply enough, we would discover that there is balance in all things and Derek and I were to discover the joy shared in each new step that he took.

The sense of achievement we felt when a new task was relearned, the laughter we shared on many an occasion but what has touched me more so than any other and brought about the greatest sense of balance to our considered loss, has been in the witnessing of the expression upon Derek's face as he re-discovered all those tiny little things we take so much for granted. The warmth of the sun on his face, the feel of the rain and the freshness he felt it brought to him. The formation of clouds which he never tired of studying, when lying on Derek's hospital bed, one could almost believe you were floating amongst them such was the view from his great expanse of window on the third floor. How his face would light up on hearing Sarah's footsteps walking along the corridor towards his room and the light which radiated from him whenever he thought of his beloved son.

Yes, there was indeed so much to bring a sense of balance into our situation, even though Derek was clinging to his mountain with all the strength that he had. My own personal inner balance was found through holding onto the very life we were actually living and the letting go of a life which had once been but was no longer, it had gone and therefore was as nothing.

I have endeavored to live my life through the teachings of a few wise words once given to me many years ago when I was asked "to live not in fear of the past, nor stand in dread of the future, but to open my heart to the 'Spirit of Simplicity' and that of 'Balance' and know that the 'Sea of Tranquility' would uphold me now and always". Those wise words of Truth have never failed to support me during my many times of weakness and self doubt, and I found that they have certainly strengthened and upheld me during this particular period of my life.

Going back to the first two months of May and June, it can be seen to be the time of a miraculous progress in Derek. I had indeed been informed that his recovery was nothing short of a miracle and had been hitherto unknown and that he was medically unprecedented. During the month of July I was informed by Derek's consulting cardiologist that because of his conditional uniqueness this, perhaps unfortunately, placed Derek in a position of the unknown.

His angiogram had shown "two-vessel disease" but generally his arteries were considered to be healthier than many men half his age. I had no idea what "two vessel disease" meant and it was further explained to me as there having been an offending site which had been the cause of a clot breaking free and travelling immediately to the heart causing the cardiac arrest. I was told how darned unlucky Derek had been and how he had been living as a ticking time bomb for what could have been years.

Derek, to all intent and purposes had died. His heart had stopped and his body had closed down, at the time of this happening Derek had made, so I am told, medical history for having survived an out of hospital cardiac arrest and being without oxygen to the brain for as long as he had been. It was finally explained to me that medical opinion was divided as to how he should be further treated and such was the dilemma of his uniqueness, it placed Derek directly in the middle of fifty percent opinion on one side advising the insertion of stents and fifty percent opinion on the other advising us of the medicinal route, and so it was that these men that both Derek and I were looking to for expert help and guidance could offer none, they could only quote medical facts, they stated percentages and statistics and then told me that I must instruct them as to what should be done next. I felt that Dr. Newall was in favour of continuing down the road of treatment by medication, although he never actually said as much.

I was thrown into a sea of confusion, how on earth could I possibly instruct this doctor, when I was truly ignorant of such matters, I say "I" as opposed to "we" for Derek simply looked to me to make the decision for him, such was his trust in me. Doing what I considered to be the only sensible thing I could do, I requested a second opinion and so an appointment was made to see a Dr.Palmer at Broadgreen Hospital whereby we discussed the insertion of 'stents', one to be positioned in the 'offending site' and a second stent to be positioned in an area of possible future concern.

Before this appointment was kept, Derek and I, after listening to Dr.Newall and all that he had had to say, talked in great detail and we reached the agreement that as we had requested a second opinion we would therefore be guided and be prepared to abide by Dr. Palmers stated opinion. For the time being Derek was happy to have had his angiogram, believing that we could now move forward in a more positive way, and so it was that we put his heart condition to one side so as to be able to concentrate on his "relearning program" as we had come to refer to it.

As the days passed by we experienced good and bad days and those days which could only be described as fantastic, such as the days when I walked Derek around the park, soaking up the hot sunshine on the few days that we had sunshine to enjoy, for most of that summer I spent having to make a fast dash from the car to the hospital entrance in torrential rain. But on looking back it is to those lovely sunny days that I am drawn, when we strolled around the park hand in hand, totally oblivious to the risk we were taking or any thought to what might have happened had Derek collapsed. Had any of his doctors looked out from the hospital windows and taken notice of this happy couple strolling by would they ever have believed one of those people to be Derek, I think not. I must add that I had been informed of what is called a crash number to ring in an emergency when Derek had first begun his walks around the hospital and as I always had my mobile phone with me, I did not consider myself to be totally irresponsible.

Whilst walking in the park or taking time to sit on one of its benches, Derek could, for a short period of time, forget that he was a hospital in-patient. Outside in the fresh-air his spirits would soar and on returning to his room he would often express a greater awareness and eagerness in carrying out his "learning tasks". As well as our visits to the park we did, on several occasions, return to visit our friend George and there enjoy afternoon tea usually on a Saturday or Sunday when all was quiet within the hospital. Derek did enjoy those times but none more than the time spent in his own home.

It had been August before he had been granted a whole weekend leave to spend at home. I had kept this as a surprise for his forthcoming birthday on the 10th August which was, as recorded in his diaries, a huge success but extremely exhausting at the same time.

After 10th August, Derek was granted permanent weekend leave, although they were to be shorter in duration than that first birthday weekend, and he grew to live for this time at home and anything, usually away from the hospital environment, which gave him back a sense of normality.

From a man who had been too afraid, on first regaining consciousness, to face his own reflection in the mirror, I found him on numerous occasions at home, looking into the mirror, as though deeply studying himself and very unsure of what he was seeing. A look of grave concern would cast a dark shadow over him which Derek was always reluctant to talk about and when questioned would quickly shrug it off as nothing. I believe that, Derek on believing himself to be only twenty five years of age when he first regained consciousness, was so shocked on first seeing his own reflection that he could not take the much older, and in his mind damaged, image looking back at him.

These home visits became the highlight of Derek's life and as reluctant as he always was to return to his room on Monday mornings, once reinstated it was never very long before he bounced back up to his ever hopeful and increasingly optimistic self. These visits, along with the planned 'one to one' visitors he was now allowed, were some of the highs that spurred Derek on in his upward climb and kept his spirit strong.

We had indeed lived through four long and difficult months but at least Derek had managed to fight off his infections and when the results finally came through that he was clear of his MRSA the relief proved too much and as the staff-nurse in charge broke the news to me I was unable to hold back the tears. I remember Clare putting her arms around me and telling me that it was good to cry and I agreed but felt I had to pull myself together very quickly incase I should never stop.

CHAPTER THIRTEEN

It was now September, our fifth month in hospital and on the advice of Dr. Palmer it had been decided that Derek's 'stents' would be inserted after his rehabilitation and we were eagerly awaiting news that a bed was available in the Neuro.unit. We felt optimistic and upbeat and thoroughly enjoyed our treasured weekends at home.

During those long stretched out months one could rise from the depths of despair to the lofty heights of happiness in such a short space of time and of course vice versa, one could never be sure of anything, we could only live for the moment and Derek and I embraced each one with all that we had.

It seemed that life in 'Arrowe Park' was coming to its end and Derek was excitedly looking forward to moving on. He believed that any day now he would be transferring to the unit which was going to complete his recovery.

Andrea Craig

Monday 3rd September 2007.

12.45p.m Derek adjusted very well coming back to hospital today, much happier than he usually is on Mondays.

He has eaten his lunch with no help whatsoever and no plate guard. He is now managing very well at meal times using both hands with knife and fork as normal, although he is still slow and has to concentrate hard.

Derek's biggest break through to-date is causing amazement to both him and myself with his ever increasing ability to recognize more and more words. This pleases him so much.

The weekend was another huge success. We enjoyed a few walks, a visit with a friend, which was the first since he had collapsed and plenty of relaxation.

I encouraged Derek to exercise both arms regularly and to instill a greater confidence in his walking. (One can definitely notice a slight deformity in his left arm which becomes noticeable causing a twist in his clothing).

Derek is trying very hard with his undressing which he can now almost manage but unfortunately he cannot manage at all with dressing himself.

We laughed several times as he believed he had it "cracked" when putting on his dressing gown to discover that he had in fact put it half on back to front.

Derek still tries to put two shoes onto one foot and claims that his brain cannot recognize two feet at the same time and added asking, "what did I expect when they were so far away from his brain." I do hope that Derek never ever loses his great sense of humour, he is my husband and I love him deeply and I also find him a sheer joy to be with.

He has, this weekend, managed to fill the kettle, (stating that his left hand and arm is definitely now a lot stronger), last week he could not manage to lift it at all.

He is also helping me to set the table and clear away after meals.

He gets very confused with drawers and cupboards. He finds it difficult to understand that handles are there to help open them.

Derek is unable to recognize the difference between fridge and freezer but is showing signs that are encouraging.

He can now manage screw tops very well but is hesitant in pouring liquid out as his hand is so shakey and I have noticed that he does not seem to be able to see water at all. We have had lots of accidents with the overflowing of water. I have tried to show him how to use his finger to feel the level as it nears the top of the cup or glass (cold water of course but have stopped this as I feel it might confuse him whenever he comes to pour hot).

The greatest area of concern is still night times, I am getting very little sleep and Derek's sleep is very disturbed. He has no problems dropping off, the trouble comes in his frequent trips to the toilet and then not being able to get himself back into bed, although he has succeeded on two or three occasions to get into bed but then could not cover himself over.

On one occasion I discovered Derek had removed all his bedding and his night clothes and was lying shivering with cold. I jokingly told him that the secret was for him to learn how to reverse the order of sequence and that he should cover himself and not strip everything off. He was not aware of what he had done and was totally confused as to what I was talking about but the following morning he remembered the incident and went on to explain that it was just a blip and that he had got a little confused with the bedding and had decided that the simplest thing for him to do was to strip everything off and start again. He went on to say that it was just unfortunate he had forgotten what he was supposed to be doing and that if I had left him a little longer then he would have done it, and in future would I not be so quick to jump in and take over!

The other area of fresh concern but is not problematic at the moment because Derek is never out alone, is the fact that he has no road sense whatsoever. This is something I have had no reason to think of before now but will have to deal with in the near future.

1.35p.m   Derek was keen to try reading after lunch and has browsed through the newspaper picking out various words. The perculiar thing is that Derek does not always pick out the same words and is yet able to recognize new ones. He says he knows this and must ask his therapist to help him to understand why.

2.00p.m   Derek has said he feels very tired and is now lying down resting.

3.30p.m   Derek got up and went to toilet and had just returned back to his room when Dr. Oates arrived. After her visit we played Connect 4, Derek is now learning the concept of the game.

4.15p.m   I took Derek for a walk down the stairs to the ground floor and out into the main car-park. I followed Derek to see how he coped with limited traffic conditions. He managed very well doing his best to concentrate on sounds of approaching vehicles but was not able to understand why he must look left or right when crossing a road and on the way back he suddenly decided take off and walk up the middle of the road on the busy approach to the main entrance.

When stopped and asked why he had decided to do that he explained that it seemed to be the shortest route back. I explained how dangerous that action had been but Derek seemed unable to grasp that fact.

He then proceeded to walk me back to his room knowing exactly where he was going and choosing to return walking up all flights of stairs which he seems to enjoy, stating good exercise. Derek now recognizes hospital and its grounds and finds his way about if it is not too busy.

He stated that he enjoyed his walk very much today and is looking forward to his dinner as he feels hungry.

5.30p.m Derek ate his meal once again unaided and has stated that he would like to watch the evening news and Silent Witness a little later on as it helps to pass the time.

Derek has been washed and changed and is ready for bed later.

Tuesday 4th September 2007.

Derek was still in bed but awake when I arrived, we had a little chat, then decided he would like his shower before breakfast. Minimal assistance was given with showering and help given with his dressing.

Derek is now sitting waiting for breakfast stating how hungry he feels! He is listening to his radio.

Derek enjoyed his breakfast and said he would try to do some writing. I wrote his name and he copied, doing very well.

We went for a stroll around the grounds but it was a bit nippy out of the sun.

Derek decided he would like to listen to his radio and have a rest and very quickly fell into a deep sleep.

12.00 noon. *Awakened and said he still felt tired but is looking forward to his lunch.*

Entered by Helen (H.C.A.)

12.30p.m *Derek was busily chatting away when I arrived with both himself and his sitter wondering what had happened to lunch. I have just been informed that breakfast had to be queried as that did not turn up either. I went to enquire and it had indeed been forgotten, someone had to be sent off to the kitchens to bring a lunch up for him. Derek has also told me that there had been no sitter last night and that he got into difficulty going to the toilet and not able to get back into bed?*

This leaves me very concerned incase of accident!

1.30p.m *Derek has been rather subdued since lunch and when asked if something was bothering him stated that he is now so fed up with it all.*

3.30p.m *In spite of a low mood to the start of the afternoon we have spent a very productive one with Derek keen to participate in everything that was asked of him.*

First of all we started off with trimming his hair and beard followed by exercising his arms, paying particular attention to his left arm which is now tremendously more flexible compared to a few weeks back.

We played throwing and bouncing the small ball and must say how good it was to see Derek's competitive streak beginning to show through once more.

He was really trying to keep me on my toes today which was good.

We moved onto the building blocks with which I marked a great improvement from the last time we used these. Derek is now able to recognize nearly all of the different colours which I think may have been previously confused due to his colour blindness and not solely down to his brain damage.

He was able to place every brick in position according to my instruction without any help or guidance.

His ability to read the notices and signs placed around the hospital has also been amazing and Derek is noticeably very pleased with this saying it gives him hope that he can return to normality.

He is continually asking for information and stating that he needs to know more detail of what has happened to him and that he must find the way back!

I find this all very sad and tragic but at the same time a very fascinating journey we are travelling with boredom being the biggest enemy.

A great deal of the time Derek feels he is wasting away or climbing the four walls of his room.

I can usually talk him out of these moods but as time marches on he feels he has been forgotten and it is becoming increasingly more difficult to keep his spirits up.

Derek stated that he would enjoy a little fresh-air so we went outside and sat in the sunshine for ten minutes before returning to his room where he is now asleep on his bed. He has fallen into a very deep relaxed sleep.

As we sat outside he told me once again of how little sleep he had last night and of how he did not know where he was and that he had been trying to find someone to help him. (Staff has already spoken to me regarding this matter, hopefully will not happen again!).

5.30p.m Derek ate his meal unaided and has stated how tired he has felt today and apologized for not being himself but that he tried to make up for this by working hard (which he has, so very hard, well done Derek).

Derek managed to take both of his socks off this evening and even put one back on but could not manage the other saying that he feels the room is too sickly hot, which it is and I have noticed that the air-conditioning unit which has been very much needed when the sun hits this room has now been removed!

Nurse kindly brought Derek a fan and I am staying with him until he has cooled down a little. I feel so reluctant to leave him this evening,

Derek seems a little lost and very vunerable.

Entered by Andrea Craig.

9.00p.m *Derek was sitting in the day room with an H.C.A. called Jenny watching the television when I arrived on duty this evening.*

Jenny tells me that they have spent a pleasant evening with a walk around the grounds and enjoyed a chat about healing which Derek seemed to enjoy very much.

10.15p.m *Derek has now settled down for the night after I had assisted with his night mask.*

00.15a.m *Derek went to toilet with minimal assistance and went straight back to sleep.*

3.00a.m *Derek requested removal of blanket as he was feeling too warm.*

7.30a.m *After falling back to sleep Derek has spent a good night.*

Wednesday 5th September 2007.

7.30a.m Derek was still asleep in bed when I arrived getting up at 7.45a.m. He showered and washed his hair with a little assistance. We then carried out some arm exercises while waiting for breakfast.

After breakfast medication was given and Derek listened to his radio and dozed on and off.

He did not wish to do any writing just yet said he would later.

11.25a.m We went for a walk around the grounds after the rain had gone off.

Derek is now sitting listening to his radio not wanting to do very much at all this morning, says he is just waiting for his lunch.

Entered by Unknown.

12.45p.m Derek was finishing his lunch when I arrived and has stated that he feels unhappy and very down-hearted.

I tried to explain that I understood his frustration but that we must be even more constructive in our endeavour to progress. He responded by saying he would do some writing practice to start with.

Derek has informed me that he has spent a good night having slept well with no problems and that he was no trouble to anyone last night, not like the night before!

He also added that he seriously doubts if anyone could ever really know how frustrated he feels right now and that he does not know how he can carry on.

We practiced writing but his heart was not in it and he was soon feeling tired and has asked if I would excuse him today as he wanted to rest.

2.15p.m *Derek is now asleep on his bed, (only he is not really asleep for I notice him peeping now and then).*

I have just received news that Derek is down for next available bed in Neuro.-rehab. (This is good news).

5.00p.m *Derek has slept, apart from a walk downstairs, for most of the afternoon saying he did not feel good today, he was fed up.*

5.30p.m *Derek ate all of his meal unaided and Sarah cheered him up.*

Entered by Andrea Craig.

Derek watched television in day-room, went to bed at 10.00p.m. He got up a few times in the night to use the toilet.

He got up at 7.00a.m
Entered by unknown.

Thursday 6ᵗʰ September 2007.

Derek was sat in his chair when I arrived this morning. He had a shower with minimal assistance needed.

Derek ate a good breakfast but said that he has never been able to eat the hospital bacon! He listened to the radio for a while, he likes to get the news, then we went for a walk around the grounds.

Coming back to his room Derek tried some writing then we had a go at a crossword.

12.00 noon *Derek was not impressed with his lunch today as the beef was too tough to chew, but has said that he has had more than enough to eat, thank-you.*

I asked Derek if he would like to do anything else and he said no that he would just listen to his radio while waiting for Andrea to arrive.

A member of Dr. Oates' team came and said will call back to see Mrs. Craig.

Entered by Helen (H.C.A.)

12.45p.m *Derek seems much more cheerful today. He claims that he feels eager to get on and has now worked for the last hour and forty-five minutes.*

He practiced writing his name using his left hand, in spite of this paining him, he says he must get over this and has stated that although still painful it does not seem quite as bad,

We went onto working with the wooden pieces board and Derek amazed me by quickly removing all the pieces and replacing each and everyone back in its rightful place. (He has never been able to do this before and as it caused him so much distress we decided to leave it out of his program).

After this we had great fun in Derek building a huge tower with the building blocks, he took great care and concentration on balancing each brick and was able to remember the correct colours. He was even able to distinquish between the different shades of colour today which was tremendous.

I also noticed today that his ability to follow my instruction was much more improved, everything appears to be registering more easily with him.

Derek insisted that I took a turn in building a tower and was amused when I succeeded in going one brick higher, he says he will beat me next time.

2.30p.m *Derek has said how much he has enjoyed himself today and is now lying on his bed resting.*

2.45p.m *Ali.(the dietitian) came in and it was agreed that Derek has now reached his ideal weight and it should now be maintained rather than gained.*

Derek did state how much he has enjoyed his food at Arrowe Park and would like to thank them.

3.00p.m Derek is resting once again on his bed.

3.40p.m Derek suddenly bounced up and said he was eager to get going again.

We exercised his arms and worked on his left wrist. *(Now showing improvement).*

I then clipped Derek's nails and gave him a hand and foot massage.

We did not leave his room as I had been informed that a doctor would be calling to have a word with me!

5.00p.m Derek is in a very up-beat mood, looking forward to his dinner and seeing Sarah, says she always cheers him up and makes him chuckle.

Entered by Andrea Craig.

21.00p.m Derek was sitting in the day-room with his sitter when I arrived on duty, they were watching television. Derek said he has spent a pleasant evening when asked how he was.

22.00p.m Derek now settled into bed after being assisted with his eye-mask.

23.00p.m I have just come on to relieve Sarah (Derek has two Sarah's taking turns to look after him this evening).

Derek has paid two visits to the toilet during the night (P.U.) other than that he has spent a good night.

6.30a.m Derek has woken up in a good and pleasant mood. He tells me he is looking forward to his breakfast.

We have enjoyed great conversation ranging from places in England, Scotland and Wales which we have both visited to aliens in outer space!

Derek tells me how much he looks forward to seeing his wife Andrea.

Derek asked for a cup of tea.

Entered by Sarah (H.C.A.)

Friday 7th September 2007.

8.00a.m Derek was sitting in his chair on my arrival, chatting to a member of staff. Derek has related to me why he is in hospital and appears to be in a very pleasant mood.

Derek ate all of his breakfast and then took his shower under supervision and was helped into fresh clean clothes.

Derek is now listening to his radio.

Entered by Katie (H.C.A.)

11.30a.m *Derek is very bright, cheery and chatty and is looking forward excitedly to his week-end at home.*

Entered by Andrea Craig.

Monday 10th September 2007.

11.30a.m *Derek enjoyed his week-end at home very much where he spent time relaxing and relearning little kitchen tasks, with which he is still struggling.*

He watched the England football game with Sarah and Max. Saturday afternoon and really enjoyed that.

Sunday morning Derek and I enjoyed a quiet stroll and then both enjoyed an afternoon nap as we were so tired.

Derek worried me Sunday evening as he walked up the stairs to bed. He was walking up ahead of me, thankfully he was holding on to the stair-rail with me right behind him when suddenly his leg started stamping involuntarily, it was over as quickly as it had begun but then he was trying to put his foot high up as though trying to clear all of the stairs in one movement. Fortunately a fall was averted but only just, although Derek maintains there was never ever any fear of him falling, this incident has left me a little concerned.

It did does not appear to have unsettled Derek in any way who claims I worry too much!

This morning Derek was loath to get up out of bed. I knew he must be feeling tired as neither of us had had very much sleep, but I also knew it was because he was reluctant to come back to hospital.

I managed to talk him into a more positive mood and he then explained it was because how of Dr. Newall had left him feeling on Friday after our meeting with him. Everyone seemed so undecided and unable to tell us what was what.

We had been walking off the ward for weekend leave when Dr. Newall met up with us and asked if we might spare him a minute or two to discuss how we had decided to proceed with Derek. Again it had been repeated that I must be the one who must make the final decision and I again said that we would abide by the decision made at our meeting with Dr. Palmer in August last.

I really do understand just how Derek is feeling, for I also feel a little lost and extremely apprehensive with it all, which is how Derek says he is feeling right now.

I have suggested that we simply cope with now and let the future take care of itself.

12.40p.m Derek enjoyed his lunch and it is heartening to see him eating normally once more, although I did have to cut up his meat for him. (He has done so well). He is now lying on his bed sleeping.

1.30p.m *Derek had a friend come to visit who cheered him up more than anyone could ever imagine. He was able to hold good conversation but got muddled when trying to talk too quickly (I believe through excitement) and he could speak his sentences back to front.*

2.30p.m *Derek's visitor has left and after taking a drink Derek has said he would rather lie down again and rest.*

4.00p.m *Derek has been going to the toilet a little more frequently than normal whilst at home and throughout today and he has just asked what I think might be wrong with him!*

4.30p.m *Doctors round and a sample is being taken of Derek's urine and quantities measured, checking his prostrate.*

5.45p.m *Derek has eaten his meal unaided and is listening to the news on his radio. He has stated that he would like to watch television in the day-room this evening from seven o'clock.*
Entered by Andrea Craig.

Tuesday 11th September 2007.

On arrival Derek was sat in bed, he was alert and very chatty. Whilst waiting for breakfast I assisted Derek to put on his jogger bottoms--- he was very confused as to which leg went where.

I found his glasses in his bed and I think he has been lying on them as one of the arms is bent. I have tried straightening it but am afraid of breaking them, I will inform staff-nurse.

Staff has fixed glasses. Derek ate his breakfast and then I assisted him with his shower.

I have been unable to obtain urine sample.

Derek and I have been for a walk around the grounds and discovered that my daughter went to the same school as Derek's daughter.

Derek's mobility is very good. He managed to fill in his own menu with some prompting from myself and he is now sitting listening to his radio.

We have spent a very pleasant morning with Derek talking a lot about his wife Andrea and daughter Sarah.

Entered by R.Jervis (H.C.A.)

12.30p.m *Derek appears to be happy but says in actual fact he feels low and down-hearted. Nevertheless he has been willing to exercise and go through various games and play cards with me which he says he can no longer see the point in.*

2.45p.m *I thought a breath of fresh-air might brighten Derek up and he said he would like to visit a garden centre, something different to the hospital which is driving him insane. I told him he would have to settle for a sit on the bench outside* but I surprised him by taking him for a walk into the park, which he said he never wanted to leave as he was enjoying it so much.

We had been out for an hour before Derek reluctantly agreed to return to his room and practice some writing.

Derek has voiced how important he considers it to be that he maintains and indeed builds up his fitness levels and this is why he enjoys walking up and down the stairs as often as he can and getting out to walk,------ he only wishes he could start jogging!------ and claims he will real soon.

It was a bit chilly outside so we enjoyed a brisk walk, well much more brisk than usual, to keep warm and feels happy to be back resting on his bed.

4.45p.m Derek requested the toilet and said that he could manage to give a sample into the bottle himself (for fluid chart), which he managed to successfully carry out, amazing me in the process and I think he was more than a little pleased also.

Stating that he now feels so much better he wishes to crack on with his writing.

Derek is showing improvement in recognizing the time, this has been a slow exercise which is now showing rewards.

6.00p.m Derek has eaten all of his dinner without any trouble or problems whatsoever. I am leaving *him listening to his radio having said he wishes to go down to the day room about seven to watch television for a couple of hours.*

Derek has been washed and changed and is ready for bed but will need to clean his teeth later.

Entered by Andrea Craig.

9.00p.m *Derek was watching T.V. in the day-room when I came on duty.*

10.30p.m *Derek was ready for his bed and used the bottle successfully for his fluid chart, before he got in.*

Derek awoke almost every hour to p.u. which was noted on his chart.

Entered by J. Rylands (H.C.A.)

Wednesday 12th September 2007.

8.00a.m *Derek was still in bed this morning as he was feeling tired after being awake for most of the night, he wishes to stay in bed until breakfast and hopefully have a little more sleep.*

8.15a.m *Derek actually wants to go to the toilet yet again (P.U.) I had to assist him to do this. He has decided that now he is up he will have a shower before breakfast arrives.*

Derek needed only minimal assistance in showering and then ate his breakfast.

9.25a.m *We are going for a walk off the ward.*

10.15a.m *We have returned to room and Derek has just had his meds. and filled in his menu. Derek and I took a long time filling the menu in as we used it to test his reading skills, he did really well and was able to read most things on the menu, although this took a lot of concentration.*

11.00a.m *We walked down to the day-room to watch the telly but sat talking most of the time.*

12.00 noon. *We are waiting back in room for lunch to be served.*
   Entered by Laura McNab.

12.30p.m *Derek was finishing off his lunch when I arrived and said how tired he felt after a sleepless night.*
   He went to the toilet (P.U.) and is now sleeping on his bed. I have no wish to push him when he is having such disturbed nights. I am anxious of overtiring him.
   (I personally believe that Derek has been over anxious of late and that this is having a direct effect upon his bladder. I feel his fear stems from the many accidents he suffered post catheter removal).
   I also know that he is extremely anxious regarding recent discussions relating to his health and Neuro-rehab delays, e.g. Dr. Pinder thinking

Derek may not be strong enough for rehab program and Cardiologists wanting rehab before any future treatment from them! I really do not think Derek knows what is going on even though Dr. Oates has done her best to explain the situation to us both and I am continually trying to allay any fears that he has.

I am very pleased that Derek is being checked out and tested for this distressing problem. I also feel it would be beneficial if his continual nose-running could be sorted, I know Derek would feel much happier if it were.

3.15p.m *Derek wished to have a little fresh-air and some exercise so we went down the stairs for a five minute sit outside, then returned back to his room walking up the three flights of stairs which present no problem to Derek whatsoever.*

4.15p.m *Derek was taken down for his bladder scan which came back all clear, also told that there was no infection present.*

4.45p.m *Derek said he was still feeling very tired and wished to lie down before dinner. (I find myself wondering how much of it is boredom with him and how much due to lack of night-time sleep!).*

5.30p.m *Derek eaten his dinner and is washed and ready for bed but I am about to walk him down to the day-room before I leave.*

Entered by Andrea Craig.

21.00p.m *Derek was in the lounge, watching T.V. when I came on duty this evening, he said that he was very happy to see me again. I am truly amazed at how well Derek has come on since I last saw him three and a half months ago, he is so different. Well done Derek, keep it up, you are well and truly on the mend.*

Derek has been very chatty. Tonight he has been telling me just how much he loves his wife Andrea and the great dinners she cooks.

Derek slept well, although he got up to use the toilet six times (P.U.), no other problems however.

Entered by Cathy Robinson (H.C.A.)

Thursday 13th September 2007.

7.30a.m *Derek was sitting in his chair when I came on duty.*

He took an early shower with minimal assistance.

He ate a good breakfast and enjoyed it, finishing off with a cup of tea.

Entered by unknown.

12.45p.m *As soon as I arrived Derek was eager to relate an experience he had had on going to bed and was generally very chatty and upbeat.*

Derek said he would like to practice some writing followed by some reading of the newspaper. (I feel he struggles with the amount of print in the newspapers).

We had greater progress with his reading than we did with his writing today.

More and more words are becoming recognizable to him.

2.30p.m *Derek is having a rest on his bed, he seems quite happy.*

3.30p.m *Derek asked if we could go for a walk as he would like some fresh-air, which is what we did. We walked down the stairs and out of the side entrance, sitting in the sunshine for twenty minutes, after which we walked the entire perimeter of all car parks and back to the seat where Derek enjoyed a lengthy conversation with another patient and his wife, who were shocked when Derek told them how long he had been in for, but not as shocked as I was in the fact that Derek could remember the correct amount of time he had indeed been in hospital, a happy moment.*

We then walked back to his room with Derek still chatting the whole way back even as he climbed the stairs, I could only nod my response I'm afraid to say, obviously not as fit as my husband!

5.45p.m Derek washed and changed ready for bed. I am about to walk him down to the day-room to watch the news.

He has been very alert today and has perked up enormously since having such a down week, even though I am fully aware that tomorrow is Friday which means home for Derek, it is so good to see him like this once again.

He actually wants me to go home so that tomorrow will seem to come more quickly!

Entered by Andrea Craig.

The experience Derek wished to share with me was thought by all the staff to have been a dream he had dreamt or the ramblings of an unbalanced mind!

Derek was definitely very excited about it and could hardly contain himself until he had related everything which had taken place.

It was during the early hours of the morning whilst Derek was asleep when he was suddenly awakened by two strange people tip-toeing around his room looking under his bed and behind the curtains as they went, they were whispering to each other but he was not able to hear what they said.

He went on to describe a light which travelled around the room with them and asked me what I thought it might have been.

"You've had a dream," I said, "You can have very vivid dreams which feel so real sometimes."

"This was no dream," replied Derek, "this really did take place and I wanted to know what was going on. I asked them what they were doing and they told me to go back to sleep and not to worry. Do you think it was perhaps a spiritual happening?" he asked.

"No I don't and although I can't say what has happened, just before you ask I don't believe it was aliens either."

"Don't be so ridiculous," says Derek, "I would just like someone to take this matter a little more seriously that's all."

Throughout the day members of staff appeared in Derek's room to listen to and give their own ideas as to what the experience might mean, most of course believing that Derek was confused, bless him, and had been awakened by a dream.

It was later that afternoon when the ward manager came in to unravel the whole incident and explain that Derek had in actual fact been quite correct in all that he had witnessed.

It had been two members of the night security team using torches so as not to disturb the patients as they searched the hospital looking for a patient who had been reported missing. Of course the day staff had come on duty knowing nothing about the matter.

I was absolutely delighted with Derek's ability to remember everything that had taken place and his knowing of what was real in spite of everyone trying to convince him otherwise.

Friday 14th September 2007.

Speech Therapy with Rebecca Smith.
I continued with Language Assessment, Derek working well despite finding some of the tasks hard.
I will provide further word packs to assist with verbal reasoning.

Monday 17th September 2007.

11.40a.m *I delivered Derek back to his room.*
Entered by George Hollis (who always had such a way with words!)

12.30p.m *I arrived to find Derek eating his lunch. He and George had been working with the blocks and writing.*
Derek wishes to continue with his writing which he is finding difficult and I see him beginning to rebel, no doubt through frustration.

1.30p.m *We are continuing with the new question sheet left by Rebecca on Friday last. (Which I have to record was Derek's best home leave to-date. Friday night he slept right through without getting up once, although Saturday and Sunday nights were back to being rather disturbed, but no way were they as bad as they have been).*

4.15p.m *Well done Rebecca! Derek enjoyed the new pack very much and found the conversations it produced very refreshing. Derek wished to keep on with them but after an hour he was getting very tired and his voice had become weak so I stopped him and persuaded him to rest. (It has been such a long time since I have seen Derek so animated, thank-you so much. I can now continue writing my own sheets out in the future).*

Derek is now having a nap before dinner.

This is the first Monday on which Derek has returned to hospital willingly and happily prepared to do so. He has worked extremely hard today. Hopefully he will manage to keep his cheery spirits up this week.

ALL STAFF PLEASE NOTE:

MY MAIN CONCERN ON RETURNING TODAY HAS BEEN THE TOILET AREA. ON THREE SEPARATE OCCASSIONS THIS AFTERNOON I HAVE TAKEN DEREK TO THE TOILET TO FIND THAT I HAVE HAD TO CLEAN NOT ONLY THE TOILET BUT A BADLY SOILED FLOOR ALSO, SOMEONE COULD HAVE EASILY EXPERIENCED A NASTY ACCIDENT BY SLIPPING IN THIS MESS, NOT TO MENTION THE RISK OF INFECTION.

THE CLEANING OF THE TOILET WAS NOT A PROBLEM TO ME BUT I WAS CONCERNED THAT HAD DEREK TAKEN HIMSELF TO THE TOILET HE WOULD NEVER HAVE BEEN ABLE TO SEE THE MESS IN THERE AND WOULD

NOT HAVE KNOWN WHAT HE WAS WALKING IN OR SITTING ON.
Entered by Andrea Craig.

21.00p.m *Derek was watching television when I came on duty this evening. He stayed up until eleven o'clock, but he went to the toilet and had his meds. before getting into bed.*

He has been very chatty to-night and seems happy.

Derek was up four times in the night to P.U. otherwise no problems.

6.20a.m *Derek got up and sat in his chair. I gave him a cup of tea and he said he was looking forward to his breakfast.*

Entered by Cathy Robinson (H.C.A.)

Tuesday 18th September 2007.

7.30a.m *When I came on duty Derek was sitting in his chair, we had a long chat about New Brighton! I asked Derek if he remembered the old swimming baths that used to be there and the Tower and the old pier! He was telling me about Heswall which is where he lives.*

We chatted about Guinea Gap baths (I used to work there at one time) Derek tells me he has been there but that he used to go to Bootle baths for a swim.

Derek ate a good breakfast.

9.0a.m Derek visited the toilet (P.U.)

9.20a.m I took Derek down to the shower where he washed himself with minimal assistance.

9.45a.m We walked down the stairs and sat in the sun outside. Derek does enjoy being outdoors.

10.45a.m Back in Derek's room where he is resting before lunch.
   Entered by Cathy (Flexibank)

12.30p.m Derek was exceptionally happy today and very eager to begin his writing.

2.15p.m. Derek has worked very hard for the past one and a half hours with one toilet break. He had wanted to be left alone to see if he could manage totally independently. I have to note that sadly he still struggles, especially with dressing himself after he has been to the toilet. Nevertheless I am pleased to note there is some definite improvement and Derek does seem quite pleased with his own progress. Although he does say that the day cannot come quickly enough when he can go to the toilet normally once more.
   (He says that he feels all fingers and thumbs and everything seems so complicated to him and yet he feels it should all be so simple).
   Derek is sitting reading through the newspaper and has just shocked me by reading out a

complete sentence. He claims that he has just shocked himself also, but we both feel as though he has just been awarded first prize, we are that pleased.

2.45p.m *We walked downstairs and out to the car-park where we practiced Derek's road drill. He was alert and bright throughout thanking drivers for stopping as we walked across the Zebra-crossing.*

He was very chatty and held good conversation as we walked.

3.30p.m *We are back in the room where Derek is resting on his bed. I have to say that Derek had wished to keep going today but from past experience I was a little afraid that he may over do things. (I am beginning to realize that Derek does not always know when he has done enough).*

He has stated that he is looking forward to going to Neuro so much as someone has told him that over there they will really work him hard, he cannot wait!

4.15p.m *Derek had a short nap and was rearing to go saying he would like to continue with the pack that Rebecca had left as he finds these very stimulating.*

5.40p.m *We were enjoying our discussion sheets so much neither of us realized how quickly the* *time had slipped by and dinner was served before we knew it.*

Derek has asked that I write in his diary just how happy he has felt today and that he feels very positive for the future.

Entered by Andrea Craig.

6.00p.m *I walked with Derek down to the day-room to watch the news, he asked he if could stay to watch the football at seven thirty, I checked with staff-nurse who said that it would be fine.*

Derek enjoyed watching television throughout my time with him.

Entered by Amanda Chapman (Flexibank)

21.00p.m *Derek was watching football in the day-room when I took over and we stayed until ten-thirty before he went to the toilet and had his meds. He has been very chatty and happy and went to bed only wakening once throughout the entire night. Derek slept well.*

Entered by Cathy Robinson.

Wednesday 19th September 2007.

Derek is cheerful this morning. He ate all of his breakfast and enjoyed it.

We had a good long chat and then he asked if we could go for a walk, which we did. We went outside for some fresh-air and continued with a walk around the hospital grounds before returning to his room.

Entered by Rachael Kennedy (Cadet)

12.30p.m *Derek was sitting alone when I arrived but quite happy. I have been asked how I felt about Derek's day-sitters being cancelled and I have agreed to come in as early as I can. Derek seems to be happy with this.*

2.00p.m *Derek has been doing some arm exercises, followed by a head and shoulder massage and is now practicing his writing.*

He is still maintaining a very positive attitude and has said how much better he is feeling within himself.

2.35p.m *Derek's concentration was short lived and after twenty minutes he was struggling so we stopped and went for a walk down to the ground floor via the lifts.*

3.10p.m *on returning to his room Derek was eager to lie down but he remained chatty and cheerful despite his tiredness.*

4.15p.m *Derek got up and went to the toilet. He told me he wished to continue with conversation as he thought this very important for him to keep practicing.*

Derek's focus has not been good today and has been very drowsy but we have continued at his insistence although I have now insisted that he should have a quiet hour before dinner.

Entered by Andrea Craig.

9.00p.m *Derek was watching T.V. when I came in tonight, he was very happy and chatty and went to bed at 10.45p.m after first going to the toilet.*

Derek slept well getting up to use the toilet twice during the night.

Entered by Cathy Robinson (H.C.A.)

Thursday 20th September 2007.

11.00a.m *Derek was sitting alone but happy when I walked into his room, he had been showered and dressed and had enjoyed his breakfast. He is now browsing through the newspaper very concerned as to why he can see to read some of it but not all. He realizes that this is due to his brain damage and gets himself terribly upset.*

I have tried to explain to him and hopefully help him to understand that he continues to improve and that he should remember that not long ago he did not even recognize what a newspaper was.

He readily accepted this explanation and became a lot more positive.

12.15p.m Derek has eaten his lunch and proved that he is able to cut up his meat and roast potatoes without any help.

I have also noticed that he is now able to place his finished dinner plate away to one side and bring his desert dish in front of himself, a great improvement.

1.00p.m Derek and I went for a walk down the stairs to the ground floor, we walked down the corridor to the side entrance and around the entire perimeter of the car-park, Derek seems to be oblivious to the traffic at times and this naturally causes me a great deal of concern.

We visited the shop to purchase a packet of biscuits before returning to his room.

2.00p.m Derek is now having a lie down before a friend arrives at 3.00p.m.

5.00p.m Derek fell into a sleep which I felt he needed but was awake before his friend came in. He enjoyed John's company very much and John was pleased to see such improvement in Derek.

6.00p.m Derek ate his dinner and is washed and ready for bed later. I will walk him down to the day-room before leaving as he enjoys watching the news.

Entered by Andrea Craig.

21.00p.m *Derek was in the day-room watching television when I came on.*

He had his meds. and went to the toilet before getting into bed at 11.10p.m.

Derek was in a very happy mood tonight and very chatty, said he was very pleased to see me again.

Derek slept well, getting up twice during the night with no other problems.

Entered by Cathy Robinson (H.C.A.)

Friday 21ˢᵗ September 2007.

9.00a.m. *I arrived early to find Derek had not been showered or washed but he had eaten his breakfast.*

I helped Derek to wash and dress and prepare for his week-end leave.

Rebecca (speech therapist) arrived for a session with Derek before we left and we were able to chat about Derek's progress which she is pleased with.

Entered by Andrea Craig.

Monday 24ᵗʰ September 2007.

11.00a.m *We arrived back in Derek's room, he is very quiet and down. I have brought in an old shirt so that Derek can sit and practice undoing and fastening buttons. He is doing this now but is far* *from happy about it and is getting very cross with the whole damned business, (his words).*

I have told him to put it down and that he does not need to do it but he is carrying on regardless, stating that he must.

The week-end was once again very enjoyable with Derek attempting to partake in whatever was taking place. (He is very limited in what he can do but it was good to see him so willing to try).

He now knows where most things are kept in the kitchen and is keen to practice his tea-making.

Sleeping is improving but his nightly trips to the toilet were more frequent than last weekend.

His getting back into bed can be successful or not, but generally this is much improved.

His walking up and down the stairs is good but can be unpredictable as he can suddenly not pick his foot up high enough and has to be accompanied at all times.

Derek is still extremely confused when undressing and even worse when dressing but again has shown a little improvement with this.

Buttons and zips cause him great confusion and frustration and he states that he wishes to practice with these much more.

Derek's conversation with myself is good and improving all the time but with others I notice him using the wrong words or even talking his sentences back to front although he realizes what he has said is wrong and apologizes and will often correct himself. I feel perhaps this may be nerves as he also tends to talk much more quickly when talking to other people.

Derek has also shown that he has no sense of direction when outside of his home or hospital environment.

1.00p.m *Derek ate his lunch and coped very well although struggled when opening and preparing his cheese and crackers.*

We went back to buttons at Derek's request but as he became very angry with his inability to perform this task we moved quickly on to other exercises.

5.00p.m *Derek has worked well this afternoon. We played Connect 4, (still struggles with this game) He managed to complete the jig-saw.*

We practiced writing and worked with the flash cards after which we went for a walk, going down the stairs, around the grounds and returned to his room coming back up the stairs.

Derek stated that he wished to continue working so we went over the conversational task sheets left by Rebecca (speech therapist). These are so enjoyed.

I insisted that Derek have a rest on his bed but he states that his afternoon naps keep him from sleeping at night and he refused to be treated like a baby.

But he did lie down and although did not sleep he was resting.

Derek expressed whilst he was lying down how he longs to undertake something new and much more challenging and how hemmed in he is beginning to feel.

He asked if he was ever going to get to Rehab.

(A visit from Dr. Oates cleared up the confusion regarding which should come first, the insertion of stents or his rehabilitation in the Neuro.unit. The way forward has now been made clear and all doctors are seemingly of one accord which has helped Derek feel a lot happier. It is to be Rehab first followed with the insertion of the stents.)

6.30p.m *Derek has washed himself and has been helped to get ready for bed. I will leave him in the day-room.*

Entered by Andrea Craig.

21.00p.m *Derek was in the day-room watching T.V. when I came on.*

He had his meds. and went to the toilet before going to bed at 11.00p.m.

Derek got up at 12.00p.m to go to the toilet and he was confused tonight.

He was up again at 2.00a.m and again at 4.00a.m. Derek has not been settled too well and said that he had a lot on his mind but would say no more.

Andrea Craig

Entered by Cathy Robinson (H.C.A.)

Tuesday 25thSeptember 2007.

12.25p.m Derek was standing at his window when I walked into his room, trying to figure out a reading tape which had been left for him. (Sadly he had no idea what to do with it). He seemed happy and pleased to see me.

He informed me that he had been alone all morning and had managed to eat his lunch alone and was so happy to have had time to himself at last.

"A sign that they must think I am growing up" he said.

1.00p.m Derek has been browsing through the newspaper, occasionally reading out the little he was able to recognize (he did exceptionally well).

He told me that he was trying to do the buttons whilst sitting alone this morning but found them impossible to do and he cannot understand why he finds it so difficult when it is such a simple thing to do and something which he has done all of his life. "I know what to do," he said, "I simply just can't do it."

1.30p.m I took Derek for a walk to enjoy a breath of fresh-air. We browsed through the shops and then walked back up the stairs to his room where he is now sitting writing out the alphabet.

2.30p.m   *Derek's focus was not good but he had worked very hard. He has seemed quite disorientated which is unusual of late.*

He is lying on his bed very worked up and agitated over something. When questioned what it was that seemed to be disturbing him he stated that he did not know, except that he feels frustrated with the lack of events (I believe not hearing anything from rehab.is what he was referring to).

4.00p.m   *Derek wished to listen to his "library tape" until dinner was served.*

Sarah came in to visit which cheered him a little and after washing and changing into his night clothes we all walked down to the day-room at 6.00pm where we left him watching the news. (I felt extremely sad leaving him this evening, more so than I normally feel.)

Entered by Andrea Craig.

21.00p.m   *Derek was in day-room when I came on, we continued to watch T.V..*

Back in his room he had his meds. and went to the toilet before getting into bed at 11.30p.m.

Derek was up twice in the night and was unsteady on his feet on both occasions.

He got up at 6.20a.m and sat in his chair. I gave him a cup of tea and we chatted with Derek saying how he faced another day of school.

Entered by Cathy Robinson (H.C.A.)

Wednesday 26th September 2007.

11.15a.m Derek was sitting alone reflecting over his past life trying, he said, to fit in all the missing pieces.

He says that he is feeling much happier because he now understands his past much more clearly and can recollect many more of his relatives. (Derek is still confused on which relatives are living and those who have died.)

11.40a.m I took Derek for a walk to get some fresh-air, we walked down and back up the three flights of stairs.

Derek has stated that he does not wish to do any exercises or tasks as he does not believe they are doing him any good and is listening to his tapes until lunch is served.

1.45p.m Derek ate and enjoyed his lunch. He is not very talkative today and I feel he is quite down. He wished to finish listening to his tape before he did anything else.

Derek's sister came in to visit and he seemed to perk up a little.

6.00p.m Derek said it was a nice surprise Elaine coming in to visit and that he had enjoyed his afternoon with the three of us together.

Derek is washed and ready for bed but I will walk him down to the day-room before I leave.
Entered by Andrea Craig.

21.00p.m *Derek was very chatty this evening and said how much he had enjoyed his day with Andrea and how each day gets better and better.*
Derek had his meds. and went to the toilet before getting into bed at 10.30p.m
He got up twice in the night to go to the toilet and each time he was a little confused as to where to go.

6.30a.m *Derek got up and sat in his chair, he said that he just had one more day of school before he was home again on Friday.*
Derek is in a lovely mood and when I told him I would see him again tonight he said that would be nice.
Entered by Cathy Robinson (H.C.A.)

Thursday 27ᵗʰ September 2007.

(Occupational Therapist)
I came to see Derek today and we went to the Occupational Therapy Kitchen on Ward 36 to make a hot drink. Derek did well although required assistance holding the kettle to pour water in.
He was able to put the plug in the wall and switch on with minimal help. He was able to collect

all of the items needed with my help in locating them.

He was able to fill the tea-pot and put the lid on properly and pour three quarter full into the cup.

Derek washed up and put cup away with minimal guidance.

Derek engaged well in conversation throughout. We discussed Everton's victory and our favourite football players.

Derek discussed his love of Capri and how he longs to go there after he has completed his rehab.

Derek was able to take us back to his room. Andrew called with the library books. Derek selected a book and held a discussion about his likes. Derek engaged well with Andrew who informed us that he has recovered from his own brain injury which was caused by a car-crash.

Andrew has said that he would like to come back and chat. We have had a nice morning's session.

Entered by Vicky Carrigan (Occupational Therapist).

11.30a.m *Derek was sat by the window reading which gave me a wonderful surprise when I came in. He actually read out the first entire sentence but said that it had hurt his brain to do so (he laughed while saying this).*

I brought in a piece of material today to which I had sewn six large buttons and made six large button holes. Derek is sitting as I write practicing how to push the buttons through the holes. He is far from happy with this exercise and is becoming very frustrated.

I brought that particular exercise to a halt and we chatted until lunch was served. He was explaining to me how much his being able to come home at week-ends means to him and that he feels quite excited when he realized that Friday is tomorrow and how quickly the week has gone by.

1.00p.m *Derek is now resting on his bed before we go for a walk and tackle our daily stair trek. (I am now becoming quite fit!).*

3.15p.m *We have just returned from our walk and am pleased to note how briskly Derek strode out with a much greater confidence than he has shown before.*

He has stated that he wishes to have a try at reading his book as he feels he must push himself with this as he is fed up with all the other aids in his room and feels they are of no further use to him! He has requested that I take them home.

(But I will leave them a little while longer).

He has also asked that I go home early today. When asked why he wished me to do this he stated that the sooner I went home the sooner tomorrow would arrive and the sooner he would be going home.

6.00p.m *Derek has eaten well and is washed and ready for bed. I will walk him to the day-room for his evening catch-up on the news and his evening with the telly.*

(Poor thing, the screen was so fuzzy and grainy last night he could hardly see it, but he did not complain).

Entered by Andrea Craig.

21.00p.m *Derek was sitting in the day-room when I came on duty this evening, he said that he had spent a very good day and that Friday was the best day of the week as school was out and it was home time!*

10.00p.m *Derek had his meds and went to the toilet before going to bed. He has been very happy and chatty.*

Derek got up to use the toilet twice. The second time at 2.15a.m he asked me what the time was. I replied that it had just gone 2a.m and he said, "Good, home to-day, it's Friday."

Derek got up at 4.15a.m to use the toilet and again at 6.15a.m but said he would stay up and sit in his chair. He is showered and ready for the day.

Entered by Cathy Robinson (H.C.A.)

Friday 28th September 2007.

Derek was showered, ready and working with Rebecca (speech therapist) when I arrived. He seemed alert and bright and had such a happy smile.

Dr, Newall called in to see Derek and a pleasant and positive discussion took place leaving Derek feeling happy.

Derek is now leaving the hospital for his weekend leave.

Entered by Andrea Craig.

CHAPTER FOURTEEN

As September turned into October it was understandable that Derek would become more and more frustrated as the days wore on. We had entered September optimistic in the belief that his transfer into rehab. was in fact only weeks away as Dr Pinder had led us all to believe that a bed was imminent, but as the days dragged on, trying to keep his spirits up became increasingly more and more difficult. The hospital staff were terrific but medically there became less and less they could do for him.

Any woman ever having had a baby will know how that last month of pregnancy seems far longer to live through than all of the previous eight months put together. Those last final weeks drag on and on seemingly never coming to an end, all you long to do is hold your baby in your arms and yet that moment, instead of drawing near, seems to fall further and further away. And so it was for Derek, the following weeks seemed almost to be without purpose for him as he waited for the day he was transferred to the unit he believed was going to be the final step on his road to recovery. Each new day to be lived through felt longer than the last and Derek states that the following month of October was to be the longest month he has ever had to live through.

I did on one occasion remind him that at least he was actually alive to be living through it, but needless to say that did not go down too well with him. Little did we realize at this time that in the days ahead we would have to battle through not the most serious of virus's there are in existence but certainly one of the most unpleasant that I have ever experienced and one that sadly we lost one of our dearest friends to in the months that followed. It is named the 'Novo virus', a virus you hardly notice you have until it has a firm hold causing sudden projectile vomiting and exhausting diorhorrea, a virus which can spread rapidly and did so on Derek's ward. Derek fell subject to it as did I, leaving me unable to visit him for several days. But thankfully we recovered from it quickly leaving us both refreshed to receive the news we had waited so long to hear.

Monday 1st October 2007.

We arrived back in Derek's room at 11.15a.m. Derek is very unhappy about being back and I would say he seems to be more angry than low in spirits, but he has said that he realizes he must accept the situation as it is for now but how he wishes his place in the Neuro unit would hurry up.

I have unpacked his belongings and spoken to the pharmacist re: Derek's eye drops being renewed. They were out of date.

Derek enjoyed his weekend. He was happy to make tea (still with guidance and he still has the habit of overflowing the cup as though he cannot see the level of fluid).

He dried dishes and said he enjoyed this as it felt like second nature to him. He carried out this task very well and was eager to learn how to put everything away so that he would know in future where everything lived. He claims that he longs to be able to wash them as he did before and I heartily agreed to that and said I could not wait!

Dining at the table is now almost back to normal for Derek and requires very little assistance except with pulling his chair up to the table.

He is undressing himself well but cannot dress himself at all, although there is significant improvement with him putting his socks on, shoes still proving difficult but he now knows what he should be doing even if he cannot quite manage it.

His focus and attention coming in and out is still a major issue although Derek himself seems to be quite unaware of this taking place.

On Sunday we experienced a little accident with Derek not managing to get to the toilet in time *and he had to be cleaned and changed. This so upset him and causes him great distress as he believes he may be becoming incontinent.*

I did try to explain to him that this sort of accident can happen to anyone when they cannot reach the toilet quickly enough and that it had happened to myself just after Sarah was born. He seemed to accept this and his upset lessened as the day wore on.

Derek was troubled with his left shoulder and states that it is now becoming much more painful, especially as he tries to turn over in bed.

1.30p.m *Derek has been working on his writing but is finding it very difficult and says that he has had enough. He went to the toilet and is now lying on his bed resting.*

As he lay he talked very quietly of how he felt it was all too much for him and that he felt he could no longer carry on. He went on to say he felt himself to be too old and weary and that he knew he could not possibly have the time to make a full recovery back to normal.

As gently as I could I went over how far he had travelled and the many obstacles he had overcome since that fateful day back in April and went on to explain that we had both travelled too far and climbed too high to give up now. Searching desperately for the right words which would give him the encouragement he so badly needed I reminded him of the time I had told him of how patient we both must learn to be in the months which lay ahead, for it would be patience that would prove to be our greatest strength and most loyal friend.

He did rally round somewhat but is still very low.

Derek then had a good cry with a sobbing which seemed to shudder from his very soul.

After he had calmed down he went on to explain how for periods of time he believes he is coming around and feels he is more like his old self again and then suddenly, like an express train hurtling out of the blue, it hits him just how damaged he really is and then the sheer impossibility of it all completely overwhelms him and he knows he will not recover and feels he cannot cope with this.

I could only ask him to lie quietly and rest and that peace would fill the space in his mind that he had just cleared of his anxieties. I talked quietly until Derek fell asleep.

2.45p.m Dr. Oates and her team arrived and discussed Derek's shoulder. He seems to be pleased that it is going to be checked out and at last something is going to be done about it.

Derek has fallen back asleep.

4.15p.m We walked down to the shop where we purchased some biscuits and returned walking back up the stairs.

4.30p.m *Derek returned to his writing with renewed energy and states that he will do a little reading after fifteen minutes.*

5.15p.m *Derek has worked very hard to try and push himself that little bit further and has done extremely well.*

He appears to be back to his old self stating that he is now determined to master buttons and will practice each and every day from now on.

(My darling Derek, ten out of ten for effort and determination).

6.00p.m *Derek is washed and ready for bed and is going to spend the evening watching television in the day-room.*

Entered by Andrea Craig.

Tuesday 2nd October 2007.

12 noon. *Derek is now spending more time alone and seems to be enjoying this space. He was sitting in his room practicing his writing having already practiced with the buttons, which he claims is impossible and fails to understand why on earth he cannot do them. (This pleased me tremendously as he had been given no prompting to carry out these tasks. He had instigated them for himself and had been able to locate them when needed).*

The only problem being was that Derek believed his writing to be correct and was thrilled with what he had done, when in fact it was not good.

12.50p.m Derek ate all of his lunch and has asked if we might have a walk to get some fresh-air.

2.30p.m We have just returned from a nice long walk around the park. Derek thoroughly enjoyed it and is much more upbeat than yesterday and has been a lot more philosophical about everything. He has been talking constantly about Rehab. and how he believes it will be so good for him.

I have trimmed Derek's hair and beard. He states that he now feels part of the human race once again. (What cheek!)

3.30p.m Derek is lying on his bed listening to his library tape of "Inspector Morse".

Derek has told me that he had his shoulder x-rayed this morning and is hoping that something will be done about it just as quickly.

4.30p.m Derek took himself to the toilet, and after washing his hands returned to his room without any problems except for his trousers having to be re-arranged. On his return he picked up the newspaper and sat reading and I could not help but be amazed how far he really had progressed from the days when he could do absolutely nothing.

6.00p.m *Derek has eaten his dinner and is washed and ready for bed. I will walk him to the day-room before I leave. (I leave him much happier than I felt last night).*

Entered by Andrea Craig.

Wednesday 3ʳᵈ October 2007.

11.30a.m *Derek was very distressed when I walked into his room this morning. He was disturbed because he could not see his reading. I called his nurse and she immediately took his blood pressure, which appeared to be alright.*

Nevertheless I have put all exercises away and will take him for a walk after he has had a little rest.

12 noon. *Derek feeling very much better after a brisk walk (and I mean a very brisk walk with Derek setting the pace every step of the way), we walked down the stairs, around the hospital grounds and back up the stairs.*

Derek picked up his paper on returning and is very pleased that his vision has returned back to normal once more.

During our walk Derek explained to me how despondent he is beginning to feel that he has been forgotten and that he feels he will never be allocated a bed in Rehab. He feels the whole situation is a bit of a mess.

1.30p.m *Derek ate all of his lunch. He is not chatting today but said he was willing to do some question and answer tasks while he lay down for his afternoon rest. After a short time he claimed he felt very tired and is now fast asleep.*

3.30p.m *Derek awoke and went to the toilet. On his return he enjoyed a cup of tea and a cream-slice and asked me to fire some more questions at him. We enjoyed this session and the conversation it prompted so much we did not notice the time fly by and were shocked as a knock on the door told us dinner was about to be served.*

5.45p.m *Derek ate his dinner and seemed cheerful stating that he had enjoyed the afternoon but then quite suddenly he told me he wanted to try and make me understand how bad things really are with him.*

He began talking of how deeply frustrated and extremely low he is feeling all of the time and how, now that the winter is drawing in, it makes him feel so trapped and very sad.

6.16p.m *Derek is washed and changed ready for bed and I will leave him watching the television but I am not happy leaving him this evening with him feeling as low as he is.*

Entered by Andrea Craig.

Thursday 4th October 2007.

9.ooa.m *Rebecca Smith (Speech and Language Therapy)*

Derek was in good spirits this morning.

He is fully orientated in person, place and time now.

We chatted about different new topics e.g. government, Burma, also the weather and the park.

We began a word finding task which Derek did well with, he needed verbal prompts to arrive at target words.

Derek was able to carry out 'Mirror' writing task.

We had a very good session. Well done Derek.

Entered by Rebecca Smith (Speech & Language Therapist)

11.30a.m *Derek was happy when I walked in this morning, very different to yesterday, although he was getting very agitated with the buttons again. I put them away and passed him the newspaper.*

The library have just been and we have changed his book for one in large print, Derek seems a lot happier with this.

12.30p.m *Lunch arrived and Derek ate well as always.*

After lunch Derek seemed very excited to show me the chapel that a nurse had taken him to. He actually remembered the floor it was on and only took one wrong turning in locating it.

We sat in silence, both of us enjoying the peace and tranquility it offered from the hustle and bustle of the hospital routine.

I had found myself wondering how many broken hearts and shattered lives had been laid bare before its' alter and how much naturally understood anger had threatened to disturb its very core of Spirituality.

As Derek took my hand I knew that he, like me, had offered up a heartfelt prayer of thanks that mere words would never be able to express.

We both long for the day when Derek will be discharged from Arrowe Park and yet we both knew as our prayers of thanks were expressed this afternoon that this hospital and its staff had forged a special place in our hearts and lives and that we will find it strange when we find ourselves no longer a part of its daily routine. (I hasten to add at this point that we wish to stay not one day longer than is necessary!)

Coming out of the chapel we went for a walk outside enjoying the fresh-air and shared with each other our feelings experienced whilst sitting in prayer.

We returned to Derek's room where Derek is now lying on his bed fast asleep. He has said that he feels more relaxed since visiting the chapel with me and is looking forward to going home tomorrow. He added that he wishes someone would give him a sleeping pill so that he could go to sleep and it would be morning that much more quickly. I told him not to be so silly, that morning would come quickly enough and he said, "Not quick enough."

3.30p.m I dropped a cup holder which woke Derek up.

He went to the toilet and then we played a game of draughts. (Much too complicated for him but he managed to keep on the same coloured squares which was an improvement on last time).

Derek has been weighed and it has been decided that his weight must now be kept in check as he is slightly over his normal weight at thirteen stone, four pounds.

4.30p.m We practiced throwing the small soft balls to each other. Derek has certainly improved I was most impressed and noticed a little more of his old competitiveness showing through.

6.15p.m Derek ate all of his dinner and is washed and ready for bed. I will leave him in day-room feeling happy and relaxed.

Entered by Andrea Craig.

Andrea Craig

Friday 5th October 2007.

10.30a.m Derek was attempting to dress himself when I came in this morning and was doing well but struggling. I helped him complete his dressing and he then cleaned his teeth.

Doctors arrived with Rheumatologist to give Derek an injection into his shoulder.

He stated that he is very pleased to have had this and he also told me that his tummy felt a little off earlier this morning but that he feels alright now.

I am taking Derek off the ward for his weekend leave.

Entered by Andrea Craig.

Monday 8th October 2007.

10.30a.m Derek is far from happy again this morning expressing that he wants no visitors at all and that even I must stay away, except for one hour a day if he should wish it, as he is now completely and totally fed up with the lot of us.

This is of course his usual Monday morning response on returning to his hospital room but this morning it began much earlier than usual when I tried to get him up out of bed and he refused to budge.

"O.K." I said, "You can jolly well stay there and when you do decide to get up you can shower and dress yourself for I am off to get myself ready and dressed."

He retaliated by shouting, "I don't bloody well need your help and in future you stay away, d'you hear, I don't need you, my nurses will look after me. God knows, what have you ever done for me, anyway!"

Foolishly I told him he first had to get himself back to hospital before anyone could look after him and that it was high time he started helping himself more or he would never be able to look after himself.

I could have bitten my tongue off but it was too late, it had been said and could not be unsaid. I was ordered out of the bedroom and told not to come back.

I left him for fifteen minutes while I got myself ready, listening all the time for movement. At last I heard him up and moving about and ventured to peep around the door only to be told to get out and stay out.

Of course I could not afford to take much notice on this occasion as time was running late and somehow I managed to persuade him to allow me to help him shower and get dressed.

He agreed to my helping him as unfortunately he had no other option but he wished me to know that all communication and any exercise activities were out from now on. (For now that is!)

Derek has not been well during this weekend. He was very much paler than usual and had *the runs for twenty-four hours. We were back to toilet visits every half-hour during the night with numerous bed changes and we are both on our knees with exhaustion.*

During the whole of this time Derek never went off his food and joined in well with conversation at small family gatherings on each of the two days. (This was his first occasion of prolonged company and he loved every moment of it).

Derek is very angry that I have informed Staff-nurse of his being unwell but I felt I needed to.

1.00p.m *Derek has eaten his lunch after a very quiet morning and is now practicing his writing without any prompting.*

2,00p.m *Derek has put his writing away and has asked if I will do some exercises with him. We did some arm stretching, balancing, following my instructions or copying my movements. He carries out these exercises with ease which is so different to a few weeks back when we had to stop because of the pain in his left shoulder.*

3.00p.m *We walked downstairs and around the perimeter of the hospital grounds. Derek was amused by the frantic goings on in the busy car-park at visiting hour, he said he had never seen anything like the madness of the drivers and how they were parking anywhere. I wondered if I had been perhaps foolish in taking him out at that time* *but it had not phased him and he said he had actually enjoyed the experience.*

I did not allow him to walk back up the stairs today as he had not had any sleep at the weekend and was tired.

He is now sleeping on his bed before dinner.

His huffiness seems to have huffed itself out and all that was said this morning seems to have been forgotten leaving him feeling very much happier and more settled.

6.00p.m *Derek has spent a good afternoon. He awoke very cheerful and stated that he feels ever so much better in himself.*

He ate all of his meal and has stated that he will push on in the morning with his reading and writing.

He is washed and ready for bed and I am about to walk him to the day-room for the evening.

Entered by Andrea Craig.

Tuesday 9ᵗʰ October 2007.

11.00a.m *Derek had just returned from an appointment in the eye clinic and was sitting alone and happy to be so. He related all that had taken place during his visit and told me of the 'Early Learning' books which had been recommended for him to help further develop his reading skills. (What a good idea).*

He seems very chatty and eager once more to crack on and learn. I have explained that this is not a good idea today as his vision is blurred with eye-drops.

Derek seems quite insistent that we crack on with something he can do then!

Before we could make a start on anything lunch was served, which as usual he enjoyed. (I bring my packed lunch which I ate with him).

Whilst eating lunch Derek explained that he had had a difficult and most uncomfortable night again last night and that he had managed to get very little sleep so I suggested he had a lie down.

4.00p.m *Derek fell into a deep sleep immediately after lunch and is still sleeping soundly.*

5.15p.m *Derek awoke at 4.15p.m and has spent the last hour working harder than he has for some time. We worked with numbers, words and shapes and Derek worked well and was very alert throughout the whole exercise.*

Dinner stopped us working and Derek states he has spent a good day, even though he had slept through most of the afternoon. (This sleep was very much needed and did him the world of good).

I will leave Derek in the day-room where he wishes to watch the evening news.

Entered by Andrea Craig.

Wednesday 10th October 2007.

Derek was bright and cheerful when I arrived and his smile beams and lights up the whole room.

He has been struggling trying to do up the buttons (unsuccessfully) and reading his menu for tomorrow.

He is thrilled with the 'Early Learning' books and colouring books which I have brought in for him.

The 'In and Around the Town' book was a little too easy for him but nevertheless he was thrilled that he did so well with it.

In all honesty Derek starts off well but he drops off quite quickly being unable to maintain his focus, although I do note an improvement with the lengthening of this compared to a few weeks ago.

Derek is now happily working with the colouring book but seems to have little control with where he wishes to put the colour and in fact the only colour which seems to exist is red.

Dr. Oates and her team called in and as always managed to cheer and uplift him enormously. (So very different to how things were last week)

2.00p.m Lunch was served a little later today after which Derek said he would like to have a rest and is now fast asleep on his bed.

Derek has worked very hard and has been full of fun creating a great amount of laughter which has been immensely uplifting.

4.00p.m *Derek awakened and asked that we might go for a walk for some exercise and fresh-air. We walked down the stairs, around the full perimeter of the grounds and back to his room up the stairs all at a brisk pace.*

When we returned to his room we found Sarah waiting to greet us.

Derek as always was thrilled to see her and said how much he has enjoyed his day. (In his own words best to date!)

We will walk Derek down to the day-room and spend a little time with him there before we leave.

Entered by Andrea Craig.

Thursday 11th October 2007.

10.45a.m *Derek was sat listening to his radio when I arrived this morning. He appears bright and chatty. He suddenly remembered that he had not cleaned his teeth after breakfast and got himself up to do so. (I thought this was brilliant that he should remember this). After he had completed this and washed his toothbrush, all without any prompting he suggested that he would like to do some more colouring. We set out the book and the pencils but Derek seemed* *very confused as to what he should actually be doing with them. He is also unable to recognize the pictures to be coloured. At least he was happy with me explaining and showing him but I knew he was unable to take any of it in so I took him quickly onto working with the flash cards for a little while. He was more sure of this exercise and did well.*

11.30a.m *We went for a walk, down the stairs, around the grounds and back up the stairs, we passed a doctor on the stairs who recognized us both and simply stood shaking his head at the speed with which Derek climbed the stairs. (The fact that Derek was climbing them at all amazed most people except Derek!)*
We returned just in time for lunch.

12.45p.m *Derek worked well with the wooden blocks and was able to sort out all the different colours, even the varying shades of the same colour, which is a major step forward from the last time we worked with them.*
He showed difficulty in distinquishing lime green from yellow but it should be remembered that Derek has always been colour blind.

4.00p.m *Derek ploughed on working this afternoon willing to tackle anything put in front of him and he did extremely well with each exercise.*

He had two visitors and was able to maintain good conversation with them which I see improving as time goes by.

We walked Derek's visitors back to their car and returned in the lifts as Derek was feeling a little tired. (He really has packed in a lot today so I am not at all surprised that he feels tired).

Derek is now resting on his bed before dinner and has said that he should be seeing visitors out from his own home and not from a hospital car-park and he wishes with all of his heart that he could come home. Then with his cheeky grin he opened his eyes and said that he did realize that it was Thursday and that he would be coming home tomorrow anyway!

We had one tiny moment when he whispered to me of how he longed to be his normal self again and why had it happened as it had. I could only reply that sadly it was life and I believed that living was about coping and turning whatever we could, whenever we could, into something positive and creative no matter how tragic the happening or dire the circumstance we found ourselves caught up in.

I saw a tear fall from beneath his closed lids and left him to wipe it away himself feeling that it was important that he should have space to himself to mourn the loss of what had once been.

Nevertheless I felt his pain within my own heart which was as strong as any form of mourning.

6.00p.m *Derek ate his dinner not quite as cheery as he has been all day but keeping up a good front I would say. He wishes to remain on his bed this evening listening to his radio but I have persuaded him to go to the day-room as I believe this will lift his spirits more than staying in his room on his own all evening.*

Entered by Andrea Craig.

Friday 12th October 2007.

9.15a.m *Speech and Language Therapy.*

We continued with word finding tasks which require Derek to provide specific examples of things e.g. things which are shiny, smooth or need tuning etc.

Derek made a very good attempt at reading his books.

Entered by Rebecca Smith (Speech Therapist).

10.30a.m *Derek was bright and cheery saying he had slept well but had been very cold and had to try and cover himself with his dressing gown.*

The morning has been spent with Derek carrying out several tasks i.e. the wooden pieces (he did very well), the flash cards (he is coming along nicely), I noticed that his focus was not as good as it has been.

We exercised with arm stretches and shoulder rotations etc.

Derek is very excited with our appointment with Dr. Chambers in I.T.U. this afternoon. He is interested in seeing for himself where he spent three weeks of his life having no recollection of. Our appointment is for 2.00p.m then home for weekend leave.

Entered by Andrea Craig.

Monday 15th October 2007.

11.45a.m *Derek was resigned to coming back this morning although he was very agitated earlier on. We are both extremely tired as we had no sleep whatsoever last night due to Derek's frequent trips to the toilet, literally every half-hour throughout the entire night. I hate myself for having at one particular moment found myself thinking how long could I cope with this and then I pulled myself up quickly by trying to imagine what it must be like for Derek.*

Friday night, his first night at home had been excellent, only one visit to the toilet during the night. Saturday night was a little more frequent counting six visits in total.

We also experienced a lot of coughing which disturbed him each night.

Our visit to I.T.U. on Friday afternoon was a great success and Derek is really so very pleased to have had the opportunity to return there.

He did mislead Dr. Chambers in the things he had him believe he could now do i.e. walk down the road to buy his own daily paper each morning, (he does not).

Derek also led him to believe that he can dress himself, which of course he cannot.

It was eventually understood that Dr. Chambers believed that Derek had already been discharged.

Derek later stated that he realized the confusion which had been caused and felt a little silly over all that business but in spite of it he had still enjoyed his visit very much because it helped to fill in a great gap in his memory.

I have to report that this weekend was an unbelievably tiring one making it very difficult for Derek and likewise for myself.

There were moments when I felt we had slipped so far back it seemed impossible that we would ever be able to move forward again but I do know that we will, given time and I feel as I do only through tiredness, (which feels more like sheer exhaustion right now!)

1.00p.m *Derek has eaten his lunch and is working willingly on the task of writing set by Rebecca Smith (speech therapist).*

3.00p.m *Derek has worked hard. He is finding the letters C and O very confusing as he cannot always see the gap in the C.*

He is still maintaining his reading level but needed a little prompting now and then today.

We worked on a new type of exercise book from which Derek had to remove a sticker and place it in the appropriate place on a map i.e. sticker of a pirate went on a ship flying the skull and crossbones. He absolutely amazed me with this as he was able to recognize and understand so well what was expected of him and the fact that he could carry it out amazed him.

He stated that he had actually had a lot of fun doing this exercise but could I get hold of a more adult book with the same type of exercise.

He claims that this has got his mind going and thinking in different ways i.e. it made him have to think and work out what went where but also it jogged his memory on so many different things.

Dr. Oates and her team arrived and we discussed Derek's frequent visits to the toilet and Dr. Oates agrees that anxiety could be the main factor resulting from his appointment at I.T.U.

Looking back over the weekend I feel this to be correct as Derek and I had held a conversation stemming from his visit and how it had forced him to look at and face up to what had happened to him and that he must stop trying to pretend that everything is alright.

6.00p.m *Derek had a rest after Dr.Oates had left the room, lying quietly on his bed but not asleep, until his dinner was served. He ate well and is washed and ready for bed later on.*

I will leave him in the day-room.

Derek states that he has had a very good day and feels that he has learnt and realized a lot which is all helping to make him feel happier and stronger within himself.

Entered by Andrea Craig.

Tuesday 16th October 2007.

10.30a.m *Derek was showered, dressed and in a happy mood. He was sitting in his chair exercising his hands using the soft balls. I assisted him with putting his jacket on (he struggles greatly with dressing still) and I encouraged him to walk ahead of me as though he were alone in this exercise. I had told him he was to go down to the shop to purchase his own paper this morning with his own money.*

I followed him down the stairs to the ground floor, where he took a wrong turn taking him away from the shop, a little later realizing that he had gone wrong he tried to correct his direction and became confused so I stepped in and set him back on course (with Derek very quickly pointing out that he knew what he was doing and if I had left him he would soon have had it sorted out for himself!)

No matter he was now back on course and heading off to the shop at a great speed.

He walked straight passed the newsagent's and into the general store where he once again became confused and disorientated, stating that he knew he was in the wrong shop and was just trying to figure it out, (which was true but he could not locate the door to go out again and was causing somewhat of a hold-up with others not realizing Derek's problem).

Once again I helped him to find his way out of the general store and led him to the newsagent where he successfully asked for his paper and handed over his money waiting for his change before thanking the lady who had served him.

With a speed which belied all that was medically wrong with him Derek took off back to his room. He walked swiftly, passing the stairway he should have taken straight down the long corridor until he had nearly reached the side entrance, determined not to interfere this time, I allowed him to carry on to go his own way and just as I thought he had forgotten where he was supposed to be going and believed that I would have to step in after all, he stopped and began to do something I found hard to take in, Derek was actually reading the hospital signs which indicated the exit, wards and various departments.

I stepped to one side and waited, before long he turned around and talking out aloud stated that he knew where he had gone wrong and was heading back to rectify his mistake. I thought it had been too good to be true when I saw him take another wrong turn, a sharp right hand turn off the main corridor which led to a side flight of stairs used by the hospital staff mostly, but stairs we had been encouraged to use as they were quieter than the main stairway, but more recently I had been taking Derek down the main stairway because it was nearer to the shops and for the zebra crossing sited just outside the main entrance which I was trying to teach him how to use.

Imagine my surprise when Derek stopped and opened the door which revealed the staircase and said, "You thought I was looking for the main stairway didn't you but this one is much quicker and a lot quieter, come on".

I was almost in a state of shock by the time we reached his room. I believed Derek had been confused when we first began this exercise but perhaps all he had needed was the time to be able to think for himself and be allowed to sort it out. When I did allow him that space he sorted it out beautifully, he realized he had gone wrong, he read the signs and then he was able to remember where the side stairway was situated, Derek I am so proud of you, well done!

11.00a.m Derek is working on his writing task sheets.

12.45p.m Derek completed a good morning's work and has enjoyed his lunch.

Derek has said he has done enough exercising for today and when I asked if he would like to have a rest he replied no and that all he wanted was to be at home.

Andrea Craig

I have suggested he do a little colouring whilst his lunch is digesting and then a few exercises with the soft balls.

2.30p.m *Derek has worked very hard today and now feels tired so is lying on his bed resting.*

I spoke to occupational therapist (Vicky) this morning and she has promised to help Derek with his dressing of himself when times permit! (He needs this help badly and I feel inadequate in helping him and feel I confuse him more than I help). Plus I feel he will respond more to a more experienced authority than he will to me.

5.15p.m *Derek has slept but kept waking saying how cold he felt. I placed his dressing gown over him which has helped.*

He got up to use the toilet (P.U.) and claims to feel unwell. He has not had his bowels opened today so perhaps this is the answer!

He went back to sleep and was awakened for his dinner. Derek had bad cramp in his foot.

I will walk Derek down to the day-room to watch the news before I leave.

Entered by Andrea Craig.

Wednesday 17ᵗʰ October 2007.

10.45a.m *Derek was sat listening to his radio which he had at last managed to switch on for himself. He is very cheerful and extremely chatty.*

He tells me that he dressed himself this morning but Staff tells me that he managed to put on his socks, underpants and trousers with a little help but could not manage his T-shirt at all. (This is what I have been struggling with for weeks, from the feet up he is managing and improving week by week but the top half of him confuses him totally. I desperately need to be shown how to help him).

Derek walked down for his paper again this morning but sadly was a lot more confused today in the shop area and had to be stopped from walking into the High Dependency Unit on the way back. He had been looking for the side stairway again and taking the wrong turning into the unit knocked his confidence.

Still his determination shone through and he asked that I take him back to the main entrance so that he could try again. This time with a little guidance he managed to find the ward and returned to his room.

Derek is finding the newspapers too difficult to read, he states there is too much to take in and his brain will not deal with it. He is now happy to sit and read his 'Early Learning' book.

12.45p.m *Derek has, as always, eaten all of his lunch and has made what I consider to be a huge discovery. As we sat eating lunch Derek mentioned how on waking up this morning he had believed it to be Wednesday 17th October and how disappointed he had felt when he looked at*

503

the notice board to discover that it read Tuesday 16th October and how long he thought the week was.

When I told Derek that he was in fact correct and it was the nurses who had forgotten to change his date board he was so visibly overjoyed it changed his entire being on every level. He felt elated because he was not as confused as he thought he was and it meant that the weekend was one day nearer.

We have shared such a good laugh over this. It was as good as a tonic.

1.30p.m Derek is now lying down resting on his bed.

3.30p.m Derek woke up and worked on his activity sheet after which we went for a walk to breathe in some fresh-air.

5.45p.m Derek has eaten his dinner and maintained his high spirits throughout the day but sadly has just sat on his glasses which meant a mad dash home for spare set.

I am a little later leaving him this evening but he can now watch the T.V. once again and see clearly so is happy.

Derek is washed, changed and ready for bed.
Entered by Andrea Craig.

Thursday 18th October 2007.

8.30a.m Occupational Therapist. I arrived to help Derek with dressing practice. Derek was already dressed except for his socks and slippers.

Derek consented to dressing practice with jumper.

Derek was able to remove jumper independently but was unable to redress jumper for the following reasons:

1) He was unable to determine inside from outside. Assistance was given showing him the correct way.
2) Derek has difficulty determining the front from the back in relation to putting the jumper on. Assistance was given showing him the correct way.
Suggestions: Only use jumper or T-shirts which have a pattern on the front.
3) Prompting was given to use left arm first. Derek was able to put left arm in but was then unable to find hole to put his head and right arm through.

We practiced this three times. Derek has great difficulty and gets himself lost in the material.
Suggestions: Only practice with T-shirts as he may find these easier.

Repetition will help him learn. Break down the task if he finds it difficult and help him with verbal prompts.

Derek did quite well. He engaged well in conversation.

Derek initiated brushing his teeth but needed prompting with using toothbrush correctly.

Derek was able to ask for comb to comb hair and helped to locate his wash-bag.

Assistance had to be given with the zip as Derek was unable to grip it.

Overall I found this to be a good session.

Entered by Vicky Carriger. (O.T.)

12.45p.m *Derek was sat eating his lunch when I arrived today. He had spent the morning after his occupational therapy in the eye clinic. He was able to inform me of all that had taken place throughout the entire morning and is very cheery and happy.*

Derek was able to put on his outdoor shoes himself but asked me to check them for him just to be on the safe side. Stated that he feels safer in his shoes on the stairs than his slippers.

He walked ahead of me today, out of his room, down the ward and knowing exactly where he was going headed straight for the stairway. He took the stairs totally independently and took all the correct turnings to the newsagents stall, where he purchased his daily paper. He tended the correct amount of money (which had been given to him before leaving his room) but alas failed to pick up the paper which the lady had left on the counter for him. With a quick prompt he recognized his mistake and quickly picked it up, laughing as he did so.

We then entered the general shop to purchase a box of tissues. Derek was able to locate these but became confused and lost his confidence handing them over to me to pay for them as he had no idea how much they were and did not wish to appear foolish.

We did our complete walk around the hospital grounds and all the way back to his room with Derek needing no help or guidance from me whatsoever.

__2.00p.m__ Derek has stated that he was left in the dayroom last night with no-one taking him to bed until after midnight and as he was up early for practice and the eye clinic this morning he feels very tired and would like to have a lie down.

__4.00p.m__ Derek awoke from a deep sleep stating that he feels quite sickly and has taken himself off to the toilet.

__5.00p.m__ On returning from the toilet Derek asked if he might practice with one of the activity books. He did well at first but his concentration was not good so I put it away.

He then said he would like to practice writing his name, again this was not a good idea.

Derek seems to be very tense and has poor focus and appears to be spoiling for an argument. Thankfully dinner was served just in time.

6.00p.m Derek is washed and changed and ready for bed but I will walk him to the dayroom before I leave.

Entered by Andrea Craig.

Friday 19th October 2007.

9.45a.m (Speech Therapy) I did assessment of Derek's reading ability today.

Derek worked well but had difficulty with his vision as well as some problems with understanding at times.

We will continue at another time.

Entered by Rachael (Speech Therapist).

10.30a.m Reading Rachael's report I question as to whether Derek had used his reading specs. or his normal sight specs!

Derek was attempting to put on his shoes when I arrived and was struggling. I told him it did not really matter and that he had almost got there but he would not be placated. He seems to be very agitated and quite disturbed over something.

After a little while of silence he explained how he had awakened this morning crying and had not *been able to shake the feeling since, saying he felt so upset and emotional but could not say why he should feel this way except to say he did not feel right somehow.*

He did seem a little flushed to me but when I asked him if he felt well in himself he stated that he felt fine that way.

Nevertheless I felt it best to mention this to Staff who came in to see him and after questioning Derek said he would be alright to go home.

Entered by Andrea Craig.

Saturday 20th October 2007.

8.30a.m *Derek had to be brought back into hospital early this morning. He had not looked too good when we arrived home but was insistent that he felt alright.*

I believed a good afternoon sleep would restore him, which it seemed to for a little while.

He did not enjoy his dinner or eat very much of it and it was then I began to know that all was not well. During the evening Derek began projectile vomiting which left him confused and exhausted. I put him to bed where he slept soundly for a few hours but was awakened with violent, uncontrollable dihorrea and continual vomiting. This continued right throughout the night making it impossible to move him anywhere.

As soon as I was able I rang the hospital and was instructed to bring him back in immediately.

Derek does now seem a little more settled but has had one more bout of diorreha

since returning. Staff on duty has tried to tell me Derek must have picked up something at home but I know this not to be the case as he was feeling a little strange yesterday morning before he left hospital.

It was as we were standing in the main corridor of the ward discussing the matter when bedlam seemed to break out on the ward. First one patient called out and then another, next there was a female patient banging on a toilet door desperate to use it but sadly it was too late, a nurse ran for mop, bucket and cleaning agent, as she endeavored to clean up the mess quickly and efficiently yet another poor soul stood before us unable to reach a toilet in time and it was quickly recognized that the ward had a major problem on its hands.

Derek is waiting to see a doctor and as there is nothing more that I can do here I must go home and clear up the mess that was left behind and try to get some much needed sleep.

I will return later in the day.
Entered by Andrea Craig.

Sunday 21st October 2007.

Derek was sat in his chair listening to his radio when Sarah and I arrived. He is aware that Andrea is poorly and unable to visit. Despite being so ill yesterday Derek is looking well and seems to be happy today.

He states that he wishes Andrea to stay at home this week and get plenty of rest.

We told Derek about our weekend away in Henley-on-Thames where the people we were staying with also had nasty tummy upsets!

Derek said he had been unable to eat all of his lunch, preferring to drink water instead.

Sarah made sure Derek was changed and ready for the evening. We have taken his dirty clothes home for washing and have left 45p on the top of his cabinet for his newspaper in the morning.

Entered by Max Payne.

Monday 22nd October 2007.

5.30p.m *I arrived to find Derek listening to his radio which he said he had only been doing for a few minutes.*

His friend John had spent an hour with him this afternoon having a good chat which he tells me helped to relieve the boredom.

I brought in some clean clothes and put Derek on the phone to mum for a little chat, he is still very concerned that she does not come in until she is completely better.

Derek seems a little frustrated that he has still not heard of his bed in Neuro. and feels he could be waiting at home rather than in hospital.

I went to take Derek for a walk to get a breath of fresh-air but we were stopped from leaving the ward. (It would seem that the ward is officially closed!)

We returned to his room where Derek got ready for bed.

I walked him down to the dayroom before I left.

Entered by Sarah Hollis.

Tuesday 23rd October 2007.

5.00p.m *I arrived to find Derek disturbed and confused about the day and date.*

Nobody had changed his date board and he knew that the day and date showing were wrong.

He is still very frustrated that he cannot leave the ward to go for a walk or down to the shops.

I found a tablet which had been left on his table which no-one seems to know what it is.

Derek spoke to mum on the phone and is now a little happier.

It transpires that the tablet is from previous evening (I am a little concerned that no-one ensured that Derek took his medication last night!)

Entered by Sarah Hollis.

Wednesday 24th October 2007.

Derek was in the toilet when I arrived this evening and was very pleased to find me waiting in his room on his return.

After washing himself he was able to get himself ready for the evening with very little assistance.

He had spent the whole day alone either listening to his radio or watching t.v. said he was so pleased to have a little company.

Nevertheless he seems to be in good spirits but is still very frustrated about the length of time it is taking to get into rehab.

6.00p.m I walked Derek down to the dayroom to watch the evening news.

Entered by Sarah Hollis.

CHAPTER FIFTEEN

I had been unable to visit the ward for three days and on the morning of my return I found myself being greeted by the friendly, smiling face of one of the nurses who, first expressing her concern for me, hoped that I was feeling very much better. I explained that I was and said that it was Derek with whom my concern lay with and how I hoped he was completely recovered.

"You need have no concerns for him", she said, "he's as right as rain now".

"That's good," I replied, "that's just what I want to hear".

"Oh yes," she continued, "in fact he couldn't feel any better than he does right now."

I walked on down the ward corridor, "Hello, Andrea, feeling better?" called another nurse.

"Yes, much better thank-you," I replied.

As I carried on walking down the corridor I became aware of the happy smiling faces on each and every member of staff I passed, were they all really this pleased to see me back?

"Isn't it wonderful news?" cried out one nurse from the sluice room.

"What news is that?" I asked.

"Don't you know," she whispered from the doorway.

"Know what?"

"Er... nothing, must dash, things to do," and with that I was left shaking my head in bemusement and wondering what on earth was going on. I began to sense something very strange in the air.

I was nearing Derek's room when Lyndsey, the charge-nurse looking after Derek that particular Monday morning, came up to me and explained that he was so looking forward to seeing me as he had something vitally important to tell me.

"What on earth is going on Lyndsey," I asked, "what is it?"

"I must let him tell you. Go on in, he can't wait to see you, he's so excited."

I hurried into his room with Lyndsey close on my heels expecting an explosion of news to greet me but was surprised to find that Derek, although obviously very pleased to see me, did not seem overly keen to impart his news, good, bad or indifferent.

I was very pleased to find him looking as well as he did for the last time I had seen him he had looked extremely poorly. As Lyndsey hovered about the room I happened to catch sight of Derek beckoning her to leave. I thought it was all

515

decidedly odd and believed by now that some test results had come through whilst I was away which he was pleased with and wished to tell me the news himself.

Once Lyndsey had left the room, Derek could contain his news no longer and with tears in his eyes he told me that he had at last been informed that he was going to rehab. the week after next and felt so happy he could hardly believe it. No sooner had the words escaped his lips when suddenly the door opened and in fell Lyndsey, who had obviously been waiting at the door for Derek to deliver his news and was just as happy and as excited as he was. The air was electric with excitement and very soon the staff one by one were all pouring in to room 23 saying how much they had all wanted to be the one to tell me as soon as I had first walked onto the ward but had realized that Derek had wanted to tell me himself. What a happy day.

Later that same day, Derek reminded me of something I had said during our conversation on the Tuesday evening when Sarah had put him on the phone to me and he had not been able to stop thinking about it since he had received his good news earlier that morning. He remembered that I had told him of a very strong feeling I had had that an announcement of his transfer to rehab was about to be made, and that not only was it imminent but it would actually take place more quickly than first planned. Derek's went on to say that he could hardly believe that the first half of what I had said had come about so quickly and that he could only hope and trust that the rest of it would follow.

Four days later the rehab unit notified the ward that they could take Derek a week earlier than first planned. The following entries show Derek's excitement and mixed emotions during his last days spent in room 23, ward 37, Arrowe Park Hospital.

Thursday 25th October 2007.

12 noon   *Derek was sat listening to his radio and was so happy to see me walk in and I was pleasantly surprised to see him looking so well.*

He asked me to sit down and fill him in on all my latest news as I have been unable to visit for the past three days. ("Norovirus" bug which has caused the entire ward to close down).

As soon as we were alone Derek excitedly gave me his own news. I have had to tether him down from floating on air.

Derek has been given the news today that he is moving to rehab. the week after next.

1.20p.m *Derek was much more willing to practice his hand writing. He is unable to cope with the letter "e" and seems unable to concentrate very well on anything and so have brought it to a halt. He seems too excited today with his good news.*

2.15p.m *Derek has said that he is not tired but would like to listen to the afternoon play on radio 4.*

3.45p.m *Derek fell into a deep sleep five minutes into the play and has just woken up and gone to the toilet saying how very happy he feels.*

Whilst waiting for dinner I cut Derek's hair and trimmed his beard. He says he can hardly wait for tomorrow to arrive.

Entered by Andrea Craig.

Friday 26th October 2007.

Derek had been showered, dressed and was eagerly waiting for his weekend leave.

Entered by Andrea Craig.

Monday 29th October 2007.

11.00a.m *Derek has just spent his best weekend to date. He enjoyed every minute of it.*

He is improving with his kitchen skills, although making tea is still very much 'hit and miss' and still needs lots of direction.

He is very good at drying dishes, ten out of ten.

Saturday we ate lunch in a restaurant and Derek coped extremely well with this. He needs assistance when visiting the toilet. (He can have trouble positioning himself correctly on the toilet but mainly the assistance required is helping him dress afterwards).

Derek enjoys company (two joined us for lunch) but does get his words and sentences mixed up. (Mainly back to front or the opposite to what he means. i.e. yes instead of no; me instead of you or vise, versa; right instead of left or can sometimes use words which have no relevance to what he is trying to say. I have noted that this occurs mainly when he is excited in company).

What I found most interesting this weekend was how much Derek had wished to discuss in depth what had happened to him on April 28th and the impairment it had left him with.

His knowing is excellent and he realizes that he struggles to express himself correctly at times and has stated that his greatest fear is of appearing foolish and having others believe that he is silly.

I have tried to reassure him that this is not so and that people will and do understand, but he will not be convinced.

Derek's excitement of transferring over to the rehab unit thankfully overshadows this fear and states that he remembers Dr. Pinder telling him that they may only be able to take him so far on his road to recovery but he says he is determined to give it his best shot whilst he is there.

He longs to be able to dress himself and to be able to read once again but has said that to be able to dress independently is more important to him.

In his dreams, Derek has described how it feels to be driving his car but has said that he understands that he will probably never drive again and that he can and does accept this.

He claims to be excited about the prospect of exercising to bring the damaged part of his body back to normality. (Exercise has played a keen part of Derek's life. Raquet sport mainly, Derek's competitive streak was always very strong, cycling, swimming and walking).

I did tell him that I personally believed that he would be better off with walking for the moment at least but he tells me that he feels sure he will be doing much more than that in rehab.and is looking forward to tackling anything they may throw at him.

Derek slept soundly this weekend in between his still frequent visits to the toilet.

He is still having to be assisted in the shower and I note that when asked to wash his hair he went to wash his feet. If I tapped his right arm to be lifted Derek would lift his left. (Opposites still).

He also appeared to be a lot more confused in the shower than on previous occasions.

2.00p.m *Derek has enjoyed and eaten all of his lunch and is now working with his activity books.*

His reading has improved a little and his colouring is more controlled.

3.30p.m *Derek is in a state of excited shock having just received the news that he is being transferred a little earlier than planned and will be moving over to rehab tomorrow at 10 00a.m.*

What strange mixed emotions Derek is expressing, indeed we are both elated and upset at the same time for ward 37 has been our life-line and security net for the past six months and we now sit facing the sudden 'leaving of it'.

I for one will never be able to express my sincerest thanks and gratitude to Arrowe Park Hospital for all they have done, not only for Derek but myself also.

Entered by Andrea Craig.

That was to be the last entry into Derek's diary during his stay in 'Arrowe Park'. I spent the rest of the afternoon collecting together and packing up to take home the many books and papers which had played their part in making up Derek's exercise program along with the contents of his locker for at last they were no longer needed here. I left only the soap bag and clean clothes that he would need for the following morning.

I made several journeys to the car with all that had been accumulated over months despite me constantly clearing out and only keeping in his room that which was needed. As I walked across the now so familiar car-park I could not stop myself from wondering how it would feel to no longer have to search for a car space each day. I would miss our secret walks in the park and our treasured moments sitting at the side-entrance enjoying the sunshine, oblivious to the coming and goings of hospital life. In spite of feeling so pleased with the news that we were to be leaving 'Arrowe Park' in the morning I felt sure there were so many little things which I was going to miss.

As soon as dinner was over that evening Derek begged me to leave, stating that the quicker I went home, the more quickly morning would bring my return and the dawn of the next phase in his recovery. The transfer, which last Tuesday I had told Derek was about to take place, had indeed come about more quickly than planned and had taken us both by surprise.

I arrived home with so many mixed emotions whirling themselves around inside of me. I felt excitement one moment, apprehension the next, with even fear and dread creeping in to cast its shadows upon our future promise, a promise of what? I had no idea but I did know that whatever it was, Derek held onto it with all that he had.

I spent the rest of the evening feeling that a major phase of our life was about to come to a close and tomorrow was to be the beginning of a whole new chapter and good, bad or otherwise I wanted to be ready for it.

Later as I climbed into bed I lay down with an ache in my heart even greater than the constant heavy ache I had lived with throughout the whole six long months Derek had spent in hospital. My heart ached when I thought if this is how I am feeling, then how much worse must it be for him. I could not even begin to imagine the many different emotions that he would be going through as he lay in his bed.

During a recent conversation with one of his speech therapists I had been asked not to put too much emphasis on his move to rehab for there would be no miracle cure or sudden awakenings and that the whole process would be a slow one. I had understood perfectly what was being said and why, but Derek could not be budged in his belief that rehab was going to put him back on his feet and no matter how I tried to convey to him that his journey would still be a slow and perhaps at times an arduous one, this was going to be the biggest if not most important part of his recovery and tonight he stood on its new exciting thresh-hold.

I hardly slept that night and when the following morning dawned I was up, showered and had finished my one round of toast before six o'clock. Feeling a little nervous and having run out of things to do to keep myself occupied, I jumped into my car and drove down to the marina for a walk which I hoped might clear my head.

It was a cold but dry morning and as I walked I remembered thinking to myself, 'How easily we allow the weather to govern our lives.' Does it really matter? Does it make a difference to what life has planned for us? Is there a certain someone looking down who declares, "Hey it's raining today, I'll just alter the course of his or her life", or "look the sun has come out, they must not be allowed to do that, they must do this instead."

I was disturbed from my ridiculous thought pattern by a shouted, "Good-morning," from a passing early morning jogger. I felt myself wanting to shout after him, "My life has changed forever, the life of my husband has changed forever and all you can do is run on by".

I felt as I had many years before when, as a young woman, I lost my dog to incurable cancer and unless you have ever shared your life with a pet then you can never know the heartbreak one experiences when losing them.

Two hours after the sad event had taken place I had needed to get out of the house for a breath of fresh air and found myself walking down the lane where I then lived. I had thought I felt strong, that I was able to cope with what had just taken place and that my dog was now in a much better place and no longer suffering, but I had no idea until then of how much the feeling of hurt is capable of isolating you.

As I walked I began to feel a strange sense of detachment, I felt invisible.

Walking passed people who seemed not to see me I suddenly found myself wanting to scream out to someone, anyone, that I had just lost my best friend. A friend I had shared my soul with. A friend who had never once told me what I could or could not do, a true and faithful friend who had never once judged me.

Now he was gone and I was hurting. I was hurting so much it caused me physical pain in my heart.

That was my first realization of coming to know that no matter how deeply you feel the pain, the rest of the world simply carries on around you and the sense of isolation you experience can be quite severe. I have come to realize that as we grow through life there are so many different happenings which cause us to feel deep heartache. Each newly inflicted wound can stem from vastly differing circumstance, yet the pain we feel can be just as hurtful. When our heart breaks we bleed from the depth of our being.

I have also come to realize that as much as we may feel ourselves injured and often isolated by the hurt inflicted upon ourselves we can and do in such times, consciously or unconsciously, shut others out for many different and personal reasons and I shudder to think of the times during my life when I may have done just that.

By the time I reached my car I had regained my balance and composed my thoughts once more enabling me to drive home in a much more positive frame of mind. Yet again a walk around the marina had saved my sanity.

I arrived at the hospital at 9.00am to find Derek showered and dressed and waiting for his breakfast although he said he felt too excited to eat very much.

Whilst he ate I took the few remaining items belonging to him down to the car so that I would be free to walk with him when he was cleared to leave. It had been agreed that I would drive Derek over to the 'Neuro' Unit as it would help to settle him in.

As we waited for his discharge and medication from the Pharmacist, room 23 became very busy with patients and staff alike, all coming in to bid their final farewells. It was a very emotional time with many tears shed and leaving was much harder than I ever believed it would be. As we walked off the ward I realized what it was I had been feeling so afraid of, our life-line had just been severed and I for one felt that I was being cast a adrift.

That was the day I came to realize how easily people can become Institutionalized, for in six months I had come to almost depend on, and can truthfully state, rely upon, the security which the hospital held for both Derek and myself.

Driving over to Clatterbridge Hospital, Derek talked of how he had begun to believe that he would never walk free of Arrowe Park Hospital ever again and that even now he felt it hard to believe that he had done so. He felt both elated and extremely excited over the next stage of his journey.

I heard the old Derek expressing his eagerness to get cracking, as he put it, on the stiff and disciplined program which lay waiting for him. Different nurses at Arrowe Park having spent time on the rehab unit all told of the programs which he would find quite tiring at first, but none of this put Derek off. He looked forward to it and relished the thought of the exercise programs he would undertake. This was the competitive Derek I knew so well.

"I won't be allowed to spend as much time with you as I have in the past", I said, "The unit will have its own program".

I thought it best to prepare him for the fact that he would not be seeing as much of me as he had grown used to and was surprised when he replied with, "You mustn't get upset, love. You know I'm really going to be too busy to miss you at all".

I could have laughed when I saw just how serious he was being but I felt so relieved that he was taking it this way.

"You really are looking forward to this adventure aren't you"? I asked. "I certainly am. It's what I need. It's one step nearer to coming home for good", he replied.

As we drew nearer to our destination I became aware that Derek had become a little subdued and was even growing a little agitated. I remained silent allowing him his own space and time to adjust to what was happening. We drove through the hospital entrance and managed to find ourselves a parking place without too much trouble.

"Well, here we are, all ready to go and face your new abode", trying to sound as light as I could.

"Before we do, there's something I want you to know Andrea", his voice was low and I could hardly hear him but I knew it was something important he wanted to say.

"I want you to know that inside I feel normal but somehow I can't do the things I once could", then getting hold of my hand he continued, "I don't want to be here at all, but they are going to help me put things right. It's very important for me to be here. You do understand that don't you".

I felt my heart breaking all over again without really understanding why. Was it the tears I saw welling in his eyes or his innocent belief in something which might prove impossible or simply the fact that he was still worrying about me and how I might be coping with it or not.

As I helped Derek out of the car I sent out a silent prayer that we would both be given the strength to shoulder whatever we had to face in the coming months. Walking across the car park, the sense of humour we both shared soon returned and after pressing the buzzer and announcing our arrival we entered the "locked unit" in high spirits once again.

We were greeted pleasantly at the desk by a member of staff who introduced us to the unit manager who in turn showed us where Derek would be sleeping and would have his own space whilst in the unit. I was allowed to stay with him as it was his first day and it was explained to me that patients often became confused and disorientated for the first couple of weeks and that I should not be worried about this as it was considered to be normal.

Two things hit me on first entering the unit, the first one being how fresh and clean everywhere looked and the other was how noisy it was in the small four bedded ward that Derek was to share with three other patients.

On our entering the ward there were no other patients present and yet three televisions were left on each competing against the other with a different channel. After six months of a quiet and controlled environment I found myself wondering how Derek was ever going to be able to cope with this situation.

I had been led to believe that Derek must have one to one conversation, not too much noise to confuse him and not too many people visiting all at once. Over six months I had taken everything on board and worked at introducing things slowly. First one visitor, then two and so on ensuring that people did not talk across each other as often happens within the company of several people. I wondered how the conflicting noise could be good for these patients when it confused myself.

No sooner had we placed Derek's belongings in his wardrobe and sorted out his drawers, he was called to go into lunch. He no longer had his meals served in his room and had to walk down to the dining room for all of his meals. He seemed happy to do this and was accompanied by one of the staff who said whilst it was his first day she would show him the way.

When Derek returned to the ward he was very quiet and down and said that he had not eaten much for lunch. I asked why that was as he had seemed so happy before. Derek explained that he had found it all too confusing. He had believed that someone would serve him his lunch but no-one had. It seemed that he had to help himself and did not know what to pick.

"I don't think I'm going to like it here after all", he whispered.

"Don't be silly", I shot at him, "It will just take a little time to get used to it. Come on we're going outside to play ball. I've spotted a net out there and we can get some exercise in".

We found a ball and for the following forty minutes we had a jolly good game and a good laugh whilst firing the ball into the net. Later that day I left Derek lifted in spirits but a little agitated at the different noises from the other televisions. I found myself home two hours sooner than normal and it made such a difference, in a strange kind of way I found myself beginning to feel a little more able to relax, especially knowing that evening visits were now being planned by Sarah, family and friends which I knew would uplift Derek tremendously.

I could hardly believe that after months of waiting Derek was at last in rehab. and would now receive the specialized help and instruction he had so badly needed.

CHAPTER SIXTEEN

Sarah rang me after visiting Derek on the Tuesday evening and explained how disappointed he was at not having received any program or exercise. We both laughed at his eagerness 'to crack on' and I explained how it would be another week before he was given a program, as he had been admitted into the unit a week earlier than planned and that this was considered to be an opportunity for him to settle in.

Otherwise Sarah had found him to be settled and quite happy. A television had been found for him but sadly was not working properly and he had stated that he must not be meant to watch television as they had never worked in Arrowe Park Hospital, which of course was true. Neither the hospital television nor the television we took into Derek, at Arrowe Park would work so he either watched the fuzzy television in the day room or listened to his radio.

Lying in bed that night I had the brain wave of how we could overcome the pandemonium of television noise in his new environment without upsetting anyone. I would purchase Derek a television with large cushioned ear muffs so that he could keep the noise of his television silent to others and keep the noise of their televisions blocked out from him at the same time. Fortunately Max was able to accompany me to a retail outlet the following morning as I set off determined to bring Derek a little light relief as he awaited his longed for program.

We were successful in purchasing the right television and Derek nearly cried when Max installed it for him, having first been told that it would have to be PAT tested by the hospital. Later that very afternoon the set was up and running and the ear muffs were a tremendous success. Derek began to relax and appeared to be happier in his new environment than he was yesterday. But once again I shall allow the diary to tell Derek's own story through his time in rehab.

Wednesday 31st October 2007.

2.00p.m *Derek was sitting happily when I arrived on the unit and was eager to chat. He proceeded to relate to me all that had gone on since I had last seen him.*

He came across as happy and settled but disappointed that he was still receiving no treatment!

I did explain that he must continue to be patient and that he should realize that he had in actual fact been admitted a week early. I dared not tell him that Max was coming in to install his television in case he was detained and unable to come. The disappointment might have proved too much.

3.00p.m Max did arrive and has installed the set and we are just waiting for it to be checked out so I took Derek for a good walk around the hospital grounds. He enjoyed the fresh-air but stated that he misses being able to walk up and down the three flights of stairs which he had been able to do previously. Said that kept him reasonably fit.

5.00p.m The occupational therapist came along and introduced herself to Derek and the prospect of starting some therapy has really cheered him up.

Derek seems to be quite settled, I was pleasantly surprised.

I said good-night as he went into dinner.
Entered by Andrea Craig.

Thursday 1st November 2007.

2.00p.m Derek was sleeping in his chair when I arrived. He excused himself to go to the toilet and then we are going for a walk to enjoy a little exercise and enjoy the fresh-air.

4.00p.m Derek enjoyed his walk and the drink of tea we had at 'Fir Trees' a coffee shop situated within the hospital grounds.

Whilst we drank our drinks, Derek explained how pleased he felt to be settling in at rehab and how positive he was beginning to feel for the future.

He was very upbeat and this was so pleasing to witness.

I could not believe that I was dismissed today at 4.30.pm as Derek stated he wanted to watch something on the television for half an hour before dinner.

Entered by Andrea Craig.

Friday 2nd November 2007.

1.30p.m Derek seems a little disorientated today but was happy at the fact he
could come home as usual for weekends.

He did tell me that he was very upset last night as no-one helped him to get ready for bed and he got himself into quite a state and was left alone. One of the other patients told me he had to go over and help him as Derek had got himself rather upset.

Entered by Andrea Craig.

Monday 5th November 2007.

9.30a.m *We are back on the unit for Dr. Pinder's ward round. I have changed Derek's clothes asking him to show me where I should put them in the hope that this will help him remember where anything can be found when he needs it.*

Derek's television controller and ear-phones have gone missing over the weekend. Nurse is looking for them as I write.

I feel I should note that Derek was more confused this weekend and did on one occasion walk into the corner of a wall which was rather an odd thing for him to do and something he has never done before. He was thankfully not hurt.

He was also a little more agitated than I have ever seen him to be, but gradually over the Saturday he settled down into a much happier frame of mind.

He is very keen to learn of a program of activity which he has been led to believe is going to be planned for him this coming week.

I have been telling him all weekend that he must be patient, more relaxed and learn how to take everything as it came along and that his program would no doubt be built up slowly.

He said that he misses our long walks that I used to take him on and the stairs he enjoyed tiring the nurses out on by walking up them each day instead of allowing them to take the lifts.

He also stated that he misses being pushed to do things and my bullying him (his words I hastened to add, not mine) when he would not have otherwise bothered.

(I must check with Dr. Pinder if the 'Epilim' drug may be causing Derek's frequent urination!)

Derek helped out a lot more in the kitchen this weekend. He managed to set the table for breakfast, made tea and put out the Weet-a-bix, sugar and milk. He still claims to prefer sugar on his cereal were as he never used to take it before.

He knew where to find all the dishes etc. (this of course was with a little help and guidance but very much improved on previous attempts).

We continued with his dressing tasks. Again much improved but still struggling with putting on his T-shirts, shirts or coats.

Derek can now undress himself totally independently but needs help with buttons, zips and the ties on his dressing gown. He is trying so hard and badly wants to be able to carry out these personal tasks for himself.

Derek's conversation continues to improve and he is showing a desire to help with jobs around the house and garden.

I had to tell him that mowing lawns and moving heavy pots were totally out of the question (these were the jobs he wished to do). His mind believed he could.

Surprise, surprise, Derek was actually eager to return to the unit this morning, saying he wished to know what his program was for the following week.

How different to Monday mornings having to return to 'Arrowe Park' when he had no desire whatsoever to return there.

I am writing this entry sitting in the day room whilst Derek is awaiting Dr. Pinder's ward round.

I am about to bid my farewell until this afternoon.

Entered by Andrea Craig.

1.00pm—1,55p.m (Occupational Therapy) *We continued with perceptual assessment.*

Derek has been looking at: matching pictures/ colours and objects.

We continued with sequencing; identifying missing parts of an object; and body image.

I discussed with Derek work over the course of this week and as we become more aware of the areas to work on I will provide worksheets for Derek to work on complete out of sessions at home.

Derek is keen to do as much as possible.

Entered by Emma (Occupational Therapist).

Tuesday 6th November 2007.

8.30a.m—9.30a.m   (Occupational   Therapy). *Personal care: Derek was able to correctly select majority of items required from his drawer.*

Moderate assistance required in shower.

Derek showed difficulty with dressing. (Identifying correct orientation of clothing, took one whole hour to dress). We will continue to work with this.

Entered by Emma & Sarah (Occupational Therapists).

1.15p.m *Derek was at first a little agitated and said that he felt upset because he thought nothing seemed to be happening.*

I explained that he must learn to be a little more patient. He replied that he was very sorry to have left 'Arrowe Park' where he had felt to be a lot more active.

I went on to say that I could understand how he felt and thought perhaps it was because he had been taken out of his comfort zone. I further added that this was what he had been heading toward so eagerly for the past several months and that he should slow down somewhat and take time to find his feet before he went hurtling forward too quickly.

(Derek then admitted it is because he believes that the quicker everything is brought on then the quicker he will be well enough to come home).

Sarah (Physiotherapist) came in and took Derek into the gym. and assessed his shoulder condition which has pleased him and also he feels uplifted with the exercise program we have been given which we are to do together, but the highlight of the session came with the opportunity for Derek to show his capability on the exercise bike. He did very well indeed and was one hundred percent improved on the last time he had been asked to get on the bike at 'Arrowe Park'

where his co-ordination and inability to take instruction had made it impossible.

3.00p.m *Derek and I went for a walk in the fresh-air and called into 'Fir-Trees' for a cup of tea.*

Derek is very upbeat and now much more positive. (He thrives on exercise).

4.15p.m *On returning we carried out a few written exercises and worked on his sheets set by speech therapist.*

Derek has worked so well this afternoon and enjoyed all that he did.

Entered by Andrea Craig.

Wednesday 7ᵗʰ November 2007.

11.30a.m—12.15p.m (Occupational Therapy)
We continued with perceptual assessment and focused on body image tasks, copying pictures, cancellation tasks.

Taking on board content of sessions and demonstrating better awareness of areas of difficulty.

Entered by Emma (occupational therapist).

1.15p.m *Derek was very upset at having broken his glasses. I drove home to collect a spare pair.*

2.15p.m *We worked on the exercise given by his physiotherapist yesterday. Derek is so keen and eager to do anything which will aid his recovery.*

I was pleased to see that Derek had begun to practice his writing once more having been encouraged he said by Joe. (fellow patient in opposite bed).

He excitedly informed me of all that Emma (O.T.) had shown him regarding dressing himself and said that we were to practice with him showing me how it was to be done. He went on to tell me that his first practice with Emma had been a huge success. (Thank-you Emma)

Entered by Andrea Craig.

Thursday 8ᵗʰ November 2007.

8.15a.m—8.45a.m *Personal care: shower and hair wash assisted by Sue.*

8.45a.m *Derek was ready to make his own breakfast.*

We held a discussion about Christmas – already! and visiting Scotland.

8.45a.m—9.30a.m (Occupational Therapy)

Function assessment: preparing breakfast. We assessed Derek's ability to plan, sequence and execute breakfast preparation.

Derek made coffee and buttered toast, he showed difficulty with orientation and holding milk accordingly, but performed well overall.

Entered by Emma Adams and Sarah Cavanagh (Occupational Therapists).

1.45p.m Derek was upset at having broken two pens, as he had wanted to show me how he was getting on with his writing when I came in.

He had unfortunately pulled off what he had believed to be the tops of the pens and had been unable to realize that one had to click them down instead.

I brought in some colouring books and coloured felt tip pens which pleased him and put him back on track.

Derek still has a long way to go but I am so pleased with his new found assertiveness and self-drive to 'crack on'.

Derek found no difficulty in copying out the letters of the alphabet today but could not manage the numbers as easily so I drew them out faintly and encouraged him to trace over them. He managed this task and said how much he had enjoyed working this afternoon, (correction as he quickly added that he had enjoyed his whole days work.)

I watched Derek go into dinner and left.

Entered by Andrea Craig.

Friday 9th November 2007.

9.30a.m We were unable to carry out planned session as Derek had already eaten breakfast.

Instead we spent the session reviewing dressing his top half using a mirror and identification of body parts.

Next week we will try different method.

Entered by Emma and Sarah (Occupational Therapists).

2.20p.m Derek was extremely disturbed and agitated when I came in over an incident which had taken place last night. He was loath to tell me about it, stating that he did not wish to get anyone into trouble.

One of his fellow patients seemed very eager to want to tell me all about it but Derek asked him not to interfere and I had no wish to encourage his involvement.

I went and asked at the desk but no-one seemed able to enlighten me further so I will let the matter drop until Derek wishes to say anymore.

3.00p.m *Derek has gone along for his speech therapy.*

I will await his return and see if he is a little more settled before I say farewell.

Entered by Andrea Craig.

Monday 12ᵗʰ November 2007.

9.30a.m *I write this entry sitting as I do each Monday morning in the day room as Derek awaits Dr, Pinder's ward round.*

Derek has spent a good weekend. It started off with Derek wanting to clear up the mystery of Friday's incident and of how much it had upset him. He had been bothered by the story Joe had been telling other people and the fact that Joe had insisted on telling me as soon as I had walked onto the ward when Derek had already asked him to mind his own business and not interfere. I tried to tell him that it really did not matter but Derek was insistent that it did to him.

Joe's story was that Derek was walking around all night with no clothes on and was left terribly upset and panicking at not being able to put on his pyjamas.

Joe claimed that he had called staff to come and assist Derek but no-one came.

(I now believe this story to be completely unfounded).

Although Joe's story had upset Derek it was not, he claimed, the real reason for his upset.

"*That was just a stupid story made up for no reason whatsoever,*" stated Derek,

"*The real reason was because my T.V. controller went missing and I was upset because the nurses believed that it was my fault it was lost, but I know where I had left the controller, I'm brain damaged, not daft. I feel as though I am in a mad house*".

Derek went on to say that he found everyone's behavior so confusing and it was not as he had imagined the unit was going to be. He told me that he was going to find it very hard sticking it out.

We talked at length of people's behavior, including that of his own, mine and so many who were considered to be normally minded people. We talked of how confused he believed the other patients in the unit were and how none of them could help their tragic condition, wereas when I or all those other supposedly normal people got confused we really had no excuse.

This he readily understood and admitted that he would try to be more understanding when he returned to the unit but insisted that he would be asking for a key to his locker as soon as he got back.

He said he felt a lot better that I now knew exactly what had gone on and that we had been able to discuss it properly. The matter was dropped and not mentioned again.

For the rest of the weekend Derek worked hard on his exercises and tasks, setting the table and helping to prepare and cook (under supervision) several meals. He stated how good it felt to be regaining some of his normal activities once more.

Derek was eager to carry out his homework set by his speech therapist and we enjoyed several walks in between the showers of rain along with a friend who had come to spend a few days with us.

I noticed a new fresh alertness in Derek, although I believe he is not getting as much rest during the day as he should. He states that his mind is too active.

His night-sleep was good, only visiting the toilet two or three times each night and returning to bed on each occasion without any assistance and then falling straight back to sleep once again. This is a tremendous improvement, long may it continue.

He amazed me on one occasion whilst doing some exercises by suddenly breaking into a Tai-Chi sequence. When I asked him how on earth had he suddenly remembered how to do that, he simply laughed and said he had had no idea but it had certainly felt good and that he had enjoyed it.

He also impressed me when I turned around in the bedroom one morning to find that he had put on his dressing gown and tied it correctly himself. He claims he had no conscious thought of doing it and has no idea how he did it but the fact that he did brought a tear to his eyes.

We were both so happy. Who was it that said, "It is the little things in life that mean the most"?

This of course would be considered by most to be one of those such, "little things" but to us it was gigantic. I hugged him until he had to beg me to stop so that he could dry the tears from his eyes.

Sadly the following morning he was confused and upset at not being able to repeat the same.

Derek still has a great deal of difficulty in getting his clothes over his head and occasionally gets into a muddle by trying to put two socks on to the same foot or two legs into the same trouser leg.

We take all of these incidents lightly with Derek fully understanding that it is only through practice that he will eventually succeed.

Entered by Andrea Craig.

1.00p.m—2.15p.m (Occupational Therapy)

We continued with perceptual assessment, looking at construction, hidden figures/shape recognition and copying.

I explained to Derek that fortunately I have been able to put in few more O.T. sessions this week, although normally this will be around five.

Where ever possible additional sessions will be included in Derek's timetable.

Entered by Emma (Occupational Therapist).

Tuesday 13th November 2007.

8.30a.m—9.30a.m (Occupational Therapy)
We reviewed dressing top half with Emma demonstrating to Derek, then Derek encouraged to practice same.

Derek benefitted from this exercise being broken down into small sequences.

Derek made coffee with Sarah.

Some difficulties were noted with object recognition.

Entered by Emma and Sarah (Occupational Therapists).

1.00p.m—1.30p.m (Occupational Therapy).
I commenced a further cognitive assessment looking at following verbal and written instructions, object recognition and verbal identification.

We will continue tomorrow.

Entered by Emma (Occupational Therapist).

1.30p.m—2.15p.m (Speech Therapy) I see from weekend entry that Derek completed his home practice but he was not sure of where it was at the moment.

We continued to work on Derek's word finding using phrase completions.

Derek tried hard but needed some prompting at times.

He has been given a new sheet for home practice.

Unfortunately there will be no Speech Therapy available next week on the unit but sessions will continue the week after.

Entered by Rachael (Speech Therapist).

2.00p.m Derek was off having his speech therapy when I arrived.

He appeared very happy on his return.

We chatted for a while, had tea and biscuits then worked with the picture cards. (Much improved on last week).

He needed a little prompting on the shaving series as he was unable to recognize the towel the man was holding. Otherwise Derek did well.

Derek stated that his head feels sluggish today and feels very bothered that he is finding it difficult to express the things he wishes to say when he knows it in his head. In spite of this I find Derek is happy and seems a lot more settled in himself.

3.15p.m Derek had a short rest on his bed then asked if we could go on the exercise bike for five minutes.

We did two minutes on the bike, five minutes gentle "physio" exercises for his shoulder and then finished off with five minutes attempted Tai-Chi movements.

4.15p.m *We spent a little time in the day room with me reading to Derek and have just returned to his area where he is now resting in his chair.*

I am about to bid him cheerio because he says he would prefer me not to leave it too late before leaving as there has been a little fog recently. (I believe he wants to watch his "telly" but is too polite to tell me!)

Entered by Andrea Craig.

Wednesday 14ᵗʰ November 2007.

8.45a.m—9.15a.m (Occupational Therapy) *We practiced dressing Derek's top half, using his red T-shirt. This was much improved from yesterday. Photographs have been taken of each stage of sequence ---- to be put into sequence chart for Derek to use.*

Entered by Emma and Sarah (Occupational therapists).

1.00p.m—1.50p.m (Occupational Therapy) *We completed cognitive assessment from yesterday focusing on auditory and visual recall, planning, problem solving and coin identification.*

Entered by Emma (Occupational Therapist).

2.00p.m *Derek is now believing that he is almost ready to come home permanently and that all he needs is a little tweaking here and there.*

I told him that would be wonderful but not to build his hopes too soon as he may still have a little while to go. He responded by telling me that I had no idea of what I was talking about and that there really wasn't very much wrong with him now except his inability in being able to dress himself.

Derek got quite agitated and said that he no longer wished to talk to me and walked off the ward.

Turned out that he went to the toilet and when he arrived back he was very apologetic. I told him that he had no reason to be sorry and that I had not meant to dash his hopes for which I was truly sorry.

Everything was forgotten very quickly and he is happy and chatty once more.

Entered by Andrea Craig.

Thursday 15th November 2007.

8.30a.m—9.15a.m (Occupational Therapy) *Dressing practice: We used the same method carried out yesterday. Derek was able to complete the first few stages with only a little help needed.*

Entered by Sarah (Occupational Therapist)

10.30a.m *Derek was lying on his bed resting when I arrived. His face lit up on seeing me and he said how happy he was feeling and that he would enjoy a walk for a breath of fresh-air and some exercise.*

We walked around the grounds and called in to have a cup of tea.

On our return we did the exercises set by his physiotherapist.

During conversation this afternoon Derek told me how confusing he finds the breakfast system and maintains that he always seems to miss out on certain things and would like to know why he can never have a drink with or after his breakfast!

He has also told me that he finds the plug for his television is always being taken out of the socket and he finds it impossible to put it back. I explained that it is probably safety procedure and that he must ask for assistance in putting the plug back. He told me that he does ask for help but has to often wait some considerable time before anyone comes. I told him that other needs must come first!

I mention these facts only to note that an explanation may help clear up Derek's confusion and ensure that he does get a cup of tea in the mornings which I consider more important than his television.

Entered by Andrea Craig.

2.00p.m—2.50p.m (Occupational Therapy) *We carried out shape recognition and matching tasks, body image tasks (Derek had some difficulty with these) although more consistent in naming body parts.*

Andrea Craig

Entered by Emma (Occupational Therapist)

Friday 16th November 2007.

8.20a.m *Derek was getting his shower bag together when I arrived to assist with his morning wash, unfortunately no showers were available and as Derek had his O.T. at 8.30a.m both Derek and I decided a bowl at the bedside would be sufficient.*

Derek suggested he would have a shower at home.

On dressing Derek was able to complete with very little assistance from me.

He was able to recognize where his arms and head were to be placed when putting on his T-shirt. He was very pleased with himself.

Entered by Pauline Brooker ST/N

8.30a.m—9.30a.m (Occupational Therapy) *We prepared a hot drink, cereal and toast. Derek coped well when only having to focus on one task. He found it more difficult when switching between cereal/toast preparation, even more difficulty with correct sequencing and object recognition.*

Derek was able to locate majority of items but had difficulty opening cupboards.

Entered by Emma (Occupational Therapist)

11.00a.m *Derek was happily sitting watching T.V. patiently awaiting his visit home.*

Entered by Andrea Craig.

Monday 19th November 2007.

9.45a.m *Derek has spent his best weekend home to date.*

He was much more alert, much more focused and his sleeping was very much improved, he averaged three visits per night to the toilet, which was excellent.

He enjoyed cooking chicken curry, with assistance from myself.

Cutting up the chicken he said that we had to be very careful as chicken could contained Salmonella poisoning.

He struggled with the frying pan, not knowing how to lift it to transfer the sealed chicken into the casserole dish. Derek is at his happiest when in the kitchen (except for when he was ever playing on a squash court that is).

I was truly amazed with Derek's recent progress in being able to now dress himself. He was so delighted and pleased in showing me this. Well done girls, you have done a wonderful job, and well done Derek I am so proud of you.

I see Derek now pushing through the barrier that I could not take him beyond. A wall I stood banging my head against for so long in frustration and at the same time feeling such a deep sense of inadequacy, I will never be able to thank you girls enough.

Derek did well at setting the table for breakfast and making the tea but did get a little confused (perhaps trying to do too much all at once but he did so want me to allow him to do it).

He also did well with the toast until he came to butter it and could not spread the butter (he seemed to be digging the knife into the toast and not understanding how to spread it across).

I still thought he did very well but Derek got quite upset by it, mainly I feel because he wanted to show me how well he was doing.

I must make note of something which I did notice and have never made note of before and that is as I watched Derek become more mentally alert and assertive in himself I could not help but notice how he began to struggle getting his words out (it was as though his brain is racing ahead and as he becomes excited his words fail to keep up).

He now seems to be doing so well and the really interesting point I notice is the fact that he has no objection to coming back to the unit as he once did going back to 'Arrowe Park' every Monday morning.

10.15a.m *As per every Monday morning I sat in the day room to write up the weekends' entry and on returning to the ward we carried out Derek's physio exercises, which he now claims are doing him no good whatsoever. Needless to say I* *insisted he did them, which he did with a great deal of reluctance!*

Derek was taken for his occupational therapy mid-morning. I was told I could wait.

Entered by Andrea Craig.

(Occupational Therapy)

Our session focused on matching cards of various colours and shapes using

"Rehacom" program on the computer.

Entered by S.Cavanagh (Occupational Assistant)

1.30p.m *Derek had a short rest after his lunch and stated that he would like to finish his exercises that we were doing this morning. We went through the exercises using the rubber band. Derek declared his shoulder to be feeling a lot better than it was.*

2.20p.m *We attended Derek's case conference which he states has now made him feel a lot more confident.*

He feels 'cock-a-hoop' with talk of a possible discharge in January or early February.

3.30p.m *Derek was taken for his 'physio' session which I was asked to join them in. He comes alive in that gym. He enjoyed it so much and said it was much needed.*

4.30p.m I am bidding farewell to a very happy man this evening. I feel a good weekend may well continue into a good week.

Entered by Andrea Craig.

Tuesday 20th November 2007.

9.00a.m (Occupational Therapy) We practiced dressing top half of body this session. Derek is becoming more confident with his dressing task and has completed first half of task without any prompting.

Entered by S. Cavanagh (Occupational Assistant)

1.30p.m—2.10p.m (Occupational Therapy) We took Derek outside around hospital site to review visual ability, road safety and ability to use visual/auditory cues.

We will repeat this session in the near future.

Entered by Emma and Mandy (Occupational Therapists)

2.15p.m Derek was very excited and as soon as I walked in he informed me that he wished to talk to me regarding family matters!

We walked down to the day room where we sat while Derek excitedly related to me how his life seemed to have at last opened up and had come flooding back to him.

He virtually described his life from being a young boy right through to his college days in London and the days before we were married.

He could at last remember his mum and dad, aunts, uncles and friends. He could remember those that had died and those still living. At times he laughed and at other memories he cried but no amount of words could possibly describe the sheer joy Derek felt at rediscovering a life he feared he had lost forever.

3.30p.m *On returning to the ward I gave Derek a large print dictionary he had been asking for and spent a little time browsing through it reading out correctly a word here and there as he was able to recognize them.*

Afterwards we worked on his task of joining dots. He was able to manage these quite easily but failed to understand why he had to do them.

(My explanation for this, and possibly an incorrect one, was so as to learn and gain control of his pen and relearn the flow movement of his hand. Whether right or wrong in my explanation, Derek could see the purpose in this and was quite happy to continue with the task).

3.50p.m *Derek has told me to go home as he wishes to watch something on the television (talk about knowing when I'm not wanted!) --- But I do feel so happy that Derek is now gaining a greater* *control and sense of independence once more. He is feeling that much more secure and it shows.*

We have quickly gone through the exercises for his shoulder which he is still claiming is improving a little more each day.

I feel I must now cut my visiting time back somewhat and allow Derek to stand on his own more.

Entered by Andrea Craig.

21.05p.m *I observed Derek undressing and organizing his pyjama bottoms and T-shirt for wearing in bed.*

He was able to dress himself without any prompts.

Entered by Pauline Brooker.

Wednesday 21ˢᵗ November 2007.

8.30a.m—9.30a.m (Occupational Therapy) *Derek chose to prepare scrambled egg on toast for his breakfast this morning.*

He showed difficulty locating and recognizing some objects.

He struggled when attempting to complete more than one task at a time and he often missed stages out.

We discussed with Derek the benefits of assessing him in his own home.

Entered by Emma and Sarah (Occupational Therapists)

1.00p.m—2.00p.m (Occupational Therapy) *We discussed with Derek and received feedback on how he felt he had performed this morning.*

We carried out matching/identification activity on the computer. Derek scored approx. 80% correctly.

Derek stated that he felt he had done better than this although he readily accepted feedback.

Entered by Emma (Occupational Therapist)

2.15p.m *Derek was once again trying to convince me that he is going to be discharged very soon, as in any day now! I explained that his earliest date was likely to be in January sometime. Once again he became so angry with me I have been and checked up that Derek had not been told something unbeknown to myself.*

I have been assured that no discharge date has been discussed as yet, so I have had a good talk with Derek, mainly out of my concern for him being so disappointed when he discovered that he was not going to be discharged after all. I think that would be too much for anyone to bear.

Derek was somewhat subdued during my conversation with him but he has accepted it and now seems a little brighter stating that he has managed to be patient for so long he feels he can remain so for that bit longer. My heart really goes out to him.

2.50p.m *We worked on Derek's 'physio' exercises and Derek is pleased that he has felt pain free today.*

3.15p.m *Derek practiced his writing and found he was struggling on most letters. I dotted several out and asked him to join them up but he was still struggling so we stopped and put everything away and went for a walk instead.*

We have to really wrap up before we venture outside now as it is so cold. We were glad to run into 'Fir Trees' for a cup of hot chocolate. Half-way through our drinks Derek suddenly asked if I could tell him the time. When I told him it was nearly four o'clock he said we had to get back quickly and that he would like me to go home. (How was I to know that he had discovered "Mid-summer Murders").

On returning I tried to show Derek how to hang his coat up but failed miserably.

Entered by Andrea Craig.

Thursday 22nd November 2007.

11.00a.m—12.00am (Occupational Therapy) *We worked on body image tasks. When discussing these Derek did appear to become a little agitated and acknowledged that he could* *dress independently now and did not have any difficulties.*

I encouraged Derek to consider his own performance on these tasks, followed by Therapists feedback.

Derek's awareness appears to be more of a problem this week, with Derek commenting on the fact that he no longer feels he needs to be in hospital.

I discussed with Derek the areas he needs to continue working on.

Home treatment session planned for Thursday 29ᵗʰ November – 9.00a.m for Derek to prepare breakfast.

Entered by Emma (Occupational Therapist. Michelle from Arrowe Park present).

Physio: practiced neck and thoracic exercises and then worked on exercises to mobilize Derek's spine more (sat on wobble cushion, curling up and then straightening).

Derek managed to take off his T-shirt independently and put it back on with only one prompt.

He then went on the exercise bike for five minutes.

The range of movement to Derek's left shoulder was only slightly less than the right and the alignment looked better also!

Entered by Sarah Goulding (Physiotherapist)

2.15p.m *Derek appeared happy and asked if we could go and have a private chat down in the day room as he wished to discuss something private.*

It would seem that Derek is still very concerned and confused over the visit yesterday morning from a woman he does not know, who apparently knew so much about his personal affairs. This is worrying Derek and I am unable to help clear the matter up. I will have a word with Mark as soon as possible.

I steered the conversation onto his work program and asked him why he feels he has been so distracted of late.

He showed no hesitation before explaining to me that it was ever since the meeting, when it was discussed that he would be discharged in January and he took this to mean that Dr. Pinder must consider that he was now better.

He went on to say that the excitement was sometimes almost too much for him

to bear and that he felt he was now better in himself and ready to go home.

I endeavored to explain, as gently as I could, that his program of recovery was far from complete and that it would go on here at the unit and at home for as long as it took but I felt sure that with our continuing patience, along with God's Grace, we would begin to pick up the pieces and learn how to put them together again when the time was right.

I noticed Derek nodding his head in agreement and I felt the frustration in him subsiding leaving a much calmer person sitting beside me.

He readily admitted behaving like an excited child (his own words) and has said that from now on he will knuckle down and continue to work hard and not waste his time here with the people who are working so hard to help him.

(There appears to be very little wrong with Derek's reasoning of the situation or his understanding of it).

Before returning to the ward, Derek has made me promise to see if I can find out who the person was who came in to see him. Before he could return back to his agitation over this matter I quickly suggested we wrap up warm and go for a walk which Derek eagerly agreed to.

Entered by Andrea Craig.

Friday 23rd November 2007.

9.00a.m (Occupational Therapy) *Dressing session: Derek displayed the ability to carry out the first part of putting on his T-shirt.*

Bottom half showed slight improvement on initial dressing session.

Entered by s. Cavanagh (Occupational assistant)

Monday 26th November 2007.

After leaving the unit on Friday, Derek spent a very good day at home. After picking him up in the morning he later helped me brush up the leaves in the garden. I brushed and he deposited the leaves into the garden sacks. (We did have a few mishaps but what the heck, they were only leaves and it was fun).

Derek held a very good and lengthy conversation with a neighbour who was very pleased to see him active once more and said what a huge difference for the better that he saw in Derek since last meeting him six weeks prior.

Mid afternoon, Derek said he was more than ready to go for a rest. He lay down and was fast asleep in no time at all. He slept for two hours.

He enjoyed his dinner and said he had never felt so happy.

We began his urine collection at 8.00p.m Friday evening (Dr. Pinder's request in response to my querying the possible side effect of 'Epilim' causing frequent urination).

Derek had no problem with using the container provided which he used three times during the night.

Saturday we spent the morning walking around the Marina and then visiting Sarah and Max who had prepared a much appreciated lunch for us.

I did notice once or twice during Saturday that Derek lost his focus and seemed a little confused

(I have not noticed this for some time) but was at all times happy within himself.

The confusion first began during his preparing breakfast, he had been doing so well but suddenly seemed to forget what he was doing and could not bring himself back to the task in hand. When the toaster popped up at the side of him Derek seemed to go into shock, dropping the knife which he had been about to butter the toast with, he stood as though completely blank not knowing what to do next. It all appeared to be too much for him to handle.

I stepped in saying how much fun it was to be working together again as we used to. I began chattering away as though nothing had happened and he soon came out of it but I could sense how disappointed he was feeling at having "messed it up", as he later described it.

Later that afternoon on returning home from Sarah's, Derek had a lie down and soon fell into a deep sleep but he did not sleep for long and remained tired throughout the rest of the day and evening.

His urine collection was completed at 8.00p.m and I commented on his being able to sleep right through as he would no longer have to use the container. He laughed at this and said "if only".

Before going to bed we did have a good talk and Derek felt able to tell me that he had felt extremely anxious all day about the O.T. girls coming first thing Monday morning to assess him at home.

I suddenly realized and immediately knew what it was all about. What an idiot I had been in failing to recognize how nervous he was. Poor Derek, he had been so eager and keen to show everyone how well he was doing. I asked if he felt able to talk about it further and he agreed it might help him to feel better.

What Derek went on to explain certainly helped me to feel a lot better about everything I had noticed throughout that day, and possible during other times previously. He explained that he had always, in the past, been a person who worried and fretted about things being correct. His exams at school and college, then later his presentations and speeches he had had to deliver during the course of his work. He had wanted to do his very best. He always wanted everything to be correct.

When I had asked him why that had been so important to him he took some considerable time before replying that he had always, he supposed, been afraid of appearing foolish in front of others. He thought this was because he lacked inner confidence but now, since he first collapsed, he always felt afraid that others would think he was mentally foolish and looked stupid in some way. This is how I now believe Derek looked to himself when he first saw his own reflection in the mirror for the first time and recoiled in shock and helps to explain his fear of how he perhaps feels his brain damage has altered his outer expression in some way.

Does Derek's brain damage cause him to feel this way because he can actually recognize something wrong with his brain or is it because he struggles to do the things he believes he can do but then finds he no longer can!

I have on several occasions walked into a room to discover Derek intently studying his reflection in the mirror as though hoping to discover something or perhaps some unexplained answer there.

This was something weighing very heavily with Derek and I had no idea how to deal with it except to simply love him and to continue encouraging him in any way I could. I put my arms about him as I had on previous occasions such as this and told him that he was still both in body, mind and spirit the boy I fell in love with.

I then brought the conversation to an end by saying that I felt he had no reason to fret or worry about next Monday as I felt sure he would show the girls and himself how at home in his own kitchen he really was.

Derek asked if I minded him having an early night as he felt very tired and I agreed we should both get a good night's rest. Sadly that was not meant to be as Derek was running to the toilet all night. (I believe it was anxiety with him!)

Sunday we spent a totally relaxed and rested day. (We both needed this after such a disturbed night).

During the afternoon Derek said he would like to practice his writing as he had a surprise for me. He sat for some considerable time trying very hard to select and copy the letters from the alphabet chart but was so terribly disappointed at not being able to write what he had wished to say.

(I believe that Derek has enjoyed a "high" over the last few weeks. A high enjoyed from experiencing a new sense of assertiveness and a newly developing confidence and after my talk with him yesterday he now realizes that he still has much further to go and is not as far along his pathway in recovery as he was believing himself to be, at the same time acknowledging how far he has already travelled. (I so often feel I might confuse Derek more than I help him and pray I could choose my words more wisely).

Derek continued to describe his past life and many of his different memories and revels in the sheer bliss he says he feels in feeling as a complete person again. He no longer feels robbed of his life, although went on to explain that it can still be somewhat jumbled in parts and this leads to confusion. It is the confusion he dislikes most of all. This is the first time he has voiced this.

Entered by Andrea Craig.

Tuesday 27th November 2007.

8.30a.m (Occupational Therapy) We focused on dressing which Derek approached confidently but still has a lot of difficulty with sequencing the whole procedure.

When only focusing on one aspect he will perform much better.

Entered by S. Cavanagh (Occupational Assistant)

11.15a.m (Speech Therapy) *We worked through orientation, Derek did well.*

He needed a little prompting for name of unit and the date but all other aspects correct.

We worked on phrase completion task, Derek completed without difficulty.

We discussed newspaper article re. teacher in Sudan.

Entered by Rebecca Smith (Speech Therapist)

1.30p.m *Derek asked me not to replace his television set as he was now more than happy with the one provided for him by the 'unit'. (The large screen television had been brought in because Derek could not focus on a small screen and so that he could use his own ear-phones and not become confused with all the different television noises. Unfortunately this set had broken down and had been taken away for repair).*

I am delighted to hear this for it shows such an improvement in just a few weeks.

For him to now be able to focus clearly on a small screen and not be confused by the goings on around him is truly amazing.

Derek appears bright and cheery, even if he is looking a little tousled and unkempt in his appearance. His hair is uncombed and full of what I believe is soap and not his shampoo (I can literally scrape it out of his hair and it smells like soap) which is causing a scalp problem. Also his skin is very dry and flaking, something quite recent and again I believe it is soap not being rinsed off.

I also notice that Derek, instead of hanging his clothes up, is shoving everything onto either the top shelf or the bottom of his wardrobe and his clothes are beginning to resemble old rags. I asked him if anyone is showing him how to hang his clothes up and he says no, no-one has ever shown him, he claims that they just say, "Put your things in your wardrobe Derek", so that is just what he does.

I will try each day to help him understand what is expected of him and hope we can succeed with a little progress in hanging up his clothes.

I am writing this entry whilst Derek is having his speech therapy. I have left the ward because the other patients are resting, I trust Derek will find me in the day room.

Derek did come and find me when he had completed his speech therapy session and informed me that a phsycologist had been to see him. He seemed agitated over this and asked why people were prying so much into his personal life and wanted to know what any of this had to do with him having a heart attack and why could he not just be left to recover from it in peace.

I managed to pacify him but he remains insistent he will take the matter up with Dr. Pinder himself.

As we were sitting in the day room we were joined by a P.A.L.S. visitor and a nurse. Derek enjoyed the shared conversation and joined in talking about travel, glasses (short sighted, long sighted etc.) and the various types and different problems arising from wearing "variafocals".

We continued with his "physio" exercises and a few simple Tai-Chi movements.

Derek is a lot happier and more settled now than a little earlier and said that he would like me to go as he wished to lie down and rest before dinner.

Entered by Andrea Craig.

(Speech Therapy).

I have come back to enter Derek's session as his diary was not on his desk earlier.

His speech session took place earlier at 1.30p.m

We went through sentence completion task, elaborating on the answers given and chatting about topics which arose.

Derek completed without difficulty.

Entered by Heather Shawcross (Volunteer)

Wednesday 28th November 2007.

a.m. (Occupational Therapy) *We focused on body image for this session as therapist is new to Derek and his needs.*

Derek became muddled between his right and left, concepts such as top of; below; beside etc. when completing body image jigsaw.

Derek was unable to recognize pictures of the body parts on each piece, he needed prompts and guidance before eventually managing to complete each task.

We sampled handwriting and free hand drawing of face and body, concluding with orientation exercises.

Entered by Mandy (Occupational Therapist)

p.m. (Physio) *We did some hand walking up the wall, ball throwing and catching, and turning from side to side. Derek needed lots of prompts to copy what I wanted him to do.*

Entered by Vicky Triggs (Physio Assistant).

3.15p.m *Derek was very down this afternoon when I came in. I asked if he was feeling alright or was anything causing him a problem and he replied that he was not at all happy with his physiotherapy today, but was reluctant to say why.*

Derek said he was not in the mood to do anything at all, thank-you!

I have felt a little concerned for Derek this week as he has seemed far from his usual self. He has not been as bright or shown any of the motivation that he was beginning to show a little while back. (I cannot as yet work out why).

We have spent a very quiet afternoon with Derek lying on his bed not wishing to talk, I could only respect his need to do so.

Entered by Andrea Craig.

Thursday 29th November 2007.

Derek was brought home this morning for his Occupational assessment in his own kitchen. After the girls had left leaving Derek to spend time at home he was concerned and at the same time eager to know how I thought he had done.

I told him how pleased I was to see his improvement in buttering the toast and that I thought we should take on board and try to remember what Emma had said about trying one task at a time and completing it before going on to the next.

He said that he knew this made good common sense and that hopefully in the future he would be able to remember this but that he also knew that throughout his life he had rushed from one thing to the next before finishing what he was doing before. (I can vouch for that!).

Derek enjoyed his time at home and helped me to look for our Christmas decorations. We had

Andrea Craig

a good laugh because we could not manage to get the box out of the attic storage cupboard and decided that Max would have to help out at the week-end.

We prepared lunch with Derek setting the table. After eating he took a short nap and said how happy he was feeling compared to yesterday.

Marlene and Glyn paid a lovely surprise visit which rounded off Derek's day before returning to the unit at 3.30p.m.

I am leaving Derek very much happier going into dinner this evening and look forward to picking him up in the morning for the weekend.

Entered by Andrea Craig.

Friday 30th November 2007.

9.30a.m (Occupational Therapy) *Our session focused on isolating each task when preparing breakfast. Derek had difficulty in locating equipment for the tasks but did show improvement in manipulating the cutlery in cutting and buttering his toast.*

Entered by S. Cavanagh (Occupational Assistant)

CHAPTER SEVENTEEN

December began with the very welcome anticipation of Christmas. In Derek's mind once Christmas was over and he returned to the unit in the New Year he considered he that he would be working on the countdown to his being discharged.

I had always been led to believe that his discharge would come towards the end of February but recently there had been mention of perhaps his discharge being as early as January. This was something I wished had never been mentioned in front of Derek as he was constantly talking about his discharge and if in fact it did come later instead of earlier, Derek was going to be very disappointed.

I was eager for Derek to come home permanently, but felt quite strongly that he still needed the expert therapy that only the unit could provide and as difficult as it would prove for me to see him go back there after spending Christmas at home, I knew that in the long run it would benefit him more.

As I began to enter December's entries into the diary I had no idea, that as well as being the last month of the year, it would be the last month Derek would spend in the unit.

It was one afternoon mid December when Dr. Pinder took me aside and asked me how I felt about Derek not returning to the unit after Christmas. I have to admit it took me a little by surprise as my mind was fixed on the therapy Derek still badly needed. He was still struggling with his dressing and although he had shown improvement with certain items of clothing he definitely had no idea with others.

I was told that Derek could now shower himself, but I had noticed recent evidence that he had not been capable of rinsing his hair or himself properly while taking a shower. Certainly when he took a shower at home Derek proved to need a great deal of instruction and assistance, especially in drying himself afterwards.

I felt afraid that Derek was being let down in some way and I could not help but feel a sense of disappointment. I shuddered at the thought of going back to a similar situation I had once found myself to be in back at Arrowe Park Hospital when left struggling to teach Derek how to do things for himself. I failed him then and dreaded the thought that I might fail him once again at home. Derek needed expert training. There are so many people like him and sadly so many more much worse than he, all in need of expert training. With it they improve dramatically in their recovery, without it unfortunately they flounder, struggle and all too often sink into despair.

Dr. Pinder had not said that Derek could not return to the unit. In fact he gave me the choice, but after further conversation with him of how cruel he believed it would be for Derek to have to return after the Christmas break, especially as there would be new therapists dealing with Derek who would not be quite as familiar with his condition, I agreed for him to be discharged.

I was later informed that his discharge date would be the twentieth of the month. What a Christmas present this was going to be for Derek, indeed for the whole family and despite any reservations that I might have it would simply be the best birthday present I could ever have wished for.

Monday 3rd December 2007.

10a.m Derek has spent a wonderful weekend. He was taken into Chester, with myself, Sarah and Max to purchase his Christmas presents and a birthday card for me. On arriving in Chester I was dispatched to go and do whatever I wished to do while Sarah and Max went off with Derek.

The trip took place first thing Saturday morning before the shops became too busy and by mid-morning we had met up to enjoy a rest over a cup of coffee with Derek claiming he could not remember when he last felt so happy and hopeful.

Back home during Derek's afternoon nap, Max retrieved the box of decorations from the loft, leaving it ready to be sorted as soon as Derek woke up. I explained that it was a little early still to put anything up but I had wanted to check if the lights were still working. Thankfully they were, "Just as well," uttered Derek, "as I could no longer fix them", but he really did not seem too upset by this at all!

Later Saturday evening he claimed that he had spent the best day ever as he had enjoyed so much fun and laughter and had said it had felt like Christmas already.

I played a silly game of trying to persuade him to tell me what he had bought me for my birthday or to please just give me a clue but no, he would not budge and told me I would simply have to wait for the surprise. But I knew he had enjoyed the teasing as this was something he was well used to my doing every year.

And as Derek had already stated, it felt so good to have a sense of normality coming back into our lives.

Sunday we relaxed and spent the day quietly.

Derek drew open four sets of curtains this morning which threw me into a state of shock as they are all cord controlled and he went straight to them, instinctively knowing what to do and exactly where to locate the cord to each set.

He said he could not help wondering why I appeared to be so surprised, as he had always been able to open the curtains. (He also keeps wondering why I keep hugging him half to death!).

Feel I must record that during Friday night Derek went to the toilet only once and so enjoyed a complete night's rest. Saturday night he went twice, enjoying yet another good night's sleep but Sunday night he paid five or six visits which broke into and prevented him from a reasonable night's sleep.

Entered by Andrea Craig.

a.m. (Occupational Therapy) *We focused this morning on dressing the whole body. Derek struggled on his first attempt and agreed to try again, second attempt showed improvement especially putting on his T-shirt.*

Derek has been given cards for top-half dressing sequence.

Entered by S. Cavanagh (Occupational Assistant)

Tuesday 4ᵗʰ December 2007.

a.m. *I assisted Derek with his shower. He needed a little prompting to wash his hair. He then proceeded to dress himself, which he had few problems with. He was able to put on his T-shirt with no problem at all.*

Entered by Pauline Brocker.

11.45a.m (Speech Therapy) *We had a good session today. Derek was very chatty. We tried some quite challenging work sheets and Derek managed them well, this task required him to draw coclusions.*

We also discussed newspaper articles.

Entered by Rebecca Smith (Speech Therapist).

a.m. (Occupational Therapy) *We focused on fastening buttons for the first half of our session and the attention card game for the second half.*

Derek had extreme difficulty with hand co-ordination as he described it!

Although the task was troublesome, Derek displayed determination and expressed wishes for further sessions to practice.

Derek's attention was poor during the second half of the session, he was aware of this and put it down to his being very tired.

Entered by S. Cavanagh (Occupational Assistant).

1.15p.m (Speech Therapy) *We attended the Christmas craft group in the day room, where Derek made a lovely card for Andrea. He chose what he wanted to put on the card and where to place it. Derek also chose what he wanted to write--- he managed well with dot to dot writing.*

Entered by Rebecca Smith (Speech Therapist).

2.00p.m *Derek was with Rebecca when I arrived this afternoon. He returned to his bedside with a beautiful Christmas card and a very happy smile.*

He stated that he would like to relax and have a rest as he had been working so hard. Derek is now sleeping on his bed.

Entered by Andrea Craig.

Wednesday 5ᵗʰ December 2007.

9.40a.m (Occupational Therapy) *We focused on full body dressing with methods for putting underwear and jogging bottoms in place. Derek was confident that he could put them on and did so correctly.*

Some difficulty was shown in trying to put on his T-shirt but after looking at method and altering accordingly, Derek feels happy that he could manage it.

(Important to remember that both arms must be placed through arm-holes at the same time before lifting T-shirt from the surface it is placed upon)

Entered by S. Cavanagh (Occupational Assistant).

a.m. (Occupational Therapy) *We worked on sequencing and preconceptive/ tactive senses.*

This will help with most functions. Derek needed prompts at times but appeared to enjoy the challenge.

Entered by Mandy (now called Milly-Molly-Mandy, as this helps Derek to remember my name!)

2.30p.m *Derek was very alert when I arrived and quickly switched off his television which he was just about to settle down to watching. He was keen to tell me all that had taken place with his therapy and sounded very positive and his actual words were, "It is now helping me to feel much more confident again".*

I took Derek down to the day room where we could sit quietly whilst I broke the sad news to him of the sudden death of a very close friend.

Derek had been told prior to this of how poorly she had been for the past few days suffering with a flu' virus, with no-one ever believing that the outcome would be so bleak. It had been discussed as to whether Derek should be informed but I felt he should be as Doreen was a friend whom we discussed and chatted about on a daily basis, with Derek always asking after her out of concern for her well being.

He took the news of her death with a sound philosophical outlook stating how very sorry he felt but at the same time asking me to remember that she would now be much happier with her husband Angus as he felt sure they would now be re-united once more.

Derek has expressed his wish to attend the funeral so as to pay his final respects and say his own personal farewell to Doreen. I will let him and the staff, know of the arranged date of the funeral as soon as I know.

3.30p.m *Derek is now lying down resting on his bed.*

As Derek was taking off his slippers to get onto his bed I noticed a distinct red, round spot on one of his slippers which I said I would try to clean off while he was resting. It was then that he told me of this wonderful idea he had come up with to help him know which slipper went on which foot. The slipper now marked with the red felt-tip went on his left foot. (We all become too clever as we grow into adulthood, or I do at least, and forget that the simple things are often the best. Well thought of Derek, I am so proud of you!) This marking technique is something so many parents do with their children to help them to tell the left shoe from the right.

Thursday 6th December 2007.

8.30a.m—9.30a.m (Occupational Therapy) *Derek advised us that he felt he would try another method of preparing breakfast, he was able to reason why.*

Derek started his task well, although as in previous sessions, he became distracted by other tasks. Derek was fully aware that he felt confused.

Entered by Emma (Occupational Therapist).

2.30p.m Derek was sitting in his chair confused as to why he could not hear his television. This was because, although he had his ear-phones on, he had accidentally pulled out the lead with his foot as he had returned to his chair.

Derek had also managed to get into a little bit of a mess with his toothpaste. Somehow the top had been left off and it had been squeezed down the front of Derek himself, over his work-top and all over the floor.

I went over the procedure of only needing to flip up the top instead of unscrewing the whole top (which of course he could not screw back on). This is a procedure Derek had become used to doing but today for some reason he had become confused with it.

3.00p.m We went for a walk around the hospital grounds with Derek leading the way showing me that he knows full well where he is and led me straight into 'Fir Trees' for a hot drink.

He wanted to talk about Doreen (our friend who had recently died) and was asking when her *funeral would take place. I am still unable to tell him.*

Entered by Andrea Craig.

Monday 10th December 2007.

9.45a.m *Derek spent a good weekend. It started off with a little Christmas shopping after we left the unit on Friday, Derek was in high spirits, he was very aware and totally un-phased by all going on around him and appeared to be more focused than I had known him to be before.*

Saturday morning was spent leisurely doing very little, then visiting friends for lunch after which we returned home, where Derek took his afternoon nap. Once again Derek had been in good spirits, amazing our friends who noticed a huge difference in his recovery.

Sunday we enjoyed a small family pre-Christmas dinner which Derek handled beautifully (everyone understanding the need to not confuse him with cross conversation, the occasion meant a lot to Derek and everyone else included).

After dinner, Derek suddenly felt so tired he almost fell asleep standing up, refusing to lie down other than in his own home we made a swift departure and within half an hour Derek was fast asleep in his own bed, where he slept for three hours.

On waking up he enjoyed a few light exercises which he keeps likes to keep going, followed by a light supper and a couple of hours television when he felt tired again and wished to have an early night.

Derek slept well whilst at home, only going to the toilet two or three times each night but on waking this morning I noticed he was not as focused as he had been. He had difficulty with dressing which frustrated him but with a little guidance he managed to sort it out.

For the first time, Derek has been talking of the deep frustration he feels in no longer being able to do all the things which he once took so much for granted. In complete contrast to how he had expressed his high spirits throughout the entire week-end, Derek's spirits had dropped and he was upset, just as his focus had been more than I had known it to be on Friday, he was now more upset than I had known him to be in a long time. Between his heart rendering sobs, I learned that buttons and zips seemed to be fixed as the biggest of the hurdles he feels he has to surmount. My response was to ask him yet again to be patient and consider that it was not so long ago that he could not even remember any of the things that he could once do and to look at all those things which he has re-learned already.

(How I wish I or someone could wave a magic wand, or be able to speak words of wisdom that could lift him out of his torment and place him at the top of the mountain he is struggling to climb. But words of wisdom failed me and I could only

help to wipe away his tears and remind him that he was not alone in his upward struggle and to remember that I was climbing right beside him every step of the way).

During breakfast Derek was very quiet and subdued but having been persuaded to help me dry the dishes he seemed to come round to his normal cheery self once again and was able to explain what it was that had really upset him so much. Yes, he admitted it was basically frustration but he went on to tell me how, over the last week, he had found himself wondering what on earth he was ever going to be able to do in the future.

"If I can't even fasten a button or do up a zip, then what will I ever be capable of doing. What future do I have?"

I suddenly recalled the words Dr. Pinder had once spoken when he explained to me, that the more Derek recovered and became able to realise what he could do, then the more he would be aware of what he could not do.

This morning Derek stopped being thankful for all that he has re-learned and realized so far, and has become overwhelmed by a somewhat dark future of all that he still struggles with and may never be able to do again.

Although the sun was streaming through the kitchen windows this morning Derek stood held in the darkness of a shadow cast from the loss of his future.

587

The day Dr. Pinder voiced those words to me he offered me no further words of wisdom then and I could impart none to Derek now, except to encourage him to not look to the future but to simply live in the reality of each moment.

It was Derek himself who managed to dispel the shadow when he announced a little later, the idea that had come to him over breakfast.

Derek has said that he would like to learn how to play the piano and that he would ask Sarah to teach him the scales. I told him I thought this was a wonderful idea and he replied that if nothing else it would help exercise his fingers so that he would be able to tackle his buttons more easily. I could only admire his logic.

We are off on our climb once more with renewed vigour and much excitement as he now feels he has solved his greatest worry of what he can do in the future. He has at last thought of something which he can do and enjoy at the same time.

He has told me that this problem was worrying him so much it was keeping him awake all of last week.

Entered by Andrea Craig.

Tuesday 11th December 2007.

8.30a.m (Occupational Therapy) *We carried out full body dressing. Derek was reminded of the methods used to put on his underwear and trousers.*

His first attempt he was given verbal clues. His second attempt Derek was to initiate independently and with a little assistance Derek managed the methods but agreed that more practices were needed.

Entered by S. Cavanagh (Occupational Assistant).

9.45a.m (Speech Therapy) *We carried out verbal comprehension and explanation task. Derek found this challenging but did well with it.*

We discussed a newspaper article about healing and the 'Benefits Agency'.

Derek was very positive to-day and was able to discuss some good things that have come out of his episode in hospital. How his whole outlook on life has changed and how a strong relationship is now even stronger.

Entered by Rebecca Smith (Speech Therapist).

Wednesday 12ᵗʰ December 2007.

4.00p.m *Derek was up most of the night running to the toilet (perhaps the excitement of being home mid-week for the funeral to-day).*

Derek became very emotional when he looked at himself in the mirror and saw himself dressed in his suit and overcoat. He claimed he reminded himself of the man he used to be. He then looked to me and asked if I would feel embarrassed at being seen out with him and did I think he would do.

I told him that I thought he would do very nicely and that he still scrubbed up very well indeed. As for being embarrassed, I had never heard such tosh in all of my life as I have always been, and always will be, so very proud of him no matter what. I consider it a privilege to be seen with him anywhere.

He coped exceptionally well with the service, indeed the whole day. So many people declared how surprised they were at the normal conversations Derek had been able to hold. He mixed and mingled with an ease which amazed me more than anyone, although I did ensure that the conversations were kept short.

It was a long day for him and he was so pleased to get home where he could lie down and rest. He deserved it for he had done so well.

On waking up, Derek once again stressed how much he was worrying about the future as he now realizes after a talk with Dr. Pinder that he will never, realistically, be able to play the piano and how he now feels that in actual fact there will be very little he can do.

I sat on the bed and listened to all that had been building up inside of him and learned of how he had once again had his hope for the future smashed into tiny pieces. He felt as though he had been smashed into a thousand little pieces and stood as nothing. He felt he had lost everything and had nothing to hold onto. Derek talked until it was almost dark and when he finally lay quiet with no more to say I took hold of his hands and praying that he would understand, I tried to explain to him that if he did hold onto anything at this stage then there was a possibility it would hold him fast to where he was at this present moment and that would not be good as he needed to go on, to continue in his climb as far up that mountain as he could possible go.

I reminded him that only a few months previously he had believed he might never walk again or be able to hold a normal conversation and yet here he was able to tell me all that was worrying him with an ease he never, ever believed possible. I asked him to look back over and recall the distance he had actually travelled in a relatively short space of time during which there had been many set-backs he had had to overcome and pitfalls which had needed careful navigation, but never once had he given up in spite of the weariness that had threatened to overtake him.

I paused giving Derek time to digest what I had said and as he remained still, I knew by the look of alertness I saw in his eyes that he had understood what I had been saying but chose to remain silent and so continuing to sit holding his hand we shared the quiet, peaceful tranquility that seemed to embrace us both.

Breaking the silence after a little while, I murmured how proud I was of the extreme effort he had applied, not only during the past six months, but to the whole passage of his life and how blessed I felt to have been able to share in a part of that journey alongside of him. Derek closed his eyes but was unable to stem the flow of tears as they slowly trickled down his cheeks.

Believing in the therapy of tears I did nothing until he quietly beckoned for a tissue with which to wipe away the last of them and to finally blow his nose. Then sitting up and swinging his legs over to sit on the edge of the bed he explained that he had understood all of what I had said and that normally he was able to look at things positively, but there were times when he simply could not.

Derek went on to claim that he is afraid that he is going to become a dreadful burden on me and he finds that too hard to bear. He then went on to explain that the concentration he has to apply every moment of every day sometimes feels too difficult and wonders just how long he will be able to sustain it.

Trying to find the right words with which to encourage him, Derek suddenly surprised me by jumping up from the bed stating that he was going to prove Dr. Pinder wrong. Without further comment he raced (with me in hot persuit) down the stairs, claiming that he felt Dr. Pinder was definitely wrong because he knew that he could move all of his fingers at the same time and had decided he was going to take lessons after all! Good for you Derek, time will tell!

Entered by Andrea Craig.

Thursday 13th December 2007.

a.m. (Occupational Therapy) *This session we focused on breakfast preparation. Derek used good reasoning behind his order of preparation (making toast and coffee).*

Derek was able to locate most of the equipment independently, although his manipulation of cutlery has not improved his ability to complete a task in isolation has.

Derek feels that the breakfast sessions are a bit repetitive but enjoys the practice.

Entered by S. Cavanagh (Occupational Assistant).

Friday 14th December 2007.

a.m. (Occupational Therapy) *Derek was able to locate button and button hole but had difficulty with co-ordinating movements to push button through.*

Derek's attention was poor during the second half of session which focused on computer card game.

Derek showed great determination in continuing with his button fastening practice.

Entered by S. Cavanagh (Occupational Assistant).

Monday 17th December 2007.

1.30p.m *Derek returned to the unit having spent a first class weekend. He was so keen and eager to know all the things he needed to brush up on i.e. how to improve his dressing, combing his hair etc.*

Walking around the village he seemed much more alert than on previous occasions and was able to take in so much more of what was going on around him. There was a most definite improvement in being aware of traffic although still not able to cross a road on his own.

Entered by Andrea Craig.

Tuesday 18th December 2007.

a.m. (Speech Therapy) *We continued with 'drawing conclusions' and language activity, Derek performed well and gave some good answers to questions and responded to prompts when they were needed.*

We also discussed his being discharged and Christmas.

Entered by Rebecca Smith (Speech Therapist).

2.45p.m *Derek was sitting quietly watching his television when I arrived*

We went through a few 'physio' exercises and the wrapped up to go for a walk and a drink at 'Fir Trees'. Derek is now more than capable of leading the way.

Entered by Andrea Craig.

Wednesday 19th December 2007.

2.30p.m *Derek was sitting at a table with three other patients in the dining room when I arrived. The unit was celebrating its Christmas party. Everyone, patients and staff alike where present and a good time was seen to be had by all.*

Later Derek asked if we might go out for a walk and a breath of fresh-air and as per usual we ended up having a hot drink in 'Fir Trees'.

As we sat I noticed that Derek was somewhat subdued and when I asked what it was he replied that he felt very tired as it had felt to be rather a long day and he had in actual fact felt a right 'Charlie' sitting there pretending he was having a good time. I found I could not respond to this and thought it best if we made our way back to the 'unit' where he is now lying down fast asleep on his bed.

Derek's stay on the 'unit' has been short in duration but during that time I have noticed a tremendous improvement in him.

He has enjoyed the atmosphere here and has grown very fond of the staff, although he found the behavior of both staff and patients a little confusing to say the least (once again these are Derek's own words!). Both Derek and myself will miss everyone, although the excitement of Derek's homecoming will, I feel sure, help us to overcome any sadness we may feel on leaving tomorrow.

I have been asked to collect Derek tomorrow afternoon after lunch as he has his last occupational preparation mid-day.

I leave him this evening praying that he will get a good night's rest and hoping that my own excitement will not keep me from sleeping. I cannot help still the slight feeling of misapprehension I have at the knowing as from tomorrow I shall have total responsibility for Derek's future progress and well-being. Please God that I am up to the task ahead of me. Derek has proved more than capable in applying his effort and so much more besides, but then he has always been so much more gracious than I and I can only pray that I will be able to show the same patience and graciousness as he.

Entered by Andrea Craig.

This was the last entry written whilst Derek was in the 'unit' and as I walked across the car-park that last evening I felt so many mixed emotions stirring within me. I found myself reflecting back over the past eight months and wondering how they seemed to have passed in the blink of an eye one moment and then seemingly stretched out for all eternity the next. I could not stop myself from wondering what life would be like from now on and discovered the newly formed question of how we were going to cope became almost overwhelming. I knew I should not dwell on this knowing that with God's Love I could and would be able to cope simply by living and dealing with one day at a time. I quickly chastised myself with the full knowing that many others were going through and coping with much worse. I felt ashamed at having allowed the question to form in the first place, but as quickly as I pushed it aside it would edge its way once again right back to the fore of my mind.

It was a dark, cold and very damp evening. Not raining as such but cold and drizzly enough to make you want to lose yourself inside of your coat and pull the collar up keeping out the cold, wet night air. I was wearing a warm grey coat, its' very colour helping me to become almost invisible and to seemingly merge as one with the night. The coat had a hood and as I walked towards my car I pulled it over my head to prevent my hair from frizzing. What nonsense we women find to fret and worry about, did it really matter if my hair went a little frizzy or not?

On reaching the car, and for some reason I cannot explain, I paused to look up at the bright, shimmering fairy-lights which decorated the trees growing in front of the hospice. These lights were growing in number with each passing Christmas, each one representing a treasured memory or a bright, glittering symbol of hope for someone's loved one. I made a conscious note to have a light lit in memory of our friend Doreen, and also one as a thank-you to all at Clatterbridge Hospital, but mainly I thought I would like one lit to simply add to the light I truly believe is Christmas.

I found it somewhat strange realizing that this was to be the last time I would leave the 'unit' and have to face going home alone. I felt strange but deliciously happy at the same time. I closed my eyes and savoured the moment.

This was another of those strange moments of seemingly no importance yet one which chooses to stand apart from the other everyday moments of daily life, imprinting itself everlastingly upon my memory.

I had walked across this car-park every evening for the last two months with people coming and going, often hearing fleeting snippets of shared conversation, which of course never really registered, between couples or small groups of people as they passed me by. But tonight, not one person or moving car could be seen entering or leaving, no cars piling up at an out-of-use barrier, as there often was, to break the eerie silence. As I climbed into my car closing the door I felt the closing of a chapter which had spanned the past eight months marking the pathway of Derek's recovery and tomorrow would herald the start of a new chapter. Who knew what that would hold in store, all I could do was be truly thankful for the many blessings which had helped to bring us both through the last long eventful chapter.

Everything at home was ready and prepared for the following day's homecoming. Derek had helped me the previous weekend to put up the evergreen garlands and a few Christmas baubles but since then I had added the wreath to the front door and adorned the house with fir branches, holly and weather-cones. As I opened the front door, I walked into the lovely fresh smell of pine and a strong feeling of Christmas. I hoped Derek would feel the same atmosphere as he walked in tomorrow.

I had sensed there to be a very strong presence with me ever since leaving the 'unit'. It had walked in unison with me as I crossed the car-park standing silently at my side as I breathed in that last moment. It had remained at my side, as if in support, as I made my way home and then finally as though having gone on ahead, it was ready waiting to embrace and welcome me as I walked through the front-door filling me with a rich warmth of happiness and contentment. If I were ever asked to state what Christmas meant to me it would be to describe how I felt that night.

Tomorrow, a day which we had both once believed might never arrive was here at last, or would be in a few short hours time. I felt like an excited schoolgirl and had to keep reminding myself that Derek had already spent so much time at home but this was different. This time he was not going to have to leave and return to the 'unit', hopefully not ever. Wondering how I was ever going to be able to sleep I decided to sit down and write him a welcoming home letter.

19th December 2007.

My darling Blue,

It is such a short time since I bid you cheerio for the night and only a few short hours away before I see you again but right now I am finding it impossible to sleep, "so what's new" I can hear you saying. I feel so excited about you coming home tomorrow, not only because we will be together for my birthday and Christmas but because you will not have to return to 'rehab'.

Eight incredible months have passed since April 28th, that beautiful, idyllic and so peaceful Saturday morning when fate took a hand in changing our lives in the most dramatic way.

Ever since that time we have travelled a journey of sadness and heartbreak but at the same time it has been a journey of strength, courage and fortitude. You, my darling, have shown a steadfastness and patience you once believed you never had and you have shown a humility that could shame nations. A journey along which we have shared moments of such deep caring and a sharing that I feel all couples should share in their own hearts, although God forbid not through the same circumstances as our own, as they travel their own particular pathway.

Our pathway led us to a mountain that sunny morning which over-powered you and almost shocked the life out of you but God, through the hands and expertise of some brilliantly exceptional people decreed that you should live. Live to climb that very same mountain which tried to claim you as its victim.

I believe we should now allow time to fall away and rest for a while, to simply breathe in and enjoy the progress you have already made. You have climbed so far up your mountain, my darling, and I want to welcome you home and say how very proud I am of the sheer effort I have watched you apply in struggling through and overcoming each obstacle which appeared before you.

You already know that I love you beyond words and we both know with absolute certainty that Love can indeed conquer mountains and cross oceans of vast distance. You, Derek have, as Doctor Oates once told you, truly steered your own course through those unchartered waters of the vast unknown.

You believed this day would never arrive. There were times when you actually trembled with fear lest some cruel twist should keep you from it. It has truly arrived, my love, you need fear no more.

Do you remember the words I once shared with you, "Do not stand in fear of the past, nor dwell in dread of the future, simply live in the security of now", then please know, my darling, that you do stand secure.

People told me that due to the brain damage you suffered you would express anger. They told me you would most certainly show extreme frustration and at times be very saddened at what had befallen you, I know that all of these emotions you have experienced, and still do at times, but the power of love has enabled you to live through it all with the graceful 'spirit of simplicity' and the all powerful 'spirit of balance' now we have a special time of rest in the calm presence of 'tranquility'. Allow the traces of fear to fall away and each day will fill your being with the fresh joy of life and simple things.

I await tomorrow with such love and excitement and great hope for the future, never ever forgetting the deeper patience we have both developed which will enable us to complete our journey when the time is right.

Goodnight, my darling Blue, as my excitement grows at the thought of seeing you tomorrow so my thoughts go out to all those other poor souls who struggle to travel their own difficult journeys. God be with them all and I pray that the light of Christmas will help illuminate each personal pathway of recovery.

My love always Andrea   xxxxxx

CHAPTER EIGHTEEN

I did in fact sleep well and spent the morning with a well planned shopping list which would hopefully free me for the next few days to spend as much time as necessary with Derek developing a new daily routine.

Derek had informed me that he would be having his Christmas dinner in the 'unit' before coming home so would I please prepare a light evening meal as he felt sure he would not be feeling too hungry. Feeling too excited to eat I skipped lunch and simply ate a piece of fruit before setting off. I believed I was going to be greeted with the equivalent excitement as I was feeling and was rather taken aback to find a very disgruntled Derek waiting at the side of his bed with what few remaining bits and pieces he had all rolled together in one bundle, which he suggested I quickly pack away so that we might escape out of the place.

Andrea Craig

This was not going as I had imagined it would. Something was wrong but on questioning Derek, I was told, "nothing," he just wanted to get out and get home.

"We have to wait a little longer," I told him and went on to explain how the pharmacy had not sent up his medication for discharge as yet.

"The organization in this place beggars belief," he muttered.

"It won't take long. Let's have one more check through all the drawers, just to make sure nothing gets left behind, shall we".

"I have done, twice", Derek firmly stated.

I was beckoned from the doorway to go to the desk where it was explained that pharmacy had sent Derek's medication but unfortunately it had not been complete and we were just waiting for them to send over the rest of it. In the meantime I was handed printed off pages describing how Derek's brain impairment had affected him. I looked them over quickly glimpsing words such as 'Dyspraxia', 'Aspasia', Cognitive Issues, Perception difficulties, the words flew off the page and I realized that I knew very little of what was really wrong with my husband. How had I spent the last eight months almost living and breathing every moment of that time at the hospital with him talking at length with his doctors and specialists, believing that I had fully understood? As I scanned the pages before me most of the words were instantly recognizable but there were several I had no knowledge of or how they affected Derek.

Suddenly the buzzer sounded and the door was opened to allow a nurse through bringing the rest of the drugs. Derek was hovering in his doorway impatient to be away and it now seemed too late to mention my lack of understanding. I stored it away, pushing it to the back of my mind, knowing that in the very near future I had some research to carry out.

Having said our brief and speedy farewells we left the 'unit' and made our way to the car-park in silence. The only words uttered by Derek during the journey home were those stating how hungry he felt, and that all he had had to eat all day was a sandwich he had made himself at lunch time. It was now turned five o'clock and he was disgusted.

I had no idea of what had really gone on and decided to wait until we were home before I tried to make sense of it. The excitement of finally walking into his own home took over and all was forgotten. He kept whispering that he could not believe it, he was actually home at last and how he never thought he would ever feel this happy ever again.

He had wanted to sit quietly and just take in the reality of it. I made a hot drink and Derek suddenly stated that he hoped we were having something good for dinner.

"We're not having dinner as such," I said, "I thought we might have a sandwhich and a bowl of homemade soup." Then realizing that this was the right moment I asked him if he could explain what had gone on today and had he really only had a sandwhich for his lunch?

"Not only for my lunch," he stated getting himself all worked up again, "I had no breakfast either." Eventually calming down, he went on, to explain that the staff believed the occupational therapists were taking Derek to prepare his own breakfast but in actual fact they did not, it was his lunch they were assessing him with. In consequence he missed out on breakfast altogether. But what upset him more was that everyone had been looking forward to their Christmas dinner, himself included, and were all called into the dining room only for Derek to be told he had to make his own sandwhich and then sit and eat it at a table while everyone else enjoyed their turkey dinner.

What diabolical planning. His O.T. session was poorly timed. Could the 'unit' be so insensitive and cruel to see such a thing carried out? No wonder Derek was feeling as hungry and incensed as he was. He was perfectly justified in feeling that way. Fortunately he was now home and within no time at all sat tucking into a good hot dinner which he enjoyed with relish, stating that he could now truly leave the 'unit' behind him.

Christmas was a mere few days away, preceded by my birthday on Christmas- eve and in spite of the problems we had to deal with it was by far one of the nicest Christmas's or birthdays I had ever spent.

The entries that follow record our first Christmas together and cover the first days up until mid-

January when I decided to close the diary in order to concentrate on other things.

Friday 21st December 2007.

5.00p.m *Derek was happy and coped very well throughout his first day at home.*

He showered with a little help but still getting very confused over washing his hair and he needs help to ensure that he rinses off all the suds all over.

He became anxious when I dressed him in a buttoned shirt, saying he is not used to them and cannot do buttons as yet, (this really does appear to disturb Derek).

We went through his exercise program which pleased him and afterwards we wrapped up (very, very cold outside) and walked around to Sarah and Max's for lunch. We arrived home late afternoon and Derek was in need of a lie down.

But now refreshed once more he is about to help me prepare a stir-fry meal for supper. All in all today has been a good day except I found it difficult coping with so many phone calls whilst I was helping to get him showered and dressed this morning. I must learn to ignore the phone.

Saturday 22nd December 2007.

Derek has been up most of the night wondering why he had to visit the toilet so often. His visits were every half an hour and at times he no sooner got back into bed then he had to go again each time passing urine.

I felt very tired this morning dressing Derek. I found I had to dress him or otherwise he would have simply sat and not proceeded with the next item of clothing. I also found it impossible to concentrate on Derek and myself at the same time for whenever I tried to leave Derek to continue unaided for a few moments so I could dress myself, he would immediately pull my attention back to helping him.

I must make a mental note not to always comply.

Derek stated this morning that he would like the luxury of being allowed a lie-in, as this was something he was never allowed to do while in hospital, whereas I on the other hand like to get up early, so perhaps this is the very solution I am looking for. In future I will get up, shower and get myself dressed and ready for the day while Derek has his coveted lie-in. I must get up and keep organized otherwise I feel I will never cope.

We got off to a bad start today but finally we were both dressed and Derek enjoyed watching the birds as we sat eating our breakfast, he said he had missed being able to do this.

Afterwards he said he would like to practice some 'Tai-Chi' but was unable to focus on any of the movements and became very confused as to which was his left foot and which one was his right. I thought it best to leave this alone.

Derek made his first phone call this morning. It took him some considerable time before he could focus on the buttons and again became confused as to how he was meant to press them in sequence. He tried several times to press all of them at once. Derek is unable to direct his fingers to do what he wants them to do. He wished to persevere with this task and was overjoyed when he eventually managed to dial the number correctly and heard the voice at the other end. (I did have to explain to him that he could not keep turning the phone upside down and he explained that it felt upside down to him and that was why he kept turning it!).

We got ready to pay our usual Saturday morning visit to George and Derek said he must just pay a quick visit to the 'loo' before we went. Because he had on his outdoor clothing he could not cope in getting his trousers down in time and had an accident wetting them and the toilet floor. This so upset him as he believed this type of thing was well and truly in the past. I fully understood the situation and how much it had upset him and hopefully was able to make light of it, but nevertheless when I had finished helping him to undress and change into clean clothes we were both exhausted and had not even gone through the front door. I was left feeling such a rung out wimp and what really worried me was this was only our second day.

George's company managed to put Derek back on track and returning from our visit we enjoyed a light lunch after which Derek slept for an hour

I must note that Derek has been a little anxious over toilet visits since his accident this morning and has stated several times that he must ensure that he gives himself enough time to get there. (And he has done so without any fuss).

Late afternoon friends called in to see him, sadly it was a difficult situation with so much cross conversation going on and a disregard for Derek's inability to keep up. I politely explained that Derek was tired and would they please excuse us. They said that they understood and were very apologetic for having stayed so long, what they had not understood was the fact it had had nothing to do with the length of time, which had been quite short in duration, it had been too much information whizzing around the room all at once and Derek's brain could not take it in.

In a way I was pleased to have experienced the situation for it made me realize just how careful I was going to have to be. Over the months Derek had been slowly introduced from 'one to one' situations to dealing and coping with small groups but on each occasion these groups had had a much fuller understanding of the importance of not speaking all at once and had been aware of the confusion it might cause Derek.

Derek has spent a full day and is resting again before dinner.

Sunday 23rd December 2007.

1.00p.m. *We have just returned from a very pleasurable visit spent with John, Paula and the boys. Derek said he felt nicely relaxed during the visit but felt a strange mixture of emotion and frustration whilst there. When asked if he could explain why, he said that he had felt foolish not being able to do certain things for himself i.e. take off his coat without help and then being a little unsure of where he should sit but mainly he said it was not being able to put his gloves on when we were leaving, he said he had really felt very embarrassed at that particular moment.*

I tried to explain that John and Paula would have understood perfectly but he said that was not the point, it was how he felt that bothered him most of all.

Back home I asked Derek if he would enjoy helping me prepare lunch but he declined stating that he would much prefer to go and tinkle on the piano for half an hour.

9.00p.m *Derek has spent a good steady day but refused to have an afternoon rest in spite of my explaining why it was necessary for him to have one, no matter how short. Derek stated he feels he no longer needs them.*

(Positioning himself on the toilet still remains a problem. Probably wearing and having to cope with different clothing is confusing him. I will go back to his wearing T-shirts and joggers for a while to see if this is any easier for him).

In spite of the above mentioned problems we have both enjoyed a lovely relaxing day.

Monday 24ᵗʰ December 2007.

Derek was again up all night running to the toilet. He says that he is becoming so fed up with it all and I keep trying to remember that although he is so excited and pleased to be home it will take him a little while to settle down. His programming is so different now to what he has been used to.

I have swollen glands and a sore throat and I have to admit I feel like hell, probably because I have had no sleep for the past four nights.

I got up early and leaving Derek fast asleep I crept downstairs to set the table for breakfast and then showered and dressed so that I could devote all of my un-divided attention to him. It was my birthday and although Derek awoke somewhat befuddled through lack of sleep he was still able to remember that he had, with the help of Sarah, bought and wrapped a birthday present for me.

He needed a little time to recall where it had been hidden but he did find it and handed it to me with such excitement, (more at having been able to find it I think!). My present revealed a lovely pair of grey slacks which I had been wanting but my greatest present was having Derek right there beside me, how could anyone have wished for more than that!

George called in after breakfast and spent the morning with us. Derek had a lie down for an hour before Sarah and Max picked us up to take us for a birthday lunch they had arranged. This was a lovely treat and enjoyed by all.

Arriving home music was played and Derek invited me to dance during which, just as once before on his own birthday, he became very emotional.

We spent a quiet Christmas-eve, but such a happy one, with Sarah and Max overseeing all preparations for the following day.

Our day has ended so much happier than it first started but I will be pleased to fall into my bed feeling just as tired as I know Derek is feeling. A happy, happy birthday!

Tuesday 25th December 2007.

Today was a peaceful, relaxed and restful day. Derek slept his first good night's sleep since coming home.

After breakfast we sat and opened our presents and the one which brought tears to my eyes (and Max's also, for he wrote the letter down as Derek had dictated it) was the most beautiful present I had ever received. It was the letter Derek had been planning to write to me as soon as he was able.

My Darling Andrea,
This year we have come through a difficult time since I had my heart attack and I know how very hard it has been for you.
We have always done everything together in such a happy way but at the time of my collapse I was unable to speak and tell you just how much
I loved you.
You told me when I was ill that I had a mountain to climb but back then I was much too frightened and could not even bear to look at it. I thought
I would never have the strength to do so and I want you to know that it is only through your wonderful love and support that I was able to face it and begin my climb. We worked so hard together in Arrowe Park Hospital and
Clatterbridge Rehab. Unit to reach my discharge and I am hugely looking forward to going to Cameron House in February with everyone. Once there we will raise a toast to say thank-you to both yourself and Sarah for all your fantastic love, help and support in helping me back to this point.
I also recognize full well how much Sarah and Max have done for us both, we could not have managed without them.

All of my love forever and ever
Your Blue xxx

Sarah and Max worked so hard to ensure that we spent a lovely day. Dinner was cooked to perfection and we all enjoyed the fun of Max's indoor firework display afterwards. Derek did not wish to lie down and insisted that he did not need treating as a child, but he did relax and thoroughly enjoyed himself throughout the whole day.

It felt to be quite the most special and enjoyable Christmas in many a year.

Wednesday 26th December 2007.

Derek slept his second night through last night. (I did too, but kept waking to check everything was alright. I felt a little edgy and did not know why. Perhaps there is so much for me to have to re-adjust to also!).

Sarah and Max got off straight after breakfast, going to visit Max's family in Derbyshire.

Weather was good so Derek and I went for a nice long walk, both of us feeling so happy, almost like going back to our second childhood. We enjoyed ourselves so much that I think maybe we overdid it as Derek was obviously relieved to arrive back home and immediately went for a lie down.

He slept for over two hours, a good deep sleep and I even managed an hour myself which felt good.

Late afternoon we joined a family gathering held at my cousin's home only a mere five minutes drive away. All were eager to meet Derek once again, many of them having not seen him since before April.

I was so very grateful and much appreciated the controlled situation which was maintained for Derek's benefit the whole time we were there. We stayed two hours before coming away.

Derek was tired but chatty during the journey home, stating how much he had enjoyed meeting up with everyone after so long and expressing how good it had felt.

We spent the remainder of the evening resting and relaxing in front of the television.

Happy days I once thought we might never enjoy again!

Thursday 27th December 2007.

Derek slept like a baby, a deep restful sleep only going to the toilet twice. (I did not sleep and I am beginning to feel desperate for a good night's rest).

How can I feel so happy and desperate at the same time and yet I do!

George, our savior came up and did some fresh food shopping for me.

Derek said he would like to have a go at some painting he had been given as a Christmas present. I agreed that would be a wonderful idea and so we set ourselves up and Derek got off to a flying start which amazed me, unfortunately *his attention lapsed very quickly and he could no longer concentrate stating that the images seemed to be blurring into each other. I thought it best to stop but no, Derek wished to continue saying he would try a more simple picture.*

He soon gave up and said he would rather play on the piano. (Again he was not able to focus or concentrate).

I quickly distracted him with lunch and then suggested we both have a lie down. Derek was asleep within minutes and followed soon after by myself.

A long lazy, restful day with both of us feeling much more refreshed after an afternoons sleep.

Friday 28th December 2007.

I cannot believe that we both slept right through the entire night without either of us waking once, hurray! We slept through until 9a.m this morning.

Derek dressed himself unaided this morning (for the last two days it has been T-shirt, sweater and joggers though!) and the fact that he has been able to do this has been a good boost to his morale.

His focus was much sharper and was once again so willing to help with breakfast after which he suggested he made a curry for dinner this evening. I said it would be fun to do it together to which he readily agreed.

Derek needed a little help peeling the onions but was able to chop them well with no help at all. The same was repeated with the apples. He then added the onions, apples and washed sultanas (washed by Derek) into the frying pan and continued stirring until softened enough to transfer into an oven dish. This he was unable to do. Completely confused he said he could not do any more and I replied that this was excellent as he had been able to recognize his limitations and stay within them. He liked and accepted this explanation.

I feel Derek is greatly improving in the kitchen but needs to be very careful with pan handles and how to hold them properly and more importantly the gas jets. Derek cannot see the flames and nearly burnt himself on several occasions and failed to understand my concern.

Once we had cleared away and the curry was already to be popped into the oven, we walked to our local supermarket. This is another area where I see a huge improvement, shopping. No longer does Derek become confused with so much going on and today he was able to find items without any help whatsoever from me. It does take time but what the 'heck' we had all day if necessary!

Derek insisted on carrying the two bags back home for me. I felt rather fraudulent allowing him to do it but it felt great to be free of them all the same and Derek did say that he felt jubilant at being able to help me once more. (That's my boy!).

With the help of Derek, the shopping was put away. I am having to get used to things becoming 'topsy-turvy' in the house, as Derek tends to put everything away upside down, (but this can be extremely messy when putting away an already opened bottle of milk in the fridge or an open packet of oats in the cupboard).

When I try to show him what he has done, he simply shrugs and states there are times when he seems to be living in an 'upside down', 'topsy-turvy' kind of world.

(What do I say to that!).

We received the written exercise sheet from Felicity (O.T.) this morning and have already been practicing the finger and thumb exercises she advised Derek to practice as often as possible. (I would like to note that Derek seems to rebel at carrying out these new tasks as he believes he is no longer in need of them, yet seemingly in complete contradiction it was he who insisted on doing them admitting that he knew he would benefit from them in the long run.)

Derek is now resting in a chair and has fallen fast asleep. (After first stating that he no longer wishes to lie down during the day as it makes him feel nauseous but did agree that he needed a rest period still).

I feel Derek is desperately trying to regain and express some form of control to his daily life which I feel is good and assertive rather than him being passive and lethargic.

Saturday 29th December 2007.

Derek still needing help in dressing, he got quite confused this morning. He could not do his hair but I did notice him watching intently as I combed it for him and then stated that he would like to have another go at it himself. He managed the front and one side without a problem but could not co-ordinate the comb properly to comb the other side or the back. (When attempting the back, instead of combing the hair down he combed it upwards and the side he struggled with, instead of combing the hair back from the face, he combed it forward onto his face. When asked to look in the mirror Derek did not seem able to recognize that his hair looked a little odd).

We worked preparing breakfast together and Derek appeared very happy and cheerful. He was keen to do whatever he could to assist.

The weather was appalling so it was a stay at home morning bringing in as many exercises as I could without Derek feeling pressurized or bored in any way.

He is still enjoying his own time at the piano tinkering away and although not very tuneful it does help him to feel he is actually doing something of his own dictate.

We worked through his physical exercises which he really enjoys and would keep going till he dropped if he could, but he has suddenly given up on his reading and simply states that he finds it too confusing to take in. Says it actually hurts his brain, so I will not force this issue at present.

We ate an early lunch and went to visit Derek's sister and family with Sarah and Max. We stayed two hours with Derek saying how much he had enjoyed himself, and therefore I found it rather strange when talking about our visit later that evening and at one point referring to 'Elaine's children', Derek suddenly and quite angrily shouted that they were not children, they were young adults and in future would I please refer to them as such. I tried to reason that I could not refer to them as 'Elaine's young adults' and no matter what their ages were, they would always be 'Elaine's children'. Derek actually stormed out of the room accusing me of being too clever for my own good!

None of this really matters except that I found the incident so totally out of character both with Derek and the pleasant conversation we had been sharing I thought I should make note of it.

He soon came back and apologized saying how foolish he had been for no reason whatsoever. The rest of the evening was spent quietly relaxing with Derek talking freely of his feelings and emotions for the first time since being discharged.

He stated that although he still felt a great sense of shock at what had happened to him and could at times, even this far into his recovery, still feel very afraid, he marveled at how happy he felt, especially now that he was home.

Sunday 30th December 2007.

Derek was sadly awake most of the night, running backwards and forwards to the toilet. I understood his frustration, especially as he was beginning to believe that this business was behind him. (He was very restless during the night and quite disturbed).

On waking this morning, Derek was still very agitated and stated that I must help him get this problem sorted out, as it was really getting him down and he did not think he could cope with it for much longer. When I asked what particular problem he was referring to, he replied his running to the toilet all night long.

He did tell me that he felt the visit to see his sister had stirred a lot of past grievances and he seems reluctant to let go of an issue regarding some family photographs. I shall endeavor to talk to Elaine about it and hopefully between us we will be able to resolve the matter.

In the meantime, Derek definitely appears to be agitated over something but is unwilling to discuss it at the moment......he has been firing question after question at me relating to his family, many of which I have not been able to answer.

I have spent most of today trying to keep Derek calm and at the same time trying to take his mind off whatever it was that was bothering him.

I did at one point mention that I believed he had thoroughly enjoyed his visit to see his sister and he agreed that he most definitely had and why would I think otherwise. I asked if anything had occurred to upset him and he replied, "Not anything which had taken place during the visit yesterday".

I have let the matter drop and if Derek wishes to talk about he will when he is ready.

I am relieved that today is almost over. I never believed, well not since nursing a teething baby, that I could feel so tired. The mental struggles can sometimes be so much more draining than the constant physical demands and I feel so ashamed of myself for feeling this way when I think of how Derek must be struggling continually, day after day.

Not a very good day today!

Monday 31st December 2007.

I had no sleep at all last night and I am feeling a little on edge, or maybe anxious, I am not quite sure, perhaps the two emotions go together.

Derek had a series of jerking spasms during the night, they did not wake him or seem to disturb him in anyway but once or twice I was a little unsure of what to do but eventually they did subside with no further occurrence but I stayed awake to observe him and to act if necessary.

Fortunately he was not up and running to the toilet, he only woke once to go.

This morning he was up and seemingly more his old relaxed self as he helped me in the kitchen. After breakfast we prepared a casserole together. He enjoyed doing this but did notice that I was a little irritable, (I was in fact very irritable but trying hard to keep it in check, obviously not as well as I thought!).

Sarah came around and Derek volunteered to make a cup of tea for the three of us. He was doing well until Sarah said she had changed her mind and would have coffee instead and proceeded to take it out of his hands believing that she was helping. Sadly it only served to confuse him but I was pleased to see that he at least had the presence of mind to walk out of the kitchen leaving Sarah to finish off.

During the afternoon we went shopping and Derek pushed the trolley round the store for the first time. He managed to steer it perfectly without incident which was quite incredible as the store was very busy. I thought perhaps there were far too many people but Derek said no, he would be alright and that I should just allow him to get on with it. I have to say he could hardly contain his excitement.

There was one anxious moment when I had turned away to pick something off a shelf and when I turned back I saw he was standing stock-still simply staring straight ahead. I moved quickly, giving a short clap of hands just in front of him, this normally did the trick of bringing him back into focus, when Derek looked at me in astonishment and asked what on earth I was doing.

"I was worried about you", I said.

"Why?" he asked again.

"Because you weren't moving, you were just standing there staring straight ahead".

"And where would you have me go with this lot all milling around. I thought I was the one supposed to be confused but this lot would take some beating. I just thought it best to wait here until they sorted themselves out."

No sooner had the words been uttered, when the way forward became clear and he was off with his trolley leaving a bemused me to follow. (I was so proud of him!).

We made a brief call on George before coming home and Derek is now resting in his chair very much happier than yesterday.

We will not be staying up seeing in the New Year as we have done in the past although Derek has said that he would like to talk over a few things before the old year disappears. The fact that he remembers this is what we always did, means so much to me.

We chose to spend each New Years' eve with just the two of us talking out the old year and welcoming in the new. We would switch off the lights and draw back the curtains, relaxing by candle-light and chatting over a glass of Champagne, we would enjoy watching the firework display which could be seen on the far side of the river along the north coast of Wales. Not very exciting to some but Derek and I had loved each New Years' eve we had spent together. Some would say how boring, too much of the same every year, but to us each one was unique in itself, for every year had been vastly different from the one preceding it, each with its own experiences and highlights and of course never forgetting the low spots. We talked and mulled over them all, our favourite memories and the holidays we had shared and last but not least and what to us was perhaps the most important of all were the lessons learnt throughout the year.

I am so looking forward to our talking out the old year this evening and I know with a sure certainty that we are both looking forward to welcoming in the new.

CHAPTER NINETEEN

A new year, a new beginning, this is really where Derek's diary comes to an end although his story and his pathway of recovery still continue. His difficult journey covers days when he had fallen down believing yet again that he would never have the strength to get up and carry on. It tells of an inner courage which made it possible for him to do so. It has been a journey we have travelled together with the help and support of a special few but with the love and prayers of so many.

My husband has always been a very special person to me and his family and now throughout a further twelve months of recovery I am able to recognize him more fully for the great man he truly is. He has expressed a gentleness and humility throughout the entire duration of his journey and shown a love and patience towards me which I am certainly not deserving of.

It has been a journey taking him back on two occasions into the very hospital where he once spent six whole months including a night when he shocked us into believing that we had lost him all over again, but one cannot climb a mountain without encountering a few pitfalls along the way and we live in the full knowing that there may well be others which cannot be avoided.

Never once, not even throughout the most difficult periods of his struggle, did I ever hear Derek complain and I feel both privileged and blessed to be walking this pathway alongside of him.

The new beginning of January 2008 was indeed the beginning of our new passage through life together and we welcomed and embraced it with hope, promise and a shared love. Life does not have a beginning or an end, and this story certainly has not. Whatever the circumstance we find ourselves up against life still goes on and somehow we are given the strength to shoulder the pain and heartbreak it inflicts upon us.

I believe love and laughter are the greatest healers, except that is for the Love and Grace of God who I truly believe has brought both Derek and myself to the point of happiness we now share. This is the Power that shall carry us forward and uphold us both when we fall, as we so often do. It will sustain us when the pathway we now walk inevitably proves too difficult and arduous for one of us, leaving the other to continue the journey, seemingly alone.

It is my unshaken belief that this same pathway will one day unite us once again in finally attaining our true freedom and reality. In my opinion that is the ever continuing journey of life. But if life has no beginning or end how then can Saturday morning 28th April 2007 be the beginning of Derek's story. It cannot be. It is merely the date that records a traumatic, heartbreaking incident that cut across our lives causing Derek to suffer the greatest struggle of his entire life and achieving what was once believed by the medical profession to be the impossible, proving that no matter how difficult the situation, miracles really do occur often changing medical opinion in the process.

In bringing about what I consider to be a more truthful conclusion to Derek's story I must go back one week before April 28th to record a more truthful beginning. Accept it or reject it as you will for what follows is my truth as experienced at that time.

It was Sunday 22nd April 2007. A warm sunny day, not too hot but exceptional for that time of year, a day when we should have been feeling on top of the world but Derek was not himself, he had not been himself for some considerable time. He had that colour about him that I hated to see. He looked grey and drained. He did not look well at all. Several times he had looked at his reflection in the mirror and asked me if I thought he looked alright.

I had on numerous occasions begged him to go for a check-up. I had tried my very best to bully him into doing just that but Derek has two faults, one he has always been stubborn and in stubbornness he refused to go and have a health check, it would have been such a simple thing to do and as it turned out he did finally go but had sadly left it too late. His second fault was his fear of all things medical and the invasion of his personal privacy. I had shared my true concern with him but what I had not been able to share with him was a sense of knowing I had held. A knowing I had shouldered for some considerable time but hoped that I had been mistaken and that it would never actually come to pass. Each and every time Derek refused to go and see a doctor I looked for any reason to explain why I might be wrong and that the time of happening had not arrived.

I go back to this Sunday not because it was the first time I suspected something to be wrong with Derek, for I had felt this to be the case for some considerable time, but because this was the day I felt that strong sense of something about to happen and try as I might I had not been able to shake it off.

Derek had been impossible to talk to that day and had spent the entire day gardening but his heart had not been in it. He was moody and wearily tired. I had even begun to wonder where the real Derek had disappeared to. The normal Derek played badminton every Tuesday and Thursday for the exercise and fun and meeting other like-minded people, but there was now another Derek who had taken his place, always insisting that everything was perfectly alright and who would thank me for not continuing to badger him. He seemed to be constantly proving something to himself, unlike the real Derek, who although always competitive by nature used to simply enjoy the game.

Over Sunday lunch I mentioned that perhaps he should take a break from the game as I thought he was beginning to take the competition of it too seriously and believed that it was beginning to do him more harm than good as he was always so tired these days. To Derek this was sacrilege and we never spoke to each other for the rest of the afternoon and after supper later that evening, Derek took himself off to spend time on his own. I told him I thought he was being silly and that his behavior was totally out of character.

He refused to be budged except to utter a little later on during the evening of how unhappy he was feeling.

"Can you explain why you feel this way"? I asked him.

"No", he replied, "except to say I feel more worried more than unhappy".

Yet again I begged him to make an appointment to have a medical overhaul.

"Won't do any good now", was all he said and took himself off to bed to sleep alone.

I rang a friend to confide how worried I was feeling regarding Derek's unusual behavior, but the shared conversation and her proffered words of wisdom did little to stem my concern of what I could now sense standing before me, growing stronger in its threat as each moment ticked by.

That Sunday night I did not go to bed and sat downstairs wishing with all of my heart that I did not live the life that I lived, for I had lived my entire life with the guidance and teachings of 'Spirit' and had known of things which could never be shared with others except when the time was right and then only within God's Will.

The burden of knowing such things very often felt too great to bear but somehow I had always discovered or been given the strength and courage to shoulder it but as I sat alone that Sunday evening I had felt the weight of the knowledge I had been carrying for some time all too much and had wanted to hand it back.

I had given my life to searching 'Truth' and its development within myself, expressing it as sincerely as I could in the 'Healing' of others, but suddenly confronted with the Truth which was about to cut directly across my life and those closest to me, like a child who suddenly found the responsibility too hard to deal with, I no longer wanted to play the game.

I sat wanting with all of my heart to pray for everything to made alright. I wanted to pray for Derek to be alright but I knew deep within my heart that to pray for such things would be selfish, that it may go against the Will of God. So as I outwardly railed against what I knew to be drawing near, I inwardly handed my life and the one person I seemed unable to help over to that same God, at the same time praying for the strength which would enable me to accept His Will. Sunday 22nd

April was most definately not a game. This was the reality of life but I did not have to like what the equation equalled.

Monday dawned and no matter how hard I tried, I tried in vain, for I could not help Derek find his peace. By mid-morning I knew that he was greatly disturbed and yet he had asked to be left alone. I could only respect his wishes and left him to it. He spent most of that day browsing through the bookcase and picking up one book after the other as though desperately searching for something causing my heart to go out to him. I could feel his torment and the icy coldness he was feeling within and around his own heart.

Derek spent Tuesday alone as I had gone out for the day. I arrived home at five o'clock and began preparing the evening meal. The atmosphere was not good, in fact it was so heavy that I suggested that I ring John and cancel our meditation group which was held every Tuesday evening at John's home.

Derek stated there was no reason to do this as he really did wish to go. I silently sent out a prayer asking that any tension between us be dissolved before we set off.

We shared small talk during the drive over but all was far from well, and as we rang the front-door bell I whispered to Derek that he should try and leave behind whatever it was that was troubling him. We spent fifteen minutes or so in social chit-chat and catching up on the previous weeks' events and by the time we walked in to sit in meditation Derek had brightened up considerably.

We sat with the warmth of the fire and the soft glow of lamp-light, each lost in our own individual, and at the same time, shared world of silence. Usually an hour would be passed in this way before I would ask each person to then focus and concentrate their minds on a given subject. Then a little later before we drew the meditation to its close each person would speak of what they had each received in thought during this period.

This particular Tuesday evening I had no sooner sat down when I suddenly became aware of a sense of panic. Realizing that this feeling did not stem from my own inner emotions I put it aside believing it to be linked to someone else and would deal with it later if necessary. I only realized that the first hour had passed upon hearing a voice asking me to invite each soul present to pass under the arch which I could now see standing clearly before me. The arch was similar in appearance to the Arc' de' Triumph in Paris, except the one before me appeared to be not as high in its structure and a little wider perhaps. Maybe the loss of height only made it appear this way, I could not be sure.

I described what I was seeing and related what had been asked of me, simply that we each should try to imagine this large arch in our minds' eye and as we passed directly beneath it we were to pause and imagine how it might feel.

I sat once again allowing the silence to envelope me and believed that I was about to walk under the described structure, instead I immediately found myself transported to a place I had often been accustomed to visiting throughout my life.

It was one of the Spiritual havens I had been introduced to as a young girl but instead of experiencing the familiar peace and sense of tranquility I enjoyed on each and every previous visit there, I felt a strange sense of agitation growing inside of me as I found myself standing upon the familiar immaculately kept lawns which rolled away into the distance as far as my vision could see. It is a place of no horizons nor hedges or fences or anything which might create a form of barrier. I stood looking out across this endless vista knowing that behind me stood a building I had only ever been allowed to enter by invitation. This was the building, known in the realm of Spirit to be the 'Hall of Learning' and within its' walls I had been taught many things by some of the wisest beings I have ever met. But there were the times when I would take myself before its great doorway believing, as I often did, that I was ready to learn whatever I was seeking at that particular moment in my life, only to find myself being left waiting outside feeling ignored and very puzzled. It took several years before the realization dawned on me that true knowledge is not given on demand but only when the student is truly ready to receive it.

I had found myself not wishing to enter the building on that occasion, in fact I did not even wish to turn around and look upon it. I felt I had to keep on the move, hoping that no soul would wish to stop and talk to me. I began to quicken my pace, walking faster and faster, something was most definately wrong and I could feel it. Was the panic I had felt my own after all? Once again I turned away from the very thought of it.

"Little One", the voice sounded soft and gentle. I ignored it and kept on walking. Again the voice called out just as gently but a little firmer in its tone.

"Please leave me", I had begged continuing to walk even faster. I desperately sought somewhere to escape to but this was a place where one could not hide and as I continued my futile pacing round and round, I began to feel something drawing closer and closer which I had wanted to push away with all of my being. And yet this had been my safe haven all of my life, where could I go to from here.

"Little one, please come and sit a while", the tone of his voice sounding a little more persistent.

"No, I must keep walking. I cannot stop", I declared. I had known that I was walking around in circles and had also felt the panic beginning to rise within me but had been afraid to stop so had foolishly walked faster still. So fast I did not notice the garden bench which suddenly appeared, seemingly out of nowhere, until it was too late for me to avoid it. Sitting on it was a gentleman I recognized dressed, as always, in a white robe. I tried very hard to look away but something in his gentleness drew me to him. I saw the truth written in his eyes and unable to find the words to speak, merely shook my head. I had felt myself begin to tremble and found that my legs had suddenly grown very weak. Patting the bench, he kindly invited me to sit down beside him and very timidly I did so.

"Little One", he had spoken so softly, "we need to talk but before we do so I would ask two things of you. The first is that you turn around to look and then tell me what it is you see".

"The Building of Learning stands there", I cried.

"Does it really, have you looked"? He asked me.

"But I know it does".

"No my child you do not know, for you have not looked and I must tell you that your limited memory will not serve you here. Here, my child, Truth serves the need and the building you believe to stand there, stood there to serve your need to learn. Now once again I ask you to look and tell me what it is you see."

I turned around slowly to see the very same building I had thought I had seen so many times before and yet as I continued to gaze upon it I began to acknowledge that it was not the building known as the 'Hall of Learning' I was looking at but another building I was not quite able to recall. This building had a familiar scent about it that stirred a distant memory.

"Well can you now describe to me what it is you see"? My companion asked.

"I realize that I am not looking at the building I thought it was, this is different and yes I do recognize it but cannot place it", I murmured thoughtfully. "It reminds me of the hospital I once saw my grandfather in just after he had died and yes, that explains the familiar smell I recognize, a smell familiar to all hospitals in our physical world."

My grandfather had never believed in life after death. He always maintained that when you were dead, that was it, you were dead. From my knowledge of Spirit it takes a little while for such people to realize that they are not dead and that they are in fact very much alive but until that realization dawns upon them they have to be hospitalized and nursed into the realization of this Truth.

As I sat dwelling on the memory of my grandfather's passing I knew with certainty that I was looking at that same hospital or one very similar to it but before I had been able to utter another word the great doors opened and I watched spellbound as several doctors, I presumed them to be doctors, accompanied by two nurses came down the steps and stood as though waiting for something or someone to arrive.

I turned to my companion with sheer disbelief filling my heart and simply shook my head, no words came. He had tried to take my hand but I had ungraciously pulled it away, not wanting anything or anyone to confirm the truth which had drawn so close I could almost reach out and touch it.

"Little One did I not say that there were two things I would ask of you. The second is that you look to your right and once again tell me what it is that you see".

I had wanted to scream out aloud how much I had loathed my life and why could I have not been left alone. I had never asked for any of this. Which of course had not been exactly true for the truth of the matter was in the fact that the very essence of who and what I was lay in discovering and expressing the truth as I experienced it.

"Do you believe that we stand unaware of how you feel right at this moment, my child, please give me your hand", and as he spoke I had placed my hand in his, feeling more fragile than I had ever felt before.

"Now look to your right".

Slowly I turned and looked out over a great expanse of countryside. Not the rolling lawns and sky of brilliant white light I had expected to see but fields, green open fields laid out with shrubberies dotted here and there beneath clear blue skies, everywhere had looked so beautiful and peaceful and in complete contrast to how I was feeling at that moment.

I was about to turn back and describe what I had seen when something caused me to pause and hesitate. Roughly somewhere in the midst of the scene spread out before me, I had noticed something happening, something was beginning to take shape. Out of nothing I witnessed a form materializing and shaping itself into the very archway I had been asked to describe as we sat in meditation. No sooner had this arch formed itself, when right before my eyes, as though switched on by some invisible hand, I witnessed on the far side of it, a light so brilliant in its intensity it almost forced me to turn away.

My gaze was fixed in dread of what was to come next. It had not been what I had seen but what I had heard that turned my dread into the beginning of a living nightmare. From out of the light I saw two arms held out as though waiting to receive someone, and a voice like no other I had ever heard which called out, "Bring him unto me".

I remember I had screamed out, but it must have been a scream from my soul for no sound had been heard although thankfully my companion in Spirit had heard my cry and held me until my trembling had ceased.

"Little One, now I must talk to you and you must listen. You have witnessed the truth and now you must be strong and brave but above all else you must be, oh so patient, so very, very patient. We shall not desert you. You shall find us here whenever you wish to talk or simply rest and when you feel alone as you surely will, then know that you are not, we will be with you. Now it is time, for you must also walk beneath the archway so that you can explain to them what you experience whilst standing beneath it".

In the split second it takes for a computer to crash, my Spirit companion was gone and as quickly as I had been transported there I had found myself back once more sitting in the silence of our group meditation. I had felt useless and inept, the whole thing had felt to be too much for me and I had wanted to cry and never stop. But how could I for I knew that I had still not completed what had been asked of me. This was not about me and I had known that I must be strong for one other person present that night. But how could I possibly tell my husband that it was him?

I walked with a heavy heart towards the archway but in spite of this I had not hesitated when reaching it to walk straight beneath its stone like structure. I had been instantly amazed by the light and instead of standing beneath the structure of an arch I had felt myself to be housed within a brightly lit chamber. I had felt myself suddenly cut off from life itself. I had no recollection of where I had been or of where I was. I had been cut off from my memory, only confusion going round and round in my head. I then had the experience of feeling as though I were floating within the chamber, tumbling over and over again. Confusion and tumbling, on and on it had gone, no beginning, no end, just on and on.

I had then found myself standing outside of the chamber once again standing back from beneath the arch and had known that it had been time to draw the session to a close and ask each person if they might describe their own personal experience of the meditation.

The archway had presented no problems to anyone other than Derek, who on approaching it in his mind's eye had felt a slight dread of entering under its arch and when about to do so had panicked and quickly backed away from it. He had stated that he had not liked the experience at all and had seemed more than a little disturbed by the whole evening.

When it came my turn to relate my own experience, I simply explained that I had found myself in familiar surroundings where I had sat and talked with Spirit for a while. I had then described the exact happenings I had experienced inside of what I had thought to be similar to that of a decompression chamber that would be used to treat divers.

Afterwards we chatted over tea and biscuits until it was time to leave and then Derek reverted back to his earlier mood so we drove most of the journey home in silence. Waiting at a set of traffic lights, Derek suddenly queried why I had not thought to relate the conversation which I had held with Spirit.

"I hadn't felt it necessary", was all I had been able to think of.

"I know what you were chatting about". The statement had been spoken without feeling but with the knowing of truth. Not wishing to elaborate, I asked him why he had felt so afraid when beneath the arch.

"I think you already know the answer to that one," he stated again without feeling.

"Derek, are you alright", I asked. "Can't you please try and tell me what it is that is bothering you?"

"Will I ever be alright again?" he murmured and as he was parking the car added, "I know that you know". Without another word he had jumped out of the car and once again behaving totally out of character had run ahead of me and disappeared into the house.

I was completely lost as to how I should be dealing with this. I had known that he was worrying over an angiogram that was coming up the following week and I had never known Derek to be intuitive in any way so how could he possibly have known. I believed that his mind was working out of fear of what the test might show up. He was having the test because of recent chest pains he had experienced and no longer prepared to take no for an answer, I had taken him straight to the surgery where our doctor had arranged for the test as soon as possible. It had been scheduled for May 2nd 2007.

Derek had gone directly up to bed without a further word leaving me to lock up. The following day he did not explain his behavior but he did apologize, and so putting it all behind us we set off and enjoyed a good walk. Out in the fresh-air Derek began to relax and was able to show his sense of humour once again. This sadly made it more difficult for me to keep a sense of balance to the situation we were experiencing and what I had experienced in meditation the night before.

Thankfully, Derek had seemingly forgotten all about it until after dinner. He had sat watching the news on television and suddenly turned towards me and stated quite simply, "I definitely know that you know."

"I have no idea what you're talking about," I said looking up from my crossword and felt a little anxious to see him rubbing his chest.

"Have you got pains in your chest"? I asked him.

"None whatsoever," he replied rather a little too quickly.

"Then why are you rubbing your chest?"

"It helps me to relax, that's all."

Silence once again. I returned to my crossword.

"Andrea", he had sounded extremely serious in his tone, "Will you please promise me one thing?"

"Yes, if I can," I replied beginning to feel a little uncomfortable.

"Will you promise to tell me if and when you know that I am going to die?"

Silence as I paused on how best to answer him, "I cannot promise you that," I said, "but what I would like to suggest is that we make a promise to each other. A promise, that when either of us dies we shall follow the light and not look back and hold onto the knowing that one day we shall stand united once more".

"I accept and make that promise."

No more was ever mentioned on the subject until that Saturday morning of April 28th when he had stood leaning against the rail at the marina and told me of how he had at last found his peace.

The medical profession had not expected Derek to pull through and having nursed the knowledge for some considerable time that the equation of my husband's life equalled him leaving this world at that allotted moment I had not expected him to live, and although it broke my heart to do so I did hand him over to his God that same morning when I bid him farewell and gently told him to follow the light.

Did Derek heed my words or remember our promise? I cannot be sure but either way in his state of unconsciousness he had remembered to look for the light and was aware of this fact when he did finally regain consciousness. The doctors consider Derek to be one hell of a lucky man but I believe it was the Love and Grace of God, and nothing to do with luck, which decreed that he should live to steer his own unique course through unchartered waters, climb a mountain almost too high and continue to walk his own pathway of recovery.

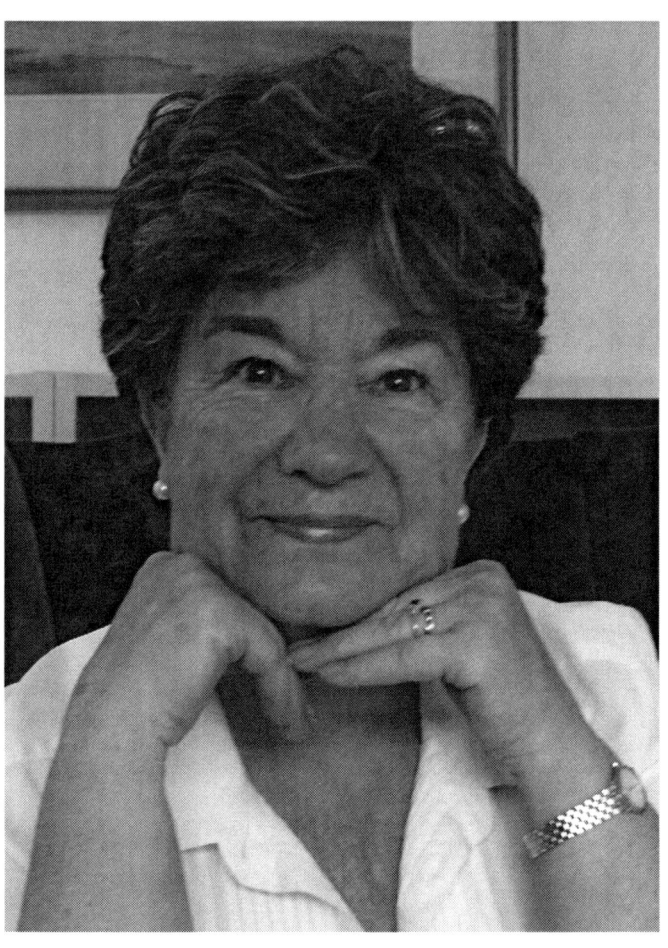

Lightning Source UK Ltd.
Milton Keynes UK
02 September 2009
143281UK00001B/2/P